Aging with a Physical Disability

Guest Editors

MARK P. JENSEN, PhD
IVAN R. MOLTON, PhD

PHYSICAL MEDICINE AND REHABILITATION CLINICS OF NORTH AMERICA

www.pmr.theclinics.com

Consulting Editor
GEORGE H. KRAFT, MD, MS

May 2010 • Volume 21 • Number 2

SAUNDERS an imprint of ELSEVIER, Inc.

W.B. SAUNDERS COMPANY
A Division of Elsevier Inc.

1600 John F. Kennedy Boulevard • Suite 1800 • Philadelphia, Pennsylvania 19103

http://www.theclinics.com

PHYSICAL MEDICINE AND REHABILITATION CLINICS OF NORTH AMERICA Volume 21, Number 2
May 2010 ISSN 1047-9651, ISBN-13: 978-1-4377-1860-7

Editor: Debora Dellapena
Developmental Editor: Donald Mumford

Reprints. For copies of 100 or more of articles in this publication, please contact the Commercial Reprints Department, Elsevier Inc., 360 Park Avenue South, New York, NY 10010-1710. Tel.: 212-633-3812; Fax: 212-462-1935; E-mail: reprints@elsevier.com.

Physical Medicine and Rehabilitation Clinics of North America (ISSN 1047-9651) is published quarterly by Elsevier Inc., 360 Park Avenue South, New York, NY 10010-1710. Months of issue are February, May, August, and November. Business and Editorial Offices: 1600 John F. Kennedy Blvd., Suite 1800, Philadelphia, PA 19103-2899. Customer Service Office: 3251 Riverport Lane, Maryland Heights, MO 63043. Periodicals postage paid at New York, NY and additional mailing offices. Subscription price per year is $230.00 (US individuals), $376.00 (US institutions), $116.00 (US students), $280.00 (Canadian individuals), $491.00 (Canadian institutions), $167.00 (Canadian students), $345.00 (foreign individuals), $491.00 (foreign institutions), and $167.00 (foreign students). Foreign air speed delivery is included in all *Clinics* subscription prices. All prices are subject to change without notice. **POSTMASTER:** Send address changes to *Physical Medicine and Rehabilitation Clinics of North America*, Customer Service Office: Elsevier Health Sciences Division, Subscription Customer Service, 3251 Riverport Lane, Maryland Heights, MO 63043. **Customer Service: 1-800-654-2452 (US). From outside of the United States, call 314-447-8871. Fax: 314-447-8029. E-mail: JournalsCustomer Service-usa@elsevier.com (for print support); JournalsOnlineSupport-usa@elsevier.com (for online support).**

Physical Medicine and Rehabilitation Clinics of North America is indexed in *Excerpta Medica, MEDLINE/ PubMed (Index Medicus), Cinahl,* and *Cumulative Index to Nursing and Allied Health Literature.*

Printed and bound by CPI Group (UK) Ltd, Croydon, CR0 4YY

Transferred to Digital Print 2011

Contributors

CONSULTING EDITOR

GEORGE H. KRAFT, MD, MS
Alvord Professor of Multiple Sclerosis Research; Professor, Department of Rehabilitation Medicine; Adjunct Professor, Department of Neurology, University of Washington School of Medicine, Seattle, Washington

GUEST EDITORS

MARK P. JENSEN, PhD
Professor and Vice Chair for Research, Department of Rehabilitation Medicine, University of Washington School of Medicine, Harborview Medical Center, Seattle, Washington

IVAN R. MOLTON, PhD
Acting Assistant Professor, Department of Rehabilitation Medicine, Harborview Medical Center, University of Washington School of Medicine; Clinical Psychologist, Department of Rehabilitation Medicine, University of Washington, Seattle, Washington

AUTHORS

RICHARD T. ABRESCH, MS
Director of Research, Department of Physical Medicine and Rehabilitation, University of California at Davis, Sacramento, California

L. BAKER, PhD, PT
Associate Professor, Division of Biokinesiology and Physical Therapy, University of Southern California, Los Angeles, California

CAROLYN R. BAYLOR, PhD, BC-NCD
Acting Assistant Professor, Department of Rehabilitation Medicine, University of Washington, Seattle, Washington

CHARLES H. BOMBARDIER, PhD
Professor, Department of Rehabilitation Medicine, Harborview Medical Center, University of Washington School of Medicine, Seattle, Washington

SOO BORSON, MD
Professor of Psychiatry and Behavioral Sciences, Director, Memory Disorders Program, University of Washington School of Medicine, Seattle, Washington

MICHELLE S. BOURGEOIS, PhD
Professor, Department of Speech and Hearing Science, The Ohio State University, Columbus, Ohio

PAT A. BROWN, EdD
Clinical Associate Professor, Department of Rehabilitation Medicine, School of Medicine, University of Washington, Seattle, Washington

GREGORY T. CARTER, MD, MS
Professor of Rehabilitation Medicine, Department of Rehabilitation Medicine, University of Washington School of Medicine, Seattle, Centralia, Washington

JOEL R. CHAMBERLAIN, PhD
Assistant Professor of Neurology, Division of Neuromuscular Disorders, Department of Neurology, University of Washington School of Medicine, Seattle, Washington

SUSAN CHARLIFUE, PhD
Research Principal Investigator, Research Department, Craig Hospital, Englewood, Colorado

ANNA MARIA DUNN, MD
Clinical Assistant Professor, University of Medicine and Dentistry of New Jersey, Piscataway-Robert Wood Johnson Medical School; Director of Services, Department of Physical Medicine and Rehabilitation, Robert Wood Johnson University Hospital, New Brunswick, New Jersey

DAWN M. EHDE, PhD
Department of Rehabilitation Medicine, Harborview Medical Center, University of Washington School of Medicine, Seattle, Washington

MARCIA L. FINLAYSON, OT, PhD, OTR/L
Associate Professor, Department of Occupational Therapy, University of Illinois at Chicago, Chicago, Illinois

S.M. FLYNN, PhD, PT
Research Scientist, Institute for Creative Technologies, University of Southern California, Marina del Rey, California

JAY J. HAN, MD
Associate Professor of Physical Medicine and Rehabilitation, Department of Physical Medicine and Rehabilitation, University of California at Davis, Sacramento, California

MARK P. JENSEN, PhD
Professor and Vice Chair for Research, Department of Rehabilitation Medicine, University of Washington School of Medicine, Harborview Medical Center, Seattle, Washington

AMITABH JHA, MD, MPH
Research Physiatrist, Craig Hospital, Englewood; Associate Professor, Department of Physical Medicine and Rehabilitation, University of Colorado at Denver, Denver, Colorado

KURT L. JOHNSON, PhD
Professor, Department of Rehabilitation Medicine, School of Medicine, University of Washington, Seattle, Washington

ELIZABETH S. KNASTER, MPH
Graduate Research Assistant, Department of Rehabilitation Medicine, School of Medicine, University of Washington, Seattle, Washington

DANIEL LAMMERTSE, MD
Medical Director of Research, Craig Hospital, Englewood, Colorado

B.S. LANGE, PhD
Research Associate, Institute for Creative Technologies, University of Southern California, Marina del Rey, California

LISA LUCIANO, DO
Clinical Assistant Professor, Department of Physical Medicine and Rehabilitation, University of Medicine and Dentistry of New Jersey, Piscataway-Robert Wood Johnson Medical School; Assistant to the Chairman, JFK Johnson Rehabilitation Institute, Edison, New Jersey

EDWARD MCAULEY, PhD
Professor, Department of Kinesiology and Community Health, University of Illinois at Urbana-Champaign, Urbana, Illinois

KELLY MILTON, MS
College of Physicians and Surgeons, New York Presbyterian Hospital, Columbia University, New York, New York

JORDI MIRÓ, PhD
Assistant Professor of Psychology, ALGOS, Research on Pain, Rovira i Virgili University, Catalonia, Spain

IVAN R. MOLTON, PhD
Acting Assistant Professor, Department of Rehabilitation Medicine, Harborview Medical Center, University of Washington School of Medicine; Clinical Psychologist, Department of Rehabilitation Medicine, University of Washington, Seattle, Washington

ROBERT W. MOTL, PhD
Associate Professor, Department of Kinesiology and Community Health, University of Illinois at Urbana-Champaign, Urbana, Illinois

ELIZABETH W. PETERSON, PhD, MPH, OTR/L
Clinical Associate Professor, Department of Occupational Therapy, University of Illinois at Chicago, Chicago, Illinois

JONATHAN P. QUEVEDO, MD
Medical Director and Clinical Assistant Professor, University of Medicine and Dentistry of New Jersey, Piscataway-Robert Wood Johnson Medical School; Medical Director, In-patient Rehabilitation, Chronic Pain Management Attending Physiatrist, JFK Johnson Rehabilitation Institute, Edison, New Jersey

P. REQUEJO, PhD
Director, Rehabilitation Engineering Program, Rancho Los Amigos National Rehabilitation Center, Downey, California

A.A. RIZZO, PhD
Associate Director, Institute for Creative Technologies, University of Southern California, Marina del Rey, California

LYSSA SORKIN, MD
New York–Presbyterian Columbia Cornell Residency Program, New York, New York

KEVIN SPERBER, MD
Assistant Clinical Professor, Department of Physical Medicine and Rehabilitation, Columbia University, College of Physicians and Surgeons, New York–Presbyterian Hospital, New York, New York

MICHELLE STERN, MD
Assistant Clinical Professor, Department of Physical Medicine and Rehabilitation, Columbia University, College of Physicians and Surgeons, New York–Presbyterian Hospital, New York, New York

BRENDA STOELB, PhD
Talaria Inc, Seattle, Washington

THOMAS E. STRAX, MD
Professor and Chairman, Department of Physical Medicine and Rehabilitation, University of Medicine and Dentistry of New Jersey, Piscataway-Robert Wood Johnson Medical School; Vice President for Medical Rehabilitation and Medical Director, JFK Johnson Rehabilitation Institute, Edison, New Jersey

F.J. VALERO-CUEVAS, PhD
Associate Professor, Division of Biokinesiology and Physical Therapy, Department of Biomedical Engineering, University of Southern California, Los Angeles, California

MICHAEL D. WEISS, MD
Associate Professor of Neurology, Division of Neuromuscular Disorders, Department of Neurology, University of Washington School of Medicine, Seattle, Washington

EVA WIDERSTRÖM-NOGA, DDS, PhD
Research Associate Professor, Health Scientist Miami Veterans Affairs, Miami Project to Cure Paralysis, Research Service, Veterans Affairs Medical Center; Departments of Neurological Surgery and Rehabilitation Medicine, University of Miami Miller School of Medicine, Lois Pope Life Center, Miami, Florida

C. WINSTEIN, PhD, PT
Professor, Division of Biokinesiology and Physical Therapy, University of Southern California, Los Angeles, California

KATHRYN M. YORKSTON, PhD, BC-NCD
Professor and Head, Division of Speech Pathology, Department of Rehabilitation Medicine, University of Washington, Seattle, Washington

Contents

> Understanding the complex trajectories of disability and aging requires a biopsychosocial approach that considers disability in the broader context of later adulthood. Although disability service researchers and gerontologists have many shared interests and a similar mission, the fields are relatively new to one another and have had little historical interaction. The purpose of this article is to increase and improve collaboration among investigators in these fields by providing some background in social gerontology to the disability researcher, and by applying key theories in aging to the issue of growing older with physical disability. The article discusses particular problem areas for older adults, including social support, and also discusses the parallel paradoxes of aging and disability.

> Aging with disabilities, such as multiple sclerosis, spinal cord injury, muscular dystrophy, and postpolio syndrome, can lead to barriers to participation, including employment barriers. Many individuals develop strategies for overcoming these barriers that may become less successful as they experience more secondary conditions concomitant with the aging process. Rehabilitation professionals can help to overcome barriers to workplace participation and should work with clients to enhance employment outcomes.

> The potential influence of age and aging on the psychological functioning of people with disabilities is surprisingly complex. In people with spinal cord injury or multiple sclerosis, depression is highly prevalent. The limited research in this area indicates that older age and greater time span since disability onset may be associated with less self-reported depressive symptoms. Posttraumatic growth (PTG) and benefit finding (BF) are also common in people with disabilities. Older age tends to be associated

with less BF and PTG. Studies that use longitudinal designs and examine multiple age-related factors simultaneously are needed. Potential mediators of age-related effects, such as historical trends, life-cycle events, maturity, and declining health, also need to be examined. There are many interesting theoretic and empiric concepts from aging research that can inform future research on the psychological aspects of aging with disability.

This article provides an overview of physical activity and its association with function, disability, and quality of life (QOL) outcomes among older adults. The rationale and the associated onset of chronic disease conditions that influence function, disability, and QOL is embedded in the "Graying of America". The literature reviewed in this article yielded 3 general conclusions: (1) there is an alarming rate of physical inactivity among older adults, particularly those aging with a disability; (2) there is strong evidence for the beneficial effects of physical activity on impairment, function, and health-related aspects of QOL among older adults, but there is less conclusive evidence for positive effects of physical activity on disability and global QOL; and (3) there is emerging support for self-efficacy as a mediator of the association between physical activity and disability, and QOL outcomes in older adults. Researchers should consider designing and testing programs that incorporate strategies for enhancing self-efficacy along with the promotion of physical activity as a means of preventing disablement and improving QOL among older adults. Such work will go a long way in identifying practical approaches that can be applied for improving the later years of life and is critical because many Americans will soon be affected by the aging of adults in the United States.

People with communication disorders form a diverse group with some experiencing long-standing disorders and others the onset of new disorders in old age. Regardless of age at onset, the burden of communication disorders is cumulative and has important implications for health care providers. Communication serves many roles for older people, not only establishing and maintaining social affiliations but also providing access to health care services. Health care providers should be aware of potential communication disorders and make provision for quiet environments, reading materials at appropriate literacy levels, and longer appointments for people with communication difficulties.

This article focuses on the role of pain and fatigue in aging people who have physical impairments and provides a brief summary of definitions, descriptions, and classifications of pain and fatigue; implications of these secondary conditions on the health and functioning; multidisciplinary assessment and treatment options; and critical gaps in knowledge and directions for future research. Central nervous system trauma, diseases of the nervous system, and degenerative muscle diseases often result in significant physical impairments and disability. People who are living and aging with these underlying medical conditions often experience pain and fatigue secondary to their physical impairment that may worsen over time, resulting in increased disability and decreased quality of life. Important areas for future research in persons who have physical impairments include identification of conditions that require age-specific considerations; identification of symptom clusters (eg, pain, fatigue, depression) and how they evolve over time; and development of interdisciplinary treatment protocols.

Using the advances in computing power, software and hardware technologies, virtual reality (VR), and gaming applications have the potential to address clinical challenges for a range of disabilities. VR-based games can potentially provide the ability to assess and augment cognitive and motor rehabilitation under a range of stimulus conditions that are not easily controllable and quantifiable in the real world. This article discusses an approach for maximizing function and participation for those aging with and into a disability by combining task-specific training with advances in VR and gaming technologies to enable positive behavioral modifications for independence in the home and community. There is potential for the use of VR and game applications for rehabilitating, maintaining, and enhancing those processes that are affected by aging with and into disability, particularly the need to attain a balance in the interplay between sensorimotor function and cognitive demands and to reap the benefits of task-specific training and regular physical activity and exercise.

Falls are a major public health problem, contributing to significant morbidity and mortality among older adults in the United States. This article summarizes and compares (1) fall prevalence rates, (2) fall risk factors, (3) consequences of falls, and (4) current knowledge about fall prevention interventions between community-dwelling older adults and people aging with physical disability. In this latter group, the article focuses on individuals with multiple sclerosis, late-effects of polio, muscular dystrophies, and spinal cord injuries.

This article reviews normative changes in cognition that are observed across the adult life span and considers how specific disabilities may interact with aging processes to increase functional decline in later life.

Disabling conditions that directly affect the brain are contrasted with those that do not. The goal is twofold: to create a framework for thinking about how cognitive changes, aging, and disability may interact to help explain individual differences in coping, and to promote the inclusion of cognition in a comprehensive approach to assessment and care.

individuals with muscular dystrophy (MD) with more functional equipment, allowing better strategies for improvement of quality of life. These advances have also allowed a significant number of these patients to live much longer. As progress continues to change management, it also changes patients' expectations. A comprehensive medical and rehabilitative approach to management of aging MD patients can often fulfill expectations and help them enjoy an enhanced quality of life.

THE CLINICS ARE NOW AVAILABLE ONLINE!

Access your subscription at:
www.theclinics.com

Foreword

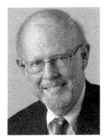

George H. Kraft, MD, MS
Consulting Editor

The combination of new medical treatments since the end of World War II in 1945 and the development of rehabilitation medicine have greatly prolonged the lives of persons with disabilities. In contrast to the previous policy of custodial care—institutional sequestration of children and adults with physical and mental disabilities—the postwar North American approach has been to develop aggressive rehabilitative strategies to improve the function and quality of life in persons with physical disabilities and restore them to productive life.[1]

Now, after many decades of this policy, there are more and more aging persons with disabilities in the population. Many, if not most, of these persons have acquired additional medical and psychological problems. These patients and their health care providers, however, often attribute their new symptoms to the natural course of the primary disability.

In the field of multiple sclerosis (MS) care, I see this frequently. Service providers tend to attribute any new neurologic symptom to MS, and in talks I give to patients and providers I continually remind them that patients with MS can also acquire other neurologic conditions. These other conditions should be treated and may be cured, and it is necessary to tease them out from the underlying MS. Several times a month I may see carpal tunnel syndrome—a curable condition—develop in MS patients. Less commonly, cervical or thoracic disc degeneration is present and produces myelopathic symptoms. Lumbosacral spinal stenosis can add to lower limb weakness, produce numbness, impair gait, and cause pain. All of these are potentially curable; they should be sought out. Although I have found it a challenge to convince surgeons to operate on these patients, with objective tests (eg, electromyograms, nerve conduction studies, MRI, and somatosensory evoked potentials) and collegial education, selective surgery can markedly improve these patients' symptoms and lives.

---

[1] An excellent source on the history of the development of rehabilitation medicine in the United States is Verville R. War, politics, and philanthropy: the history of rehabilitation medicine. Lanham, Boulder, New York, Toronto, Plymouth (United Kingdom): University Press of America; 2009.

Phys Med Rehabil Clin N Am 21 (2010) xiii–xiv
doi:10.1016/j.pmr.2010.02.002
1047-9651/10/$ – see front matter

Even though the population of disabled persons is aging, there has been too little research on the impact of aging on disabilities. This is why I was so pleased to see my colleagues, Dr Mark Jensen and his co-researchers of the Rehabilitation Research and Training Center on Aging with Disabilities, University of Washington in Seattle, Washington, awarded a 5-year center grant from the National Institute on Disability and Rehabilitation Research. This issue of the *Physical Medicine and Rehabilitation Clinics of North America*, entitled "Aging with a Physical Disability," is the first major dissemination effort of this Center.

Mark Jensen, PhD, and Ivan Molten, PhD, the guest editors of this issue, have drawn together a large number of rehabilitation researchers, representing a variety of disciplines, who have been active in aging research in several diseases. Aging with common specific diseases are discussed. Drs Carter, Chamberlain, Abresch, and Jensen review aging with muscular dystrophy, and Drs Charlifue and Jha discuss aging with spinal cord injury. Aging with MS is presented by Drs Stern, Sorkin, and Sperber, and Drs Strax, Luciano, Dunn, and Quevedo present aging with developmental disabilities.

Moving from specific diseases to transdisability symptoms, discussion of falls is by Drs Finlayson and Peterson; psychological function by Drs Bombardier, Ehde, Stoelb, and Molton; physical activity and quality of life by Drs Motl and McAuley; pain and fatigue by Drs Widerstrom-Noga and Finlayson; communication by Drs Yorkston, Bourgeois, and Baylor; and cognition by Dr Borson.

Vocational impacts of aging with a disability are presented by Drs Johnson, Brown, and Knaster, and biopsychosocial perspectives are discussed by the guest editors. Finally, the future applications of virtual reality and gaming interventions and how they might promote successful aging are presented by Drs Lange, Requejo, Flynn, Rizzo, Valero-Cuevas, Baker, and Winstein.

In summary, "Aging with a Physical Disability" is a useful and accessible source of information on the wide variety of problems that persons with disabilities may (or will) encounter as they age. I am confident that it will continue to be a useful reference for clinicians and researchers for years to come. I want to thank the guest editors and article authors for the uncounted hours they have spent to bring this volume to fruition.

George H. Kraft, MD, MS
Department of Rehabilitation Medicine
Department of Neurology
University of Washington, Box 356490
1959 NE Pacific Street, Seattle
WA 98195-6490, USA

E-mail address:
ghkraft@uw.edu

Preface
Aging with a Physical Disability

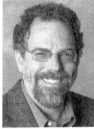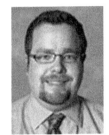

Mark P. Jensen, PhD   Ivan R. Molton, PhD
Guest Editors

It has been 5 years since the last *Physical Medicine and Rehabilitation Clinics of North America* special issue on aging with physical disability.[1] At that time, it was already well known that, owing to rapid medical and technological advances, individuals with physical disabilities were living much longer than at any other time in history. This increasing longevity means that larger numbers of adults will face both the general processes and problems that can come with growing older, along with a range of additional medical, social, psychological, and vocational concerns associated with aging with a physical disability. The many topics covered in that issue, ranging from basic age-related changes in physiology to topics associated with specific symptoms such as fatigue and basics of elder law, provided a state-of-the science review of the key topics important to geriatric rehabilitation.

The goal of the current special issue is to provide an update on many of the topics covered in that important first issue, and to introduce the reader to some new areas associated with scientific advances in the field. Themes covered in the current issue that overlap and update the previous issue include reviews of aging with specific disability conditions: spinal cord injury (Charlifue, Jha, and Lammertse), multiple sclerosis (Stern, Sorkin, Milton, and Sperber), cerebral palsy (Strax, Luciano, Dunn, and Quevedo), and post-polio syndrome (Carter, Weiss, Chamberlain, Han, Absresch, Miró, and Jensen). Also covered is the matter of aging with symptoms such as pain and fatigue—and, in this issue, sleep (Widerström-Noga and Finlayson); and topics associated with exercise (Motl and McAuley) and mobility and falls (Finlayson and

Support for this special issue was provided, in part, by a grant from the Department of Education, National Institute on Disability and Rehabilitation Research (H133B080024). The contents of this article do not necessarily represent the policy of the Department of Education and the reader should not assume endorsement by the Federal Government.

Phys Med Rehabil Clin N Am 21 (2010) xv–xvi
doi:10.1016/j.pmr.2010.02.001
pmr.theclinics.com

Peterson). In addition, the current issue introduces some new topics that are of vital concern to individuals aging with disabilities including a broad theoretical review of psychosocial concepts relevant to the field of geriatric rehabilitation (Molton and Jensen), discussions of employment, benefits, and insurance (Johnson, Brown, and Knaster), psychological functioning (Bombardier, Stoelb, Ehde, and Molton), communication (Yorkston, Bourgeois, and Baylor), the use of technology to improve quality of life (Lang, Requejo, Flynn, Rizzo, Valero-Cuevas, Baker, Ragusa, and Winstein), and cognitive functioning (Borson).

Our hope is that the information provided in this special issue will provide important information that clinicians will find useful when working with individuals aging with disabilities. We also hope that scientists will use this information to inspire new discoveries in the burgeoning field of geriatric rehabilitation. We hope that through a better understanding of this complicated area, we will ultimately make it easier for people to maximize their overall quality of life as they age with disability.

Mark P. Jensen, PhD
Department of Rehabilitation Medicine
Box 359612
University of Washington
Harborview Medical Center
325 Ninth Avenue
Seattle, WA 98104-9612, USA

Ivan R. Molton, PhD
Department of Rehabilitation Medicine
Box 356490
University of Washington
1959 NE Pacific Street
Seattle, WA 98195-6490, USA

E-mail addresses:
mjensen@uw.edu (M.P. Jensen)
imolton@uw.edu (I.R. Molton)

REFERENCE

1. Cristian A. Physical medicine and rehabilitation clinics of North America: aging with a disability. Philadelphia: Elsevier; 2005.

Aging and Disability: Biopsychosocial Perspectives

Ivan R. Molton, PhD[a], Mark P. Jensen, PhD[b],*

KEYWORDS

• Aging • Disability • Geriatrics

> "True terror is to wake up one morning and discover that your high school class is running the country."
> ~ Attributed to Kurt Vonnegut Jr

The term "older adult" has a complicated history, and is associated with more than a little political and public health controversy. Although in the broadest sense of the word, aging is a process that begins at birth, most researchers who describe aging are really talking about changes that come about after physical maturity and in later adulthood. In this sense, growing older is often seen as a time-dependent series of irreversible and progressive declines in functioning that manifests at reproductive maturity and eventually ends in death.[1] In this purely biological model of aging, these processes are seen as normal, cumulative, and inevitably associated with loss and decline.

Given the historical dominance of this conceptualization of aging and later adulthood, it is no wonder that researchers and health care professionals have for many years associated being older with sickness, frailty, and depression. Media and popular opinion contribute to this view by emphasizing the losses that occur with age, which include loss of spouse, friends, relatives, sensations, cognitive functioning, finances, independence, work, and physical ability. Younger adults, caregivers, and families project their own fears onto their elders, and presume that in the face of such overwhelming losses, older individuals must experience depression and chronic grief. Older adults are therefore often depicted either as isolated and depressed, or paradoxically, as gentle and noble creatures who somehow transcend suffering and

This research was supported, in part, by a grant from the Department of Education, National Institute on Disability and Rehabilitation Research (H133B080024). The contents of this article do not necessarily represent the policy of the Department of Education and the reader should not assume endorsement by the Federal Government.

[a] Department of Rehabilitation Medicine, University of Washington School of Medicine, 1959 Northeast Pacific Street, Box 356490, Seattle, WA 98195-6490, USA
[b] Department of Rehabilitation Medicine, University of Washington, Harborview Medical Center, 325 Ninth Avenue, Box 359612, Seattle, WA 98104-9612, USA
* Corresponding author.
E-mail address: mjensen@uw.edu

Phys Med Rehabil Clin N Am 21 (2010) 253–265
doi:10.1016/j.pmr.2009.12.012

dispense timeless wisdom. Between these extremes, there is little room for an older adult to be a genuine person, and to experience the wide range of emotions and social changes associated with living into old age. Even more importantly, such stereotypes downplay the incredible heterogeneity of the older adult population; older individuals have tremendous variability in terms of physical, cognitive, and emotional functioning, and adequate approaches to aging must take into account this heterogeneity.

One place that this vast variability manifests is in physical disability. Older adults vary greatly in their abilities to perform activities of daily living and instrumental activities of daily living, and in their responses to disability. Concurrent to the trajectory of aging (in chronologic years) is the trajectory of disability, and these trajectories interact in complex ways across the life span. People who are free of disability until late in life experience disability with age.[2] This group includes individuals who experience sudden disability resulting from stroke or spinal cord injury (SCI) late in life and those who experience a more gradual decline in function associated with the cumulative effects of multiple health conditions (eg, osteoarthritis, diabetic complications, complications from cardiovascular or pulmonary disease). At the same time, those growing older with long-standing, early-onset disabilities (such as polio and multiple sclerosis) are said to age with disability.[2] In fact, owing to improvements in the medical care and rehabilitation of persons with disabilities, individuals with physical disabilities acquired in early adulthood are now living a near normal life expectancy, and this group is representing more and more of the older adult population. These individuals also face a unique array of stressors. For example, there is evidence that the organ systems of persons with physical disabilities age faster than in their nondisabled peers, and that this increase in aging rate results in faster and more severe onset of health conditions (such as heart disease and obesity), mobility limitations, perceived symptoms (such as pain and fatigue), and other secondary conditions (such as depression). These secondary conditions can have profound negative effects on the quality of life, including community participation and employment.

Individuals aging with disabilities and those aging into disability may therefore ultimately arrive at similar places in terms of physical functioning, but take vastly different routes to get there. These individuals vary in terms of age at disability onset (including whether this disability was on time or off time in terms of expectation), age cohort (including the available medical treatments and the social environment at the time of disability onset), biologic age (because long-standing disabilities are often associated with early organ decline), and duration of disability (which includes the sum of experiences an individual has acquired in terms of managing disability). In a sense, older adults with long-standing disabilities (ie, those aging with disability) may have much to teach their age cohort in terms of coping with declines in physical functioning and generally getting around as a disabled person. Despite this, although a large body of research has now investigated a range of topics within aging into disability, little attention has been paid to older adults with long-standing physical impairments.

Although it is increasingly clear that the fields of social gerontology and disability services research have considerable overlap, the research and service networks of these groups typically have been fragmented and loosely organized.[3] In disability research, investigators have focused on describing disabilities in certain specific age groups (eg, children or the very old) and have focused on cross-sectional methodologies with short time frames. On the other hand, gerontologists are interested primarily in understanding the experience of older adults, which includes (but is not limited to) disability. Neither group has traditionally emphasized that age and disability are trajectories that interact across time, requiring research that looks forward for children with disability and looks back for older adults with new impairments.[2]

The purpose of this article is to tackle this disconnection from the perspective of the disability services researcher, by providing researchers and clinicians working in this area with a primer in aging and gerontology as they relate to disability. By doing so, the authors hope to provide some tools to better understand the complex interaction of biologic, social, and psychological factors for older adults living with long-term and newly acquired disabilities.

To accomplish this, this article first describes the social environment of the older adult, with an emphasis on social support, grief, and bereavement. There follows a discussion on the primary theories on aging, with special relevance to aging with disability, including a review of what is known about coping with chronic illness in older individuals. Finally, the authors use these theoretical approaches to confront an important (and on the surface puzzling) finding in aging and disabilities literatures, which is the reported high quality of life in the context of poor physical function and decline.

SOCIAL SUPPORT, BEREAVEMENT, AND THE OLDER ADULT

Human beings are social creatures, and having a group of people who can consistently provide reciprocal emotional and tangible support is an essential part of quality of life. Although the desire for meaningful relationships does not appear to change with age, the availability and flexibility of the available network does.

Changes in social support network size and organization are one of the best-documented effects in the aging literature. However, although younger people are more likely to have larger social support networks than older adults,[4] it is important to remember that among older people, quality is more important than quantity in terms of preserving well-being.[5] Although earlier work in this area tended to emphasize an involuntary decrease in social network size due to the loss of loved ones and isolation associated with physical decline,[6,7] more recent work has proposed that older adults may also intentionally restructure and downsize their social support networks,[8,9] such that there is an age-related decrease in the number of peripheral social partners, while the number of close social partners remains essentially stable throughout the life span.[10] Essentially, older adults appear to be more selective in their choice of social partners, and prefer to be with people who are like themselves and who provide information that is consistent with their beliefs.[11]

This process of downsizing is most pronounced from early to middle adulthood, suggesting that (contrary to popular belief) whatever emotional distress may exist in later adulthood is not clearly related to involuntary changes in social support.[12] Rather, as people grow older they become more aware of mortality and reductions in time left, and appear to become increasingly thoughtful about who they want to spend their time with.[13,14] In support of this hypothesis, recent studies have shown that social selection is influenced by perception of time restraint.[15,16] For example, in one series of studies, participants of all ages were asked to imagine that they had half an hour of free time with no pressing time commitments and that they had decided to spend that time with another person. The subjects were given 3 potential choices: a close family member (ie, an emotionally close connection), an acquaintance with whom they seem to have much in common (ie, a potential new social partner), or the author of a book they had just read (ie, a novel and exciting social partner). Older adults were more likely to prefer the familiar social partner, whereas younger adults showed no preference. This finding has also been shown to generalize in samples of adults in China, Hong Kong, and Taiwan.[17] Importantly, these effects disappeared when all participants experienced a sense of foreshortened future (ie, when they were asked to imagine that they would soon be moving across the country); individuals of all ages preferred an emotionally close partner (a family member) to novel or potential social partners.

Gender differences are also well documented in older adult social support networks, with women tending to have larger networks and being more likely to receive support from multiple sources.[18] Across the life span, women tend to base friendships on intimacy resulting from emotional sharing, whereas men tend to base friendships on shared activities.

In summary, normally aging older adults appear to change their social networks through an intentional process and have networks typified by fewer members, but greater emotional closeness to social partners. Moreover, networks based on emotional intimacy are associated with greater social satisfaction, more frequent exchanges of tenderness, and less loneliness.[19]

Although the kind of social network trimming described earlier does not appear to be a function of involuntary factors (such as the death of friends), it does leave older adults at greater risk for absorbing tremendous social support losses when a member of this (now smaller) social support network passes away. Thus, bereavement is a real issue for older persons. Over the age of 65, 51% of women and 13.6% of men in the United States have been widowed at least once.[20] Although grief reactions in older adults tend to be more flat or subdued, particularly if the partner died of an illness that was lingering,[21] there is little evidence to suggest that the loss of a partner is less distressing for the elderly compared with younger adults. In fact, normal bereavement is associated with a broad range of poor outcomes in the elderly, including chronically decreased mood,[22] increased use of prescription medicine,[23] greater likelihood of being placed in a nursing home,[24] and even risk of mortality.[25] One famous set of studies[26] from 1988 to 1989 followed 503 elderly men for 6 years after the loss of their spouses, and found that the death rate for widowers over the age of 75 years was significantly higher than for their same-aged, nonbereaved peers. In addition to the painful loss of the loved person, a bereaved individual also loses an important source of interaction and tangible support. Perhaps because these losses can be so impacting, the remaining social network of bereaved older adults appears to take on greater importance at the time of bereavement.[27,28] Given that many older adults reduce their social network to a few key friends, the remaining social support structures can become strained, leaving older adults at risk for social isolation.

THE SOCIAL SUPPORT NETWORK IN OLDER ADULTS LIVING WITH PHYSICAL DISABILITY

Individuals who are aging with or into disability have unique social support needs. Although little research has been done in this area, the general literature on disability documents the importance of social support in fulfilling a range of important needs. These include providing instrumental help (physical assistance such as help with meal preparation, bowel or bladder management, transfers), emotional support, anxiety reduction through empathic interactions, and a measure for progress and comparison to others.[29] Furthermore, the literature on individuals with long-standing disabilities such as SCI emphasize the importance of the disabled person's spouse in fulfilling many of these needs,[30] often to the exclusion of other forms of support. For example, in one study by Decker and colleagues,[30] 41% of the sample with SCI reported only a single source of support, and that support was a spouse. Research has also found that individuals with disabilities, such as SCI, are more likely to remain unmarried after injury and have higher than average divorce rates (eg, 21.2% compared with 12.6% in the general population).[31] Therefore, individuals aging with disabilities can face several interrelated problems in terms of social support; they are more likely to be unmarried or divorced because of their disability, and for those with a spouse, they are more likely to rely on that person exclusively for care. In terms of aging, this latter tendency leaves individuals with disabilities vulnerable to losing virtually all of their tangible support networks when their spouses develop age-related health problems or pass away.

In a series of focus groups involving disabled older adults conducted by the authors' research team, social support emerged as a key factor in qualitative analyses (Yorkston and colleagues, unpublished data, 2009).[32] As expected, the participants in this study often referred to the aging of their own social support network. For example, one participant (with post-polio syndrome) had a husband who had developed advanced Parkinson disease, and this had a dramatic effect on his ability to care for her. Another man (with SCI) reported: "As I'm getting older, so is my spouse and my friends. Every friend I have lives upstairs and they haul you up the steps. They're getting older and they have their aches and pains and say, 'My back's out, I can't help'." Individuals with long-standing disabilities may also feel frustrated by friends and family who are now developing their own limitations, and are working to "push through" them. A comparison process may begin, in which those with more normative limitations (ie, those aging into disability) may misunderstand disability resulting from conditions such as multiple sclerosis or post-polio syndrome, and put unfair expectations on the aging disabled person. Normally aging individuals may not understand that issues such as fatigue, memory problems, and chronic pain are subjectively different for individuals with a long-standing disability. One participant in the authors' group described this process of comparison by saying, "You're doing things they want you to do, maybe not as much, maybe not as often, but they don't quite understand the fatigue and the fact that the pain is always there". From these qualitative data and published studies, it would seem that the normal trimming process of aging intersects with increasing disability for these individuals, such that social support may be more limited, more vulnerable, and at times more stressful for the adult aging with disability. However, there are to date virtually no quantitative studies investigating this area.

THEORETICAL PERSPECTIVES
The Life Span Developmental Approach

Perhaps the most dominant theoretical model of aging in contemporary Western thought is the life span developmental approach, a theoretical orientation of aging that is concerned with the description, explanation, and modification (optimization) of developmental processes in the human life course from conception to death.[32] This theoretical orientation was based on early work of several investigators, including Carl Jung, but really took shape after the coinciding publication of several important longitudinal aging studies that began before World War II and the resulting inception of gerontology in the 1950s.[32] This orientation provides a biopsychosocial framework for understanding the aging process, and is often described as a counter model to more traditional approaches based on loss, decline, and the abnormal psychology of aging.

In brief, the life span developmental approach proposes that development occurs throughout the life span, and not just during the formative years of childhood and adolescence. Individuals are seen as continually making adaptations to changing external demands, including (but not only to) physical and mental decline. As a result, the magnitude of individual differences and the variability of functioning are seen to be greatest during infancy and then again in older age. The life span developmental model also emphasizes the interaction of biologic, social, and psychological factors, and takes into account the influence of cohort effects (ie, the impact of shared experiences that occurred at a set point of time and during a particular period of development for a group of people).

In the life span developmental perspective[33] the following propositions about the nature of human aging have been described:

1. There are major differences between normal, pathologic, and optimal aging, the latter defined as aging under development-enhancing and age-friendly environmental conditions.
2. The course of aging shows much interindividual variability.
3. There is much latent reserve capacity in old age.
4. There is aging loss in the range of reserve capacity or adaptability.
5. Individual and social knowledge can compensate for age-related decline in fluid intelligence.
6. With age, the balance between gains and losses becomes increasingly negative.
7. The self in old age remains a resilient system of coping and maintaining integrity.

Key to the life span developmental model are 2 concepts: successful aging and the notion of on-time/off-time events. Successful aging in itself is thought to involve 3 elements: (1) selection, or an increasing restriction of one's life to fewer domains of functioning due to of age-related losses in adaptability; (2) optimization, or the engaging in behavior that enrich and augment life; and (3) compensation, or the use of adaptive behaviors to compensate for losses in functioning. Therefore, one can be seen to have aged successfully when one is able to continue to perform life tasks that are personally meaningful and important despite decreases in skills, memory, and performance. On-time/off-time events refer to the sequence of experienced life events as compared with individual expectations. For example, if an event occurs at a time or at an age that is considered normal for most people, then it is on time. A woman giving birth to children in her late twenties is an example of an on-time event. Alternately, events are considered off time when they occur out of the expected sequence or at a time or chronologic age that is unusual; the same woman giving birth to children in her late forties might be considered off time. Importantly, the use of the terms on and off do not imply that being different from the expected time schedule is "good" or "bad", merely that these events have unique impacts on the psychosocial trajectory of aging based on when in the life span they occur. It has been suggested, for example, that older adults are less bothered by physical health problems such as chronic pain if they perceive them as occurring on time or being normal.[34–36]

Clearly, the orientation or model described earlier was developed in normally aging individuals, including those aging into disability, and has rarely been applied to adults aging with disabilities acquired in young adulthood. For these individuals, physical impairments and limitations have occurred off time with expectation. Although difficulties in ambulation might seem normal (and be therefore less threatening) in an 80-year-old individual, the same impairments are not expected to occur in a person's thirties and forties. The effect of this off-time disability is not well studied. Does having significant physical limitations in younger adulthood inoculate or prepare one for the kinds of limitations that are inevitable in later life? Successful aging is said to occur when an individual is able to compensate for limitations in losses of functioning, actively selects activities that are within his or her realm of abilities, and actively seeks behaviors that enrich quality of life. Clearly, these same processes are present in younger and middle-aged adults facing disabilities. If that is the case, are these individuals better prepared for later adulthood? If so, then the trajectory of adults aging with disabilities would likely include stable or increasing quality of life despite rapid declines in functioning, and this would be greater than would occur in adults aging into disability. However, little research has applied this well-known aging model to adults with disabilities.

Socioemotional Selectivity Theory

A second major model designed to account for age-related changes in social support, coping, and engagement is socioemotional selectivity theory (SST).[37] SST posits that with increasing age, perceived limitations on time lead to reorganizations of goal hierarchies, such that goals related to here-and-now emotional meaning are prioritized more than goals associated with an improved future. Generally speaking, individuals are guided by the same set of social and emotional goals throughout life, such as feeling needed, seeking novelty, and expanding one's horizons.[14] However, the relative importance of these goals changes as a function of perceived time left to live. For those with decades ahead of them, goals aimed at knowledge acquisition, career planning, the development of new social relationships, and other endeavors that will pay off in the future are adaptive. On the other hand, for older adults (or those who perceive little time left) it is thought to be more adaptive to emphasize the positive emotional aspects of here-and-now situations and to prioritize emotion-focused strategies more than problem-focused strategies. Older adults are hypothesized to therefore focus more on emotion regulation, on the pursuit of emotionally gratifying interactions with social partners, and other pursuits whose benefits can be realized in the present. These individuals will emphasize alleviation of present suffering to maximize emotionally meaningful activities, including quality time with loved ones.

According to SST, it is time perspective (ie, perceived time left as an independent being), rather than actual chronologic age, that drives this reorganization. In fact, in several studies of younger people with presumably limited futures (eg, young males with symptomatic HIV infections), a reorganization of goals similar to that seen in older people occurs.[38] Additional support of SST comes from studies that have shown that older adults have a distinctive bias in attention and memory, such that older people attend to and remember positive information more than negative information.[39]

APPLICATION: THE PARADOX OF AGING MEETS THE PARADOX OF DISABILITY

Given that older adults often experience multiple losses, occurring simultaneously and within a short period of time, it would be logical to assume that old age would be associated with decrements in well-being. Similarly, given the myriad challenges and social and physical limitations faced by individuals with disabilities, such as SCI and multiple sclerosis, it would be logical to expect that individuals with disability would also live lives of suffering and difficulty. Surprisingly, the majority of empirical evidence does not support either assertion. In terms of aging, well-being is relatively stable throughout adulthood and does not show large negative age changes even in very old age.[40–42] Moreover, in terms of disability, research has shown that the majority of individuals with a range of disabling conditions report high quality of life despite significant physical impairments.[43] Although little research has investigated emotional well-being in the nexus of aging and disability, published studies describe a decreased impact of physical symptoms (such as pain) in later adulthood for individuals with disability.[44]

This is not to say that adults with disabilities have the same quality of life as those without them; in fact several major studies[45] suggest that adults with disabilities report lower satisfaction in areas such as health, finances, and work, and that health problems in the elderly are associated with greater negative affect and pessimism.[46]

Rather, it can be said that overall life satisfaction is not clearly or <u>consistently</u> related to disability or age. Put succinctly, older individuals and individuals with disability do appear to suffer, but not as much as would be expected given significant limitations. Such paradoxes demonstrate the complexity of concepts such as quality of life and well-being in these populations, and emphasize the relative importance of other factors, including social connectedness, attainment of personal and professional goals; and a sense of life purpose.[47] The aging and disability fields have worked simultaneously to provide adequate theoretical explanations for this phenomenon, and several prominent theories have been offered.

Perhaps the oldest explanation for relatively high quality of life in older adults with increasing physical limitations (ie, those aging into disability) comes from the coping literature. Much research over the past several decades has examined the ways that older adults cope with stressors, and has noted differences in the process and the content of coping as compared with younger adults. In general, these differences have favored older adults, suggesting more effective coping in later life. For example, from the psychodynamic/developmental perspective, Vaillant[48] reported that middle-aged men used fewer neurotic and immature defense mechanisms compared with their younger selves. More recently, Diehl and colleagues[49] reported that a group of older adults reported a combination of coping strategies indicating greater impulse control and positive appraisal of conflict situations as compared with younger adults and adolescents. Studies of standardized measures of coping have also supported these findings, suggesting that older adults generally use less escapism and avoidant coping.[50–52]

However, findings of more effective or positive coping in older adults have not been consistent across stressors or populations. For example, Folkman and colleagues[53] found that older people used more escape avoidance, although this effect could not be replicated by Aldwin.[51] Further, small[54] or no differences[55] in coping across age groups have been reported by several investigators, particularly in the area of problem-focused coping.[56] One finding in several studies is that older adults appear to use fewer strategies, but use them as or more effectively than younger adults.[51,57] Older adults also tend to use the same strategies for managing stressors across life domains.[58]

The dual process model of coping[59] states essentially that 2 coping tendencies are thought to mitigate depressive symptoms and foster positive adaptation to age-related losses: the assimilative mode (tenacious goal pursuit) and the accommodative mode (flexible goal adjustment). In the assimilative mode, an individual makes persistent efforts to actively adjust life circumstances to his or her preferences. This mode is characterized by direct action and problem solving, by attempts to modify the relationship between person and environment.[60] By contrast, the accommodative mode is associated with adjustment of goals, preferences, and expectations to situational constraints (eg, acceptance). The accommodative mode is seen as an unintentional process of restructuring goal hierarchies to achieve the best possible match between what is expected and what is possible. This mode may involve effective detachment from obstructed goals or emotional reappraisal of bad situations through attempts to derive meaning from them.[60] These modes of coping are not mutually exclusive, and sometimes operate simultaneously or in rapid succession. However, this model predicts that in a healthy individual, assimilative processes tend to dominate when situations are changeable, and that accommodative strategies tend to be activated and are most appropriate when assimilative efforts become ineffective. Given the multitude of changing environmental factors (and losses) associated with aging, one would hypothesize a shift toward greater accommodative coping in the elderly, and in fact the data generally support this notion.[59,61] However, important in this is the notion of on-time versus off-time changes in physical function. For older adults, there is probably a certain expectation of disability and activity restriction,[62] and this expectation of disability as being on time is important in terms of a shift to accommodative coping. For example, older adults with functional impairments may show more flexibility in terms of readjusting priorities than middle-aged adults, if these impairments are expected.[63] Conversely, analyses from one major study of aging[40] suggests that aspects of disability that cannot be explained by a person's age appear to have greater negative effects on subjective well-being than those that are expected in aging.

Given the findings presented earlier, one would expect that the perception of disability as off time (or unexpected given age) would contribute to greater negative effect initially, followed by an inoculation effect that better prepares individuals aging with disability for greater losses of physical function in later adulthood. However, available data also refer to the great complexity of these issues in people aging with and into physical disabilities. In one recent study of older adults aging into disability, Paul and colleagues[46] assessed functional limitations and quality of life in 999 people aged 65 years or older. Results partially confirmed disability and aging paradoxes, as people in the oldest age group (80+) reported good perceptions of quality of life despite high prevalence of health and mobility problems. However, the more disabled, the more pessimistic participants were about their futures. Also, the relationship between disability and well-being varied with age, such that among the oldest old, those reporting poorer health were also less optimistic (which is the opposite of what would be expected from the aging or disability paradox models).

Boerner[64] analyzed cross-sectional data on accommodative versus assimilative coping, chronologic age, and depressive symptoms in a group of middle-aged and older adults with significant vision loss. As expected, increasing age was associated with a decrease in assimilative coping (although not an increase in accommodative coping). A significant accommodative coping × functional disability × age interaction also emerged, such that the beneficial effects of accommodative coping (in terms of buffering depression) were much stronger for middle-aged adults with more significant visual disability. However, for older adults, the benefit of accommodative coping was present regardless of disability level. These data can be interpreted to suggest that for persons with disabilities that occur off time (ie, vision loss at middle-age), the shift toward accommodative coping happens sooner and is of greater benefit than to those who experience disability in later life (ie, those aging into disability).

SST (described earlier) may also contribute to explaining the paradoxes reported in aging and disability literatures. According to this model, the relative importance of life goals change as a function of perceived time left to live. For individuals with long-standing disabilities, aging is typically associated with increases in secondary symptoms such as fatigue, pain, and weakness, and with greater rate of decline in independence than has been experienced in the prior decades. Therefore, an adult experiencing a rapid decline of hard-won gains in independence may become aware that their time is limited, and therefore begin to prioritize emotion-focused strategies more than problem-focused strategies, and focus on emotionally gratifying interactions with social partners and other pursuits whose benefits can be realized in the present, rather than in the uncertain and shifting future. Hypothetically, these strategies would lead to greater emotional well-being, and thereby buffer the expected effects of age and disability on quality of life.

In relation, SST researchers also point to a greater experience of poignancy or the simultaneous (or closely related) experience of positive and negative effect in later adulthood.[65] Poignancy is thought to result from the simultaneous experience of positivity (eg, being generally satisfied with life) and an awareness or anticipation of future losses.[66] Theoretically, perceived limitations on time increase appreciation for life, eliciting positive emotions such as happiness. Simultaneously, an awareness of death or loss of independence leads to an awareness that these positive experiences will soon come to an end.[66] Although the literature on poignancy is somewhat new and controversial in older adults, its application to older adults with physical disabilities is clear. By the same processes described earlier (eg, age-related increase in the rate of physical decline), aging with disability may trigger a poignant experience of effect that could mask unidimensional depression and anxiety expected by researchers, which could create what seems to be a paradox: high quality of life at a time of declines in physical health. This complexity is also seen in cross-sectional literature, where age and functional health constraints have been shown to relate differentially to positive and negative effect.[40] In essence, it is not that older adults with disability experience significantly lower rates of negative effect, but that their experience is more complicated and multifaceted than in younger adults.

The trajectory of aging and disability must also be considered. Based on the findings from available research, it may be inferred that if health constraints were not a problem, we would expect consistent increases in emotional well-being as we age.[67] However, in later life, functional limitations inevitably begin to manifest. The rate at which these limitations appear varies as a function of many factors, including chronological age and duration of disability. However, it would also appear that when physical health decreases beyond a certain level, it offsets the stability of positive effect in aging, leading to an increase in negative effect that is associated with serious disability.[40]

SUMMARY

Greater collaboration and communication is needed between the fields of aging and disability. In many ways, geriatrics has paved the way for disability researchers, as the graying of the disabled population makes theoretical models of aging salient for persons growing older with disability. The trajectories of aging with disability are vastly complicated, and when considering clinical and research questions in this area one must consider the reciprocal interactions among factors such as duration of disability, current social support, biological aging, and quality of life. Further, longitudinal work is needed to better understand these interactions and to provide appropriate care for this population.

REFERENCES

1. Arking R. Biology of aging: observations and principles. 2nd edition. Sunderland (MA): Sinauer Associates; 1998.
2. Verbrugge LM, Yang L. Aging with disability and disability with aging. J Disabil Pol Stud 2002;12:253-8.
3. Putnam M. Moving from separate to crossing aging and disability service networks. In: Putnam M, Campbell M, editors. Aging and disability: crossing network lines. New York: Springer; 2006. p. 5–17.
4. Lee DJ, Markides KS. Activity and mortality among aged persons over an eight-year period. J Gerontol 1990;45:S39–42.
5. Antonucci TC. Personal characteristics, social support, and social behavior. In: Binstock RH, Shanas E, editors. Handbook of aging and the social sciences. 2nd edition. New York: Reinhold; 1985. p. 94–128.

6. Cumming E, Dean LR, McCaffrew I. Disengagement: a tentative theory of aging. Sociometry 1960;23:23–5.

7. Maddox GL. Activity and morale: a longitudinal study of selected elderly subjects. Soc Forces 1963;42:195–204.

8. Lang FR. Endings and continuity of social relationships: maximizing intrinsic benefits within personal networks when feeling near to death. J Soc Pers Relat 2000;17:155–82.

9. Carsentsen LL. Evidence for a life-span theory of socioemotional selectivity. Curr Dir Psychol Sci 1995;4:151–6.

10. Levitt MJ, Weber RA, Guacci N. Convoys of social support: an intergenerational analysis. Psychol Aging 1993;8:323–6.

11. Brown SL, Asher R, Cialdini RB. Evidence of a positive relationship between age and preference for consistency. J Res Pers 2004;39:517–33.

12. Carstensen LL. Social and emotional patterns in adulthood: support for socioemotional selectivity theory. Psychol Aging 1992;7:331–8.

13. Cavanaugh JC. Friendships and social networks among older people. In: Nordhus IH, VandenBos GR, Berg S, et al, editors. Clinical geropsychology. Washington, DC: American Psychological Association; 1998. p. 121–38.

14. Lockenhoff CE, Carstensen LL. Socioemotional selectivity theory, aging, and health: the increasingly delicate balance between regulating emotions and making tough choices. J Pers 2004;72:1398–424.

15. Fredrickson BL, Carstensen LL. Choosing social partners: how old age and anticipated endings make people more selective. Psychol Aging 1990;5:335–47.

16. Fung HH, Carstensen LL, Lutz AM. Influence of time on social preferences: implications for life-span development. Psychol Aging 1999;14:595–604.

17. Fung HH, Lai P, Ng R. Age differences in social preferences among Taiwanese and Mainland Chinese: the role of perceived time. Psychol Aging 2001;16:351–6.

18. Rawlins WK. Friendship matters. Hawthorne (NY): Aldine de Gruyter; 1992.

19. Lang FR, Staudinger UM, Carstensen LL. Perspectives in socioemotional selectivity in late life: how personality and social context do (and do not) make a difference. J Gerontol B Psychol Sci Soc Sci 1998;53:21–30.

20. Larue A, Dessonville D, Jarvik L. Aging and mental disorders. In: Birren J, Schaie KW, editors. Handbook of the psychology of aging. New York: Van Nostrand; 1985. p. 664–702.

21. Wisock PA. The experience of bereavement by older adults. In: Hersen M, Van Hasselt VB, editors. Handbook of clinical geropsychology. New York: Plenum Press; 1998. p. 431–45.

22. Pasternak R, Reynolds C, Miller M, et al. The symptom profile and two-year course of subsyndromal depression in spousally bereaved elders. Am J Geriatr Psychiatry 1994;2:210–9.

23. Avis N, Barmbilla D, Vass K, et al. The effect of widowhood on health: a prospective analysis from the Massachusetts Women's Health Study. Soc Sci Med 1991;33:1063–70.

24. Wolinski F, Johnson R. Widowhood, health status, and the use of health services by older adults: a cross-sectional and prospective approach. J Gerontol B Psychol Sci Soc Sci 1992;47:8–16.

25. Mendes le Leon CF, Kasl SV, Jacobs S. Widowhood and mortality risk in community sample of the elderly: a prospective study. J Clin Epidemiol 1993;46:519–27.

26. Bowling A. Who dies after widow(er)hood? A discriminant analysis. Omega J Death Dying 1988;19:135–53.

27. Norris F, Murrell S. Social support, life events, and stress as modifiers of adjustment to bereavement of older adults. Psychol Aging 1990;4:150–65.
28. Siegel J, Kuykendal D. Loss, widowhood, and psychological distress among the elderly. J Consult Clin Psychol 1990;58:519–24.
29. Holicky R, Charlifue S. Ageing with spinal cord injury: the impact of spousal support. Disabil Rehabil 1999;21:250–7.
30. Decker SD, Schulz R, Wood D. Determinants of well-being in primary caregivers of persons with spinal cord injury. Rehabil Nurs 1989;14:6–8.
31. National Spinal Cord Injury Statistical Center. Annual report for the model spinal cord injury care systems. Birmingham: Alabama: NSCISC; 1996.
32. Baltes PB, Reese HW, Lipsitt LP. Life-span developmental psychology. Annu Rev Psychol 1980;31:65–110.
33. Baltes PB. Theoretical propositions of life-span developmental psychology: on the dynamics between growth and decline. Dev Psychol 1987;23:611–26.
34. Cook A, Thomas M. Pain and the use of health services among the elderly. J Aging Health 1994;6L:155–72.
35. Greenlee K. Pain and analgesia: considerations for the elderly in critical care. AACN Clin Issues Crit Care Nurs 1991;2:720–8.
36. Parmeless P. Pain and psychological function in late life. In: Mostofsky DI, Lomranz J, editors. Handbook of pain and aging. New York: Plenum Press; 1997. p. 207–26.
37. Carstensen LL, Isaacowitz DM, Charles ST. Taking time seriously: a theory of socioemotional selectivity. Am Psychol 1999;54:165–81.
38. Carstensen LL, Fredrickson BL. Influence of HIV status and age on cognitive representations of others. Health Psychol 1998;17:494–503.
39. Charles ST, Mather M, Carstensen LL. Aging and emotional memory: the forgettable nature of negative images for older adults. J Exp Psychol Gen 1993;132:310–24.
40. Kunzmann U, Little T, Smith J. Is age-related stability of subjective well-being a paradox? Cross-sectional and longitudinal evidence from the Berlin aging study. Psychol Aging 2000;15:511–26.
41. Diener E, Suh ME. Subjective well-being and age: an international analysis. In: Schaie KW, Lawton MP, editors, Annual review of gerontology and geriatrics, vol. 8. New York: Springer; 1997. p. 304–24.
42. Horley J, Lavery JJ. Subjective well-being and age. Soc Indic Res 1995;34:275–82.
43. Albrecht GL, Revenson T. Age differences in stress, coping, and the attribution of responsibility. Paper presented at the 93rd Annual Meeting of the American Psychological Association. Los Angeles, August 23–27, 1985.
44. Molton IR, Jensen MP, Ehde DM, et al. Phantom limb pain and pain interference in adults with lower extremity amputation: the moderating effects of age. Rehabil Psychol 2007;5:272–9.
45. Kemp BJ, Krause JS. Depression and life satisfaction among people with postpolio and spinal cord injury. Disabil Rehabil 1999;21:241–9.
46. Paul C, Ayis S, Ebrahim S. Disability and psychosocial outcomes in old age. J Aging Health 2007;5:723–41.
47. Koch T. The illusion of paradox: commentary on Albrecht, G.L. and Devlieger, P.J. (1998). The disability paradox: high quality of life against all odds. Soc Sci Med 2007;50:757–9.
48. Vaillant G. Adaptation to life. Boston: Little, Brown & Company; 1977.

49. Diehl M, Coyle N, Labouvie-Vief G. Age and sex differences in strategies of coping and defense across the lifespan. Psychol Aging 1996;11:127–39.
50. Aldwin C, Revenson T. Age differences in stress, coping, and the attribution of responsibility. Paper presented at the 93rd Annual Meeting of the American Psychological Association. Los Angeles, August 23–27, 1985.
51. Aldwin CM. Does age affect the stress and coping process? Implications of age differences in perceived control. J Gerontol 1991;46:174–80.
52. Irion JC, Blanchard-Fields F. A cross-sectional comparison of adaptive coping in adulthood. J Gerontol 1987;42:502–4.
53. Folkman S, Lazarus RS, Pimley S, et al. Age differences in stress and coping processes. Psychol Aging 1987;2:171–84.
54. Aldwin CM, Sutton KJ, Chiara G, et al. Age differences in stress, coping and appraisal: findings from the normative aging study. J Gerontol 1996;51: 179–88.
55. Blanchard-Fields F, Sulsky L, Robinson-Whelen S. Moderating effects of age and context on the relationship between gender, sex role differences, and coping. Sex Roles 1991;25:645–60.
56. McCrae RR. Age differences and changes in the use of coping mechanisms. J Gerontol 1982;44:161–9.
57. Meeks S, Carstensen L, Tamsky B, et al. Age differences in coping: does less mean worse? Int J Aging Hum Dev 1989;28:127–40.
58. Moos RH, Brennan PL, Schutte KK, et al. Older adults' coping with negative life events: common processes of managing health, interpersonal, and financial/work stressors. Int J Aging Hum Dev 2006;62:39–59.
59. Brandftstadte J, Renner G. Tenacious goal pursuit and flexible goal adjustment: explication and age-related analysis of assimilative and accommodative strategies of coping. Psychol Aging 1990;5:58–67.
60. Brandtstadter J. Personal self-regulation of development: cross-sectional analyses of development-related control beliefs and emotions. Dev Psychol 1989; 25:96–108.
61. Heckhausen J. Developmental regulation across adulthood: primary and secondary control of age-related challenges. Dev Psychol 1997;33:176–87.
62. Williamson GM, Schulz R. Activity restriction mediates the association between pain and depressed affect: a study of younger and older adult cancer patients. Psychol Aging 1995;10:69–78.
63. Brandtstadter J, Rothermund K. Self-percepts of control in middle and later adulthood: buffering losses by rescaling goals. Psychol Aging 1994;5:58–67.
64. Boerner K. Adaptation to disability among middle-aged and older adults: the role of assimilative and accommodative coping. J Gerontol B Psychol Sci Soc Sci 2004;59:35–42.
65. Ong AD, Bergeman CS. The complexity of emotions in later life. J Gerontol B Psychol Sci Soc Sci 2004;59:117–22.
66. Ersner-Hershfield H, Mikels JA, Sullivan SJ, et al. Poignancy: mixed emotional experience in the face of meaningful endings. J Pers Soc Psychol 2008;94: 158–67.
67. Lawton MP, Kleban MH, Rajagopal D, et al. Dimensions of affective experience in three age groups. Psychol Aging 1992;7:171–84.

Aging with Disability in the Workplace

Kurt L. Johnson, PhD*, Pat A. Brown, EdD,
Elizabeth S. Knaster, MPH

KEYWORDS

• Disability • Workplace • Employment • Aging

Individuals with disability, such as multiple sclerosis (MS), spinal cord injury (SCI), muscular dystrophy (MD), and late effects of polio (LEP), often develop a range of skills and strategies that when combined with environmental and social accommodations compensate for barriers they encounter to participation. As their function changes with age, however, these strategies and accommodations may not serve as effectively, especially at work.

Today, many individuals with disability live into later adulthood because of advances in medical knowledge and practice. For example, in 1940 the average life expectancy after SCI was just 18 months. In 2005, the same individual with SCI is expected to live approximately 85% of a normal life span (approximately 68 years).[1] By way of comparison, in the past 50 years the survival rate for individuals with SCI has increased 2000%, as opposed to only 30% for people in general.[2]

Although individuals with disabilities are living longer, they also are confronting higher levels of secondary conditions and barriers to participation than people in general. Increases in pain, weakness, fatigue, and other secondary symptoms may influence their work performance and their ability to remain in the workforce. For example, cardiovascular data from individuals with SCI indicate that they may "age faster" than those without SCI.[3,4] Moreover, older individuals with disabilities report higher rates of unemployment than older individuals who do not have a disability.[5] It is not surprising that given the high levels of unemployment, one of the significant risks associated with disability is poverty.[6]

In addition to the financial challenges that come with shifts in employment status, maintaining employment has been repeatedly linked with improved quality of life.[7,8]

This research was supported, in part, by a grant from the Department of Education, National Institute on Disability and Rehabilitation Research (H133B080024). The contents of this article do not necessarily represent the policy of the Department of Education and the reader should not assume endorsement by the Federal Government.
Department of Rehabilitation Medicine, University of Washington School of Medicine, Box 356490, Seattle, WA 98195, USA
* Corresponding author.
E-mail address: kjohnson@uw.edu

Issues around employment can be paramount as people age with increasing functional limitations.

Little is known about the impact of aging on employment for individuals with MS, SCI, MD, or LEP. Approximately 90% of individuals diagnosed with MS are employed before their diagnosis.[9] As few as 30% remain in the workplace 5 years postdiagnosis,[10] however, despite the fact that many (40%) who are unemployed want to return to work.[9] There have been few studies about vocational rehabilitation and individuals with MS. In a study in the United Kingdom, Sweetland and colleagues[11] concluded that individuals with MS need assistance with managing the interaction between the impairments caused by MS, the physical environment, and the demands imposed by the work. Studies conducted in the United States have found that interventions to preserve employment are more successful than those returning people to work, and that issues impacting employment are both related to the disease and to the work environment.[12,13] A few recent studies have examined issues around aging with MS, concluding that individuals with MS leave work earlier than the national average because of disability.[14] There are very little data, however, specific to the impact of aging and secondary conditions related to MS on employment or on the potential role of vocational rehabilitation interventions to prolong worklife.[15]

About 60% of individuals with SCI were employed before their injury, yet only 20% to 40% are employed 10 years and more postinjury.[16] Those individuals with SCI who do return to work require assistive technology, job placement, support services, and counseling.[17] As with individuals with MS, however, little is known about the impact of secondary conditions on continued employment as they age. Krause[18,19] found that it is extremely unlikely for those with SCI injured after the age 55 to return to work unless they are returning to their preinjury job. Those who do return to employment are not likely to remain until the traditional retirement age. Krause and others[20–22] also found that employment rates after age 50 continued to decline for those returning to work, although the reasons for this decline in employment rate and early retirement are not clearly determined beyond the relationship between employment and personal factors, such as increased education and functional status, and decreased medical complications.

As with individuals with MS, those with LEP experience early educational and professional options at the same level as their nondisabled siblings.[23] A total of 80% of the more than 1,000,000 survivors of poliomyelitis living in the United States experience symptoms consistent with LEP after age 40.[24] These symptoms, which include increased weakness, fatigue, and pain, are frequently severe enough to result in significant employment loss.[5,24,25] Most people with LEP have significant fatigue and 40% report that fatigue interferes with their ability to work.[26] To date there is no literature that investigates the role of vocational rehabilitation interventions addressing these symptoms and extending participation in employment for those with LEP.

No recent literature is available on the impact of aging with MD, secondary conditions related to MD, and participation in the workforce. Fowler and colleagues[27] found that employment decreased as individuals aged. Of the 157 people with MD that they interviewed, 40% were currently employed and 50% had previously been employed. Gagnon and colleagues[28] found that more than 45% of those surveyed with MD had experienced disruption in employment because of disability-related factors.

BARRIERS TO EMPLOYMENT

There are both individual and programmatic facilitators and barriers to employment for people with disabilities. The interaction among these facilitators and barriers form a personal economy of energy and resources. As barriers increase, the resources within the personal economy decrease, and as this happens individuals must make difficult decisions about resource allocations: whether to continue allocating increasingly scarce personal resources to employment at the expense of applying those resources to family and leisure. In several studies[29,30] subjects described that as their secondary conditions worsened, they found that when they arrived home from work, they often did not have enough energy to participate in family or leisure activities, and felt caught between valuing work, income, and health care benefits and missing out on important non–work-related quality of life. It is not just the progression of secondary conditions but rather the interaction of that progression with social and environmental barriers that takes a toll on the available economy.

Individual disability factors contributing as barriers to employment include secondary conditions, such as pain, fatigue, changes in mobility, depression, changes in cognition, changes in vision, and bowel and bladder control. Individual factors can also include characteristics of the individual that may or may not be related to disability, such as educational level, level of social support, and assertiveness.[31]

Societal and environment variables also can serve as barriers to employment for people with disabilities. Societal variables, such as the lack of universal health care coverage and the lack of portable health care coverage that follows an individual from job to job, are significant barriers. For example, people with disabilities may find themselves in the "disability trap" where their only viable option for health care coverage is associated with disability income subsidy. Similarly, they may have limited options, even with federal work incentive programs, to work while on subsidy. Environmental variables may include lack of accessible physical environments, such as restrooms and curb cuts, or inaccessible information technology, such as lack of usable computer interfaces.

To assist people with disabilities to retain or gain employment, informal or formal accommodations are often useful. Under many circumstances an employer is required by federal and state laws to provide accommodations for disability if asked.

KEY LEGISLATION

Because societal barriers have been so profoundly disabling, people with disabilities advocated unsuccessfully for disability status to be included as a protected class in the civil rights legislation of 1964 to 1966. In the 1974 amendments to the Rehabilitation Act of 1973, civil rights for people with disabilities were protected with respect to employment, education, and access if the entity (eg, school or employer) received federal dollars. It was not until the passage of the Americans with Disabilities Act (ADA) in 1990 that true disability civil rights legislation was enacted.[32–35]

The ADA provides true civil rights protection under most circumstances. The ADA prohibits discrimination in employment against qualified individuals with disabilities who are able to perform the essential functions of the job with or without accommodation. It also prohibits discrimination against individuals with disabilities in the areas of transportation, public accommodations, state and local governments, and telecommunications. Title I of the ADA, which took effect on July 26, 1992, prohibits private employers, state and local governments, employment agencies, and labor unions from discriminating against qualified individuals with disabilities in job application procedures, hiring, firing, advancement, compensation, job training, and other terms, conditions and privileges of employment. Because of recent federal and US Supreme Court decisions limiting the scope of ADA by finding that individuals may not sue state governments for discrimination in federal courts (although they may still file a complaint and the federal government could chose to sue a state government) and that "treatable" disabilities are not covered (eg, if the disability related to low vision is eliminated by eyeglasses, then the disability is not covered), Congress passed what was known as the "ADA Restoration Act," or the ADA Amendments Act of 2008. In the Act, Congress clarified its intent that the ADA covers a broad range of people and conditions and contexts.

ADA does not extend protection to every individual with a disability. Protection is limited to those individuals with disabilities that limit major life activities. Under ADA, a qualifying disability is defined as physical or mental impairment that substantially limits one or more of the major life activities of such an individual, record of such an impairment, and being regarded as having such an impairment. Reasonable accommodation may include but is not limited to making existing facilities used by employees readily accessible to and usable by persons with disabilities; job restructuring, modifying work schedules, reassignment to a vacant position; and acquiring or modifying equipment or devices, adjusting or modifying examinations, training materials, or policies, and providing qualified readers or sign language interpreters.

An employer must make an accommodation to the known disability of a qualified applicant or employee if it does not impose an undue hardship on the business. Undue hardship is defined as significant difficulty or expense in light of such factors as the employer's size, financial resources, and the nature and structure of its operation. Employers are not required to lower quality or production standards to make an accommodation, or to provide personal use items, such as eyeglasses or hearing aids.

Even though it is common practice, employers may not legally ask job applicants about the existence, nature, or severity of a disability but may ask about the applicant's ability to perform specific job functions. This can place the applicant in a difficult position because some disabilities, such as SCI, may be obvious to the employer, whereas for some people with MS or LEP, disability may be hidden. Strategies with respect to disclosure are discussed later in this article. A job offer may be contingent on the results of a medical examination only if the examination is required for all entering employees in similar jobs. Medical examinations of employees must be job-related and consistent with the employer's business needs. Similarly, qualifying tests must be clearly related to the demands of the job, and if accommodations are necessary for the employee to have a fair take on the test, they must be provided.

The US Equal Employment Opportunity Commission has issued regulations to enforce the provisions of Title I of the ADA for employers with more than 15 employees. Many states have laws that complement or exceed ADA requirements.

THE VOCATIONAL REHABILITATION PROCESS

Many people with SCI, MD, MS, and LEP are currently employed, or have a history of employment, and may even have a job to which they may return. The vocational rehabilitation process may be applied by individuals seeking to preserve their employment or find employment. It should not be viewed as a lockstep process but rather as a flexible set of interventions and tools that can be tailored to the needs of an individual. For individuals newly injured with SCI, this process may begin on the day of admission on the inpatient rehabilitation unit, if such services are provided. For people who have lived with SCI, MD, LEP, or MS, the vocational rehabilitation process can be initiated in the outpatient clinic or by the individual themselves. Whenever the process begins, it includes the following steps discussed next.

Referral

Health care providers are often in an ideal position to make referrals for vocational rehabilitation services. Note that many individuals also self-refer. Not only should individuals who are not working be considered for referral, but so should individuals who are working if there is an indication that they are dissatisfied with their employment or are at risk for losing their job. The vocational rehabilitation process should be driven by the person with the disability and supported by the rehabilitation counselor and others.[36]

Assessment

The assessment begins with a review of records and an interview with the client, significant others, family members, and other key informants. The assessment process includes a review of functional limitations and strengths, and an investigation of current and potential barriers to employment. A careful review of educational, vocational, and avocational history yields a list of transferable skills and an employment history (eg, a resume). An appraisal of the career interests may be useful either through the counseling process or with career assessment instruments. Generally, people are more satisfied in employment that is consistent with their career interests, for example preferences for working with data versus people, or in activities requiring creative problem solving versus routine activities. Similarly, it may be useful to understand an individual's temperament or personality style. This can be evaluated by a review of history, interview with the client and other key informants, observation, or psychologic assessment.[37]

If potential rehabilitation goals include return to school or pursuit of occupations that require certain levels of educational attainment, then it is necessary to evaluate achievement by a review of educational records, interview, and perhaps through achievement testing. An assessment of readiness for education can often be obtained by the client by taking the placement tests at community colleges and vocational training programs.

When possible, the best assessment involves review of actual performance, interview, and real world tryouts. The validity of paper and pencil tests is limited. Another approach to vocational evaluation involves the use of work samples.[38] Work samples are either organized along various tasks common to many jobs or tasks thought to represent a specific job. For example, one might have activities that sample the individual's ability to manipulate small objects or demonstrate eye-hand coordination. Commercially available vocational evaluation systems using work samples often include norms that purport to allow the evaluator to compare the performance of the person being evaluated with a standard necessary for successful occupational performance. These predictions do not hold up well; however, the vocational evaluation systems may provide a useful way for people with disabilities to try out a variety of occupational activities and for the evaluator to collect observational data about the way the client engages in the task.

Situational Assessment

Situational assessment is the generic term for using real-life situations to assess performance. In vocational rehabilitation, job stations or paid employment may serve this purpose. Job stations may be created by collaborating with employers to have the client try out elements of a job for a period of time. For example, consider a 55-year-old woman with LEP who has worked as a telephone reservations clerk for an airline for 20 years. Because of increasing fatigue and pain, she simply cannot keep up with the demands of the job despite accommodations. She is uncertain what else she could do. She has excellent public interaction skills and good computer skills. A job station is set up for her at the medical center where she performs the work of a patient care coordinator. Here she is able to change positions frequently, take breaks as necessary, and there is less focus on production speed. She is able to use this experience as a job tryout, and can get a recommendation from the supervisor and perhaps an introduction to a potential open position.

Labor Market Analysis

As part of the assessment process, the outlook for employment in various occupations is evaluated. The US Department of Labor and State Departments of Employment Security maintain statistics on trends in occupations including the number of people currently employed part time and full time in each occupational group, and the percent growth or decline predicted during the next 5 years. Clients can identify the number of jobs currently available in an occupational group within their immediate geographic area. They can also find out the wages, tasks, educational preparation, and other characteristics of occupations. This information is readily available on the US Department of Labor and other governmental Web sites.

Counseling

Many clients with disabilities find counseling useful to help them re-evaluate their expectations, enhance their personal adjustment, and understand and react to the perceptions and biases of others around them including family members, potential employers, and coworkers. As part of the counseling process the clients may take stock of the resources they bring to bear on the issues, the barriers they confront, and compensatory strategies to which they have access or can learn.

Selecting a Goal

Through the counseling process, the client evaluates the assessment data and develops a terminal goal and intermediate steps. For example, a 45-year-old woman with relapsing remitting MS who is having increasing difficulty with fatigue and cognition might set as her long-term goal to try and work until she is 55 and then go out on medical retirement. To reach that goal, she may need to develop intermediate steps that could include (1) improving accommodations in her job; (2) putting aside more savings in anticipation of reduced earnings in retirement; (3) engaging in careful estate planning to ensure that she preserves assets for herself and her family if her health deteriorates and she requires assisted living or skilled nursing; and (4) as her fatigue increases, she may need to either negotiate with other family members to pick up household chores, such as cleaning and shopping, or hire outside help.

Educational or Vocational Re-entry

Once the goal setting and planning is completed, the next step in the vocational rehabilitation process is intervening to preserve employment; vocational re-entry if a new job is the goal; or if additional education is the outcome, then educational re-entry. To preserve employment, individuals may be able to self-initiate informal accommodations in the workplace and negotiate necessary changes outside the workplace independently. Often, however, consultation from a rehabilitation counselor or other professional is useful. In vocational re-entry, the client may be able to secure a job independently, but often may require assistance in job development and placement from the rehabilitation counselor. Although discrimination against qualified individuals with disabilities is illegal, discrimination at the point of hiring is difficult to prove and may not be intentional on the part of the employer. Employers may not have experience interacting with people with significant disabilities and may not be able to imagine them working productively. Advocacy and assistance in obtaining employment is often an appropriate role for the rehabilitation counselor.

Supported Employment

Some people with disabilities require ongoing support in the workplace to sustain employment. For some, such as persons with high-level tetraplegia, support may involve assistance in positioning in relation to a task, manipulating materials, and so forth. They may also require personal care assistance in the workplace. Others, such as individuals with MS who have advancing cognitive difficulties, may require ongoing support in the form of job coaching from a coworker or paid assistant.

Job Placement

When the rehabilitation counselor is assisting with the job placement process, he or she begins by searching for jobs that meet elements of the client's goal. When potential jobs are identified, the rehabilitation counselor conducts a job analysis to determine the actual kinds of work done in that particular job; the cognitive, social, and physical demands of the job; and potential accommodations. Incidentally, this is the same process conducted to assist an individual to preserve employment. Then, in collaboration with the client and the employer, the fit of the job with the client is evaluated:

- Is this job a good match for what the client was seeking in terms of interest, skills, distance from home, social environment, pay, and benefits?
- Can the client do the essential functions of the job with or without accommodation?
- Given the size of the employer and the employer's resources, are the accommodations reasonable?
- If the client cannot perform the essential functions of the job, is the employer willing to modify the job or create a job the client could do by merging components of other jobs?
- Could the client do the job with additional accommodations not paid for by the employer, such as the support of a job coach?

Job Accommodation

Dowler and colleagues[39] reviewed the requests for information on accommodation made by 1000 people with SCI who called the national Job Accommodation Network. They reported that callers with tetraplegia most frequently reported difficulties with gross and fine motor skills, such as keyboarding, manipulating small parts, holding pens, and sorting. Those with paraplegia reported difficulty with driving, heavy lifting, carrying objects, reaching work areas, and so forth. Job accommodations can include modification in work schedules; modification of tasks; and modification of the environment to make it more accessible (eg, installing electric door openers or a ramp). Some accommodations are as simple as removing a desk drawer or raising the height of a desk with four wood blocks to permit wheelchair access. Other accommodations are high technology and involve designing computer interface software and hardware, or writing scripts to allow a user to control multiple applications using voice recognition. Still other accommodations are practical, such as providing a private changing area and storage for a change of clothing for a male employee with tetraplegia who uses a condom catheter in case of bladder accidents when the condom becomes disconnected during transfers. In many cases, the need for additional accommodations becomes apparent as the employee begins settling into the job.

Accommodations for fatigue include modifying schedules so that the employee can take rest breaks. Teaching the client pacing skills may also be useful and working with the employer to allow the client to maintain control over the pace of activity is a reasonable accommodation. Accommodations for cognitive changes include allowing the employee to begin the work day early before others arrive so he or she can focus on more difficult tasks before the environment becomes more distracting. Also, using common tools, such as email, electronic calendars, office computers, and smart phones, as "cognitive prosthetics" may be useful.

LONG-TERM EMPLOYMENT ISSUES

Employment rates for individuals with disabilities in general and individuals with SCI, MD, LEP, and MS in particular decline with age. This represents the accelerated morbidity associated with aging with disabilities. It is critical that vocational rehabilitation not be considered to be complete once a job has been preserved or obtained. Proactive, strategic planning with periodic intervention reduces the occurrence of additional disability and employment problems in the future.

VOCATIONAL REHABILITATION SYSTEMS

In the past, vocational rehabilitation counseling services at some inpatient and outpatient rehabilitation programs were provided as part of the program fee. Increasingly, hospital-based rehabilitation counselors and those in the private sector provide fee-for-service rehabilitation counseling to address employment concerns. Some services can be paid for by health insurance policies and others are paid directly by the recipient. It is not unusual for personal injury policies and long-term disability policies to provide for vocational rehabilitation benefits. For people with disabilities who are employed, the employer may pay for some services to meet their obligation to provide reasonable accommodations or simply because it is good business to keep a good employee on the job. Finally, many legal settlements rising from traumatic SCI include funding for vocational rehabilitation. In addition to these individual options, there are several major social service systems that provide vocational rehabilitation.[40]

FEDERAL-STATE VOCATIONAL REHABILITATION PROGRAMS

The Rehabilitation Act of 1973 funds a vocational rehabilitation program in each state with four federal dollars for each dollar appropriated by the state. Some Native American groups have also established federally funded vocational rehabilitation programs. State vocational rehabilitation programs are designed to help people with disabilities prepare for, obtain, and retain employment. The goal is not simply to obtain employment, but to assist the person with a disability to maximize his or her employment potential. The state vocational rehabilitation agencies work in collaboration with program participants, employers, and the community. To be eligible for services, applicants must have a significant disability that limits their ability to work. Services include the following:

- Medical evaluation: determination of a person's strengths and vocational limitations through expert medical, psychiatric, social, and psychologic evaluation.
- Vocational assessment: identification of a person's interests, readiness for employment, work skills, and job opportunities in the community.
- Counseling and guidance: rehabilitation counselor and participant establish an ongoing relationship in which they explore evaluation results and labor market opportunities, and develop a realistic plan for employment.
- Restoration: increase work potential and ability to retain a job through use of medical and assistive technologies.

- Job preparation: build work skills through services, such as volunteer experience, on-the-job training, vocational and technical education, and higher education.
- Support services: support the participant through services, such as transportation assistance; the purchase of tools, equipment, books, or work clothing; job coaching; and independent living support.
- Job placement: develop work opportunities and obtain and maintain a job suited to the participant's interests and capabilities.
- Follow-up: follow the progress of the participant for at least 90 days to ensure that employment is satisfactory.
- Postemployment: provide short-term services from time to time necessary to help a participant sustain employment.

STATE WORKER'S COMPENSATION PROGRAMS

Each state has a worker's compensation program for workers who sustain work-related injuries. It seems obvious that some people may have work-related injuries resulting in SCI, but people with SCI, MD, MS, and LEP may sustain work-related injuries that "tip the scale" on the resource economy described earlier and require vocational rehabilitation. In many states, the program is regulated by a state agency but implemented by commercial insurance carriers that cover the employer. Larger employers may often be self-insured. In some states, all phases of the process are conducted by the state agency or its contractors. Worker's compensation programs in most states include a vocational rehabilitation component. In worker's compensation rehabilitation, the goal is to return the injured worker to his or her previous job, or a similar job. If neither of these is possible, then depending on the state, the goal may be to return the injured worker to any suitable employment. Covered services are similar to those described for the federal state system, but usually services are only provided with respect to the work-related injury. Worker's compensation vocational rehabilitation programs typically have two phases. The first is characterized by the continuing recovery and rehabilitation of the injured worker. The second phase begins when the injured worker reaches "maximum medical improvement." Wage replacement is typically paid during both phases. When the injured worker cannot return to previous employment or a similar job, and does not have the transferable skills necessary to perform other suitable work, retraining can be authorized. If a worker is determined not to have the potential to resume employment, he or she is typically awarded a settlement or pension.

VETERANS ADMINISTRATION

Individuals with MS and SCI who are eligible for services through the Veterans Administration have access to vocational rehabilitation services at many comprehensive Veterans Administration system rehabilitation centers and through other community access points. Veterans Administration services are similar to those provided through the federal state system.

OTHER VOCATIONAL REHABILITATION SYSTEMS

A variety of other systems with similar features exist for workers who sustain disabling work-related injuries in federal government, off-shore, maritime, and railroad settings.

KEY DISABILITY BENEFIT SYSTEMS

For some people with disabilities, an extended period of education, retraining, or reha-bilitation may be necessary before return to work and they are considered totally disabled for at least a year or two. Others need to retire from employment or will never return to work. These include people who cannot resolve health insurance issues or who live in rural areas without access to transportation or employment, older workers who had relied on their ability to perform physical labor or cognitive effort and who do not have sufficient transferable skills to work in another field, or people who as their secondary conditions advance simply cannot sustain employment. Under these circumstances, it is the responsibility of the rehabilitation professionals to advocate for disability benefits and assist in the application process. Some individuals have long-term disability insurance policies where the premiums have been deducted from their pay but most do not and rely on various state and federal programs.

SOCIAL SECURITY ADMINISTRATION

The Social Security Administration (SSA) pays disability benefits under two programs: Social Security Disability Insurance (SSDI) and Supplementary Security Income (SSI). The medical requirements for disability payments are the same under both programs and a person's disability is determined by the same process. Eligibility for SSDI bene-fits is based on history of employment covered by SSA, however, whereas eligibility for SSI disability payments is determined by financial need. SSDI is a federal long-term disability insurance program funded by payroll taxes, whereas SSI is a federal welfare program for, among others, people with disabilities who are unable to work and are poor.

The SSA considers a person disabled if he or she is unable to perform any kind of work at a level of "substantial and gainful" activity, and the disability is expected to last at least a year or to result in death. Applicants should contact a Social Security office as soon as they become disabled because there is a waiting period before some types of disability benefits begin. This waiting period starts with the first full month after the onset of the disability as determined by SSA. Filing for disability bene-fits can be done online, by telephone, by mail, or in person at any office. Spouses and children who are financially dependent on the disabled worker may also qualify for disability benefits under certain conditions.

Newly injured individuals with SCI should consider applying for SSA benefits imme-diately if it seems likely that they will not return to work for at least a year. Once eligi-bility is established, depending on the program, recipients are immediately eligible for state Medicaid benefits, or after a waiting period, federal Medicare benefits. Under the Ticket to Work legislation of 2000, many recipients of SSA benefits are able to continue their Medicare coverage after they return to work. SSA also has several work incentive programs where a person with a disability who must purchase services or goods to work can deduct those expenses from his or her income to remain below the threshold and continue eligibility for subsidy and Medicare. Individuals with SCI, LEP, MS, or MD who find that they are unable to work should apply for SSDI or other disability benefits, such as long-term disability insurance, as soon as possible.

CONCLUSIONS AND RECOMMENDATIONS FOR HEALTH CARE PROVIDERS

People with disabilities have high rates of unemployment in general and unemploy-ment increases as they age, and yet many prefer to work and can work with accom-modations. There are occasions, however, where it is no longer feasible for people to work. Rehabilitation health care providers are in an ideal position to help people with SCI, LEP, MS, and MD make and support decisions about employment. This assistance can be in the form of counseling about options, making referrals for assistance, and helping to collect data about functional strengths and limitations to inform the accommodation process or to establish the basis for disability subsidy.

It is recommended that providers routinely ask patients about their employment status and preferences, and whether they have any concerns about employment. For patients who are working and experiencing difficulties at work, early intervention is a key to preserving employment status.

REFERENCES

1. Sasma G, Patrick C, Feussner J. Long-term survival of veterans with traumatic spinal cord injury. Arch Neurol 1993;50:909–14.
2. Kemp BJ. What the rehabilitation professional and the consumer need to know. Phys Med Rehabil Clin N Am 2005;16(1):1–18, vii.
3. Adkins RH. Research and interpretation perspectives on aging related physical morbidity with spinal cord injury and brief review of systems. NeuroRehabilitation 2004;19(1):3–13.
4. Bauman WA, Spungen AM. Disorders of carbohydrate and lipid metabolism in veterans with paraplegia or quadriplegia: a model of premature aging. Metabolism 1994;43(6):749–56.
5. Mitchell JM, Adkins RH, Kemp BJ. The effects of aging on employment of people with and without disabilities. Rehabil Couns Bull 2006;49:157–65.
6. She P, Livermore G. Long-term poverty and disability among working-age adults (Research Brief) in rehabilitation research and training venter on employment policy for persons with disabilities. Ithaca (NY): Cornell University; 2006.
7. Johnson K, Amtmann D, Yorkton KM, et al. Medical, psychological, social, and programmatic barriers to employment for people with multiple sclerosis. J Rehabil 2004;70:38–50.
8. Hess DW, Meade MA, Forchheimer M, et al. Psychological well-being and intensity of employment in individuals with spinal cord injury. Top Spinal Cord Inj Rehabil 2004;9:1–10.
9. Larocca N, Kalb R, Scheinberg L, et al. Factors associated with unemployment of patients with multiple sclerosis. J Chronic Dis 1985;38(2):203–10.
10. Kornblith AB, La Rocca NG, Baum HM. Employment in individuals with multiple sclerosis. Int J Rehabil Res 1986;9(2):155–65.
11. Sweetland J, Riazi A, Cano SJ, et al. Vocational rehabilitation services for people with multiple sclerosis: what patients want from clinicians and employers. Mult Scler 2007;13(9):1183–9.
12. Gordon PA, Lewis MD, Wong D. Multiple sclerosis: strategies for rehabilitation counselors. J Rehabil 1994;60(3):34–8.
13. O'Connor RJ, Cano SJ, Ramió i Torrentà L, et al. Factors influencing work retention for people with multiple sclerosis: cross-sectional studies using qualitative and quantitative methods. J Neurol 2005;252(8):892–6.
14. Phillips LJ, Stuifbergen AK. Predicting continued employment in persons with multiple sclerosis. J Rehabil 2006;72(1):35–43.
15. Johnson K, Bamer A, Fraser R. Disease and demographic characteristics associated with unemployment among working age adults with multiple sclerosis. Int J MS Care 2009;11(3):137–43.

16. Lidal IB, Huynh TK, Biering-Sorensen F. Return to work following spinal cord injury: a review. Disabil Rehabil 2007;29(17):1341–75.
17. Marini I, Lee GK, Chan F, et al. Vocational rehabilitation service patterns related to successful competitive employment outcomes of persons with spinal cord injury. J Vocat Rehabil 2008;28(1):1–13.
18. Krause JS, Sternberg M, Maides J, et al. Employment after spinal cord injury: differences related to geographic region, gender, and race. Arch Phys Med Rehabil 1998; 79(6):615–24.
19. Krause JS, Broderick L. A 25-year longitudinal study of the natural course of aging after spinal cord injury. Spinal Cord 2005;43(6):349–56.
20. Anderson CJ, Vogel LC. Employment outcomes of adults who sustained spinal cord injuries as children or adolescents. Arch Phys Med Rehabil 2002;83(6): 791–801.
21. Krause JS, Anson CA. Employment after spinal cord injury: relation to selected participant characteristics. Arch Phys Med Rehabil 1996;77(8):737–43.
22. Krause JS, Kewman D, DeVivo MJ, et al. Employment after spinal cord injury: an analysis of cases from the model spinal cord injury systems. Arch Phys Med Rehabil 1999;80(11):1492–500.
23. Farbu E, Gilhus NE. Education, occupation, and perception of health amongst previous polio patients compared to their siblings. Eur J Neurol 2002;9(3): 233–41.
24. Elrod LM, Jabben M, Oswald G, et al. Vocational implications of post-polio syndrome. Work 2005;25(2):155–61.
25. McNeal DR, Somerville NJ, Wilson DJ. Work problems and accommodations reported by persons who are postpolio or have a spinal cord injury. Assist Technol 1999;11(2):137–57.
26. Bruno RL, Frick NM, Cohen J. Polioencephalitis, stress, and the etiology of postpolio sequelae. Orthopedics 1991;14(11):1269–76.
27. Fowler WM Jr, Abresch RT, Koch TR, et al. Employment profiles in neuromuscular diseases. Am J Phys Med Rehabil 1997;76(1):26–37.
28. Gagnon C, Mathieu J, Jean S, et al. Predictors of disrupted social participation in myotonic dystrophy type 1. Arch Phys Med Rehabil 2008;89(7):1246–55.
29. Johnson KL, Yorkston KM, Klasner ER, et al. The cost and benefits of employment: a qualitative study of experiences of persons with multiple sclerosis. Arch Phys Med Rehabil 2004;85(2):201–9.
30. Yorkston KM, Johnson K, Klasner ER, et al. Getting the work done: a qualitative study of individuals with multiple sclerosis. Disabil Rehabil 2003;25(8):369–79.
31. Beatty WW, Blanco CR, Wilbanks SL, et al. Demographic, clinical and cognitive characteristics of multiple sclerosis patients who continue to work. J Neurol Rehabil 1995;9(3):167–73.
32. Pennell F, Johnson J. Legal and civil right aspects of vocational rehabilitation. Phys Med Rehabil Clin N Am 1997;8(2):245–62.
33. Rehabilitation Act of 1973, 87 Stat.355, 29 U.S.C § 701 et seq.
34. Rehabilitation Act Amendments of 1974 89 Stat.2.
35. Americans with Disabilities Act of 1990, Stat.327, 42 U.S.C § 12101 et seq.
36. Fraser R, Johnson K. Vocational rehabilitation. In: Frank R, Elliott T, editors. Handbook of rehabilitation psychology. 2nd edition. Washington, DC: American Psychological Association; 2009. p. 357–64.
37. Innes E, Matthews LR, Johnson K. Assessment of occupational functioning. In: Mpofu E, Oakland T, editors. Assessment in rehabilitation and health. Boston: Allyn & Bacon; 2009. p. 480.

38. Brown C, McDaniel KR, Couch R. Vocational evaluation systems and software. Menomonie (WI): Stout Vocational Rehabilitation Institute, University of Wisconsin-Stout; 1994.
39. Dowler ID, Batiste L, Whidden E. Accommodating workers with spinal cord injury. J Voc Rehabil 1998;10:115–22.
40. Johnson K. Vocational rehabilitation. In: Lin V, editor. Spinal cord medicine: principles and practice. New York: Demos; 2009. p. 715–22.

The Relationship of Age-Related Factors to Psychological Functioning Among People With Disabilities

Charles H. Bombardier, PhD[a],*, Dawn M. Ehde, PhD[a],
Brenda Stoelb, PhD[b], Ivan R. Molton, PhD[a,c]

KEYWORDS

• Multiple sclerosis • Growth • Aging • Depression

In this article the authors examine the intersecting influences of age-related factors and disability on psychological functioning. The scope of this study has been restricted to people with multiple sclerosis (MS) and people with spinal cord injury (SCI) because there is a well-developed research literature on psychological factors in these 2 groups. Furthermore, this article focuses on depression, as it is arguably the most commonly studied psychological condition in persons with disability. However, this review also includes a discussion of positive psychological concepts such as posttraumatic growth (PTG) and benefit finding (BF), which are particularly important given that most individuals achieve healthy psychological adjustment despite the challenges of aging and disability. In addition, a better understanding of healthy functioning may help improve the lives of people with disabilities at least as much as understanding less adaptive functioning.

This research was supported, in part, by a grant from the Department of Education, National Institute on Disability and Rehabilitation Research (H133B080024). The contents of this article do not necessarily represent the policy of the Department of Education and the reader should not assume endorsement by the Federal Government.

[a] Department of Rehabilitation Medicine, Harborview Medical Center, University of Washington School of Medicine, 325 9th Avenue, Box 359612, Seattle, WA 98104, USA
[b] Talaria Inc, 1121 34th Avenue, Seattle, WA 98122, USA
[c] Department of Rehabilitation Medicine, University of Washington, 1959 Pacific Street NE, Box 356490, Seattle, WA 98195-6490, USA
* Corresponding author.
E-mail address: chb@uw.edu

Phys Med Rehabil Clin N Am 21 (2010) 281–297
doi:10.1016/j.pmr.2009.12.005
1047-9651/10/$ – see front matter © 2010 Elsevier Inc. All rights reserved.

It would be optimal if researchers consistently used widely accepted nosology[1,2] and valid diagnostic interviews, such as the Structured Clinical Interview for Diagnostic and Statistical Manual of Mental Disorders IV (DSM-IV),[3] to identify specific pathologic conditions such as major depressive disorder (MDD). In most cases, however, self-report measures are used to measure constructs or identify cases. Even well-developed, widely used, self-report measures usually lack proven diagnostic accuracy, especially in the context of disability.[4] Therefore, in this article, terms such as "depression" and "depressive symptomatology" are used to refer to non-diagnostic approaches and self-report measures of negative affect. The use of these terms should not be misconstrued to indicate the presence of a diagnosable psychiatric condition. The authors have used diagnostic terminology such as "major depressive disorder" only when the assessment is based on widely accepted diagnostic criteria, and a reliable and valid evaluation process.

Age-related concepts are surprisingly complex and merit some explanation. Age factors addressed in the disability literature to which we refer include age at the onset of diagnosis of the condition, time since diagnosis or onset, chronologic age at the time of assessment, and the historical era (eg, the "cohort"; the early 1900s, the 1960s). In addition, aging can represent different phenomena, especially with regard to depression.[5] Aging can represent larger historical trends when, for example, a higher rate of depression is associated with lower education among older cohorts who tended to have lower educational achievement. Aging may also represent life cycle events. For example, depression may be higher in older adults because older age is associated with retirement, widowhood, and other possible depressogenic loss experiences. Aging may represent a decline in health. Depression in old age may be attributable to poorer health and functional decline than in chronologic age. Older age may also represent differential survival. Because survival into old age may be lower because of depression, a lower rate of depression in older adults may represent preferential survival of more healthy individuals. Alternatively, women tend to survive longer than men and women are characterized by higher rates of depression. Consequently, a higher rate of depression in older adults may be attributable to differential survival of women. Finally, aging may represent greater maturity, psychological integration, or improvements in coping. Lower rates of depression may be associated with older age to the extent that old age–related improvements in insight, self-integration, and self-esteem buffer depression risk. For example, socio-emotional selectivity theory[6] posits that when one perceives that one has less time left to live, one reorganizes one's goals to more closely conform to what one can realistically accomplish. A similar process may influence adjustment to and aging with disabilities.[7]

This complexity means that age-related theoretic influences may operate differently based on study design. Cross-sectional aging studies may be confounded by historical trends. In the case of aging with disability, an important historical trend is the changes in the nature and length of rehabilitation programs over the past 50 years.[8] Longitudinal studies may be confounded by differential survival. In people with SCI, a salient fact is that there has been a 2000% increase in life expectancy over the past 50 years.[8] Depression-related risk factors, such as low education, loss events, poorer health, accelerated functional decline, differential survival, and the wisdom of maturity, may complicate studies of aging with disability because these risk factors may be more common, more salient, or occur earlier in people with disabilities. The trajectories of key variables, such as functional impairments, are specific to the type of disability, for example, immediate decline plus aging effects in people with SCI versus variable decline plus aging effects in people with

MS. Finally, these age-related theoretic factors may operate differently with regard to the various psychological concepts such as depression versus posttraumatic growth or resilience. Clearly, the literature on psychological adjustment in persons aging with disability is complex and multifaceted, which may in part explain the few studies published in this area.

DEPRESSION AND AGING FACTORS IN THE GENERAL POPULATION

Overall, global measures of subjective well-being improve through adulthood.[9] Most older adults adjust well to aging, and most older adults with disabilities, such as SCI, do not report significant depressive symptoms.[8] Similarly, older adults tend to have lower rates of MDD compared with younger adults[10] or about the same prevalence.[11] Prevalence rates of DSM-IV MDD are 1% to 3% in the general elderly population.[1,12,13] Among older people sampled in primary medical care, settings rates of MDD are 5% to17%.[1,14] Nevertheless, older adults are more likely than younger adults to report subclinical symptoms of depression (about 16% in the community,[15] or 29% in primary care settings).[14] Older adults tend to have a different presentation of depression,[16] including more anhedonia and lack of energy, lower prevalence of dysphoria, less guilt, less passive suicidal ideation, and more prominent somatic symptoms, such as fatigue and poor appetite. This presentation has been called "depletion syndrome" and "nondysphoric depression."[17] When older adults are clinically depressed, prognosis and impairment are worse compared with younger persons. Among clinically depressed older adults undergoing treatment as usual, at 24 months 33% were well, 33% remained depressed, and 21% had deceased.[18] Depressed adults (with or without MDD) have poorer overall functioning, comparable or worse than that of people with heart and lung disease, diabetes, and so forth.[19] Depression increases the perception of poor health,[19] which is one of the most salient predictors of mortality in older people.[20,21]

DEPRESSION AND AGING IN PEOPLE WITH SCI

Depression is thought to be the most prevalent and disabling psychological condition associated with SCI. Depression is not considered a stage in the process of healthy adaptation to catastrophic injury, but a comorbid condition that merits assessment and treatment.[22] The overall prevalence of major depression is 15% to 23% in most studies that use diagnostic interviews.[23] Moreover, depressive symptoms are linked to a myriad of negative outcomes including poorer subjective health, poorer community integration, more secondary conditions, and higher rates of suicide.[22,24,25]

The authors searched PubMed and PsychLit for papers with the key words such as SCI, depression, and age or aging. Study reference lists were also searched for additional papers that mentioned these 3 topics. **Table 1** displays the subset of studies that analyzed depression and age-related factors in people with SCI. Studies are difficult to compare because of the use of diverse measures of depression ranging from psychometrically sound instruments to single item indicators. Studies also focused on different age-related concepts and used several designs. One study by Tate and colleagues[26] excluded people with major depression and therefore was not included in this review. Glass and colleagues[27] used an unfamiliar depression measure and reported depression prevalence that was inconsistent with the rest of the studies.

Among studies reporting rates of depression in people living 10 or more years after SCI, depression prevalence ranged from 17% to 33%. Although depression prevalence in these samples is certainly higher than rates of MDD in nondisabled aging samples, it does not appear different from the average prevalence rate observed in

Table 1
Depression and age-related factors in SCI

Author, Year	Number	Mean Age	Mean Years Since SCI	Results
Schulz & Decker,[34] 1985	100	56	20	Cross-sectional study; mean CESD scores = 9.74 among persons at an average of 20 y post SCI; 22% scored in the depressed range
Holicky & Charlifue,[35] 1999	225		≥26	Cross-sectional study; mean CESD scores = 11.5 among unmarried versus 10.1 for married; among married, CESD scores are highest for those aged 50–59 y and lower in earlier and later age cohorts; for unmarried, CESD scores decline in each successive age cohort
Kemp & Krause,[8] 1999	177	40	14	Cross-sectional study in people at an average 14 y after SCI; 17% scored in depressed range on GDS
Glass et al,[27] 1999	287	35	6	Cross-sectional study; 66% scored in depressed range on IDA scale; those older than 50 y had higher depression scores but greater time since injury was associated with lower depression scores
Krause et al,[28] 2000	1391	42	10	Cross-sectional study; 24% scored in the probable major depression range on the OAHMQ; the percentage with probable major depression levels increased with greater age and age at injury onset; higher rates of probable major depression were observed in cases with the most years post injury (26 y or more) and those with the least years post injury (1–5 y)
Charlifue & Gerhart,[32] 2004	178	59	36	6-y longitudinal study; trend toward increased depression on CESD over 6 y (means = 9.4, 10.2, 11.5 in years 1993, 1996, 1999, respectively)

Charlifue & Gerhart,[32] 2004	189	59	36	6-y longitudinal study of quality of life; lower quality of life was associated with greater subsequent depression on CESD
Bombardier et al,[23] 2004	849	37	1	Cross-sectional study of people 1 y post SCI; rate of probable MDD on PHQ-9 was significantly higher among people aged 25–49 y (15.0%), compared with older (8.7%) or younger (6.5%) age groups
Saikkonen et al,[29] 2004	76	~51	~10	Cross-sectional study with 31% scoring in depressed range on BDI; higher BDI scores were correlated with age at time of injury (r = 0.35) and year of injury (r = 0.52). Those injured between the age of 46 and 60 y had a mean BDI score of 11.6 vs a mean of 9.4 among those more than 60 y old. Those injured in the 1990s had higher BDI scores than those who had been injured earlier
Richardson & Richards,[31] 2008	Total n = 2570	38–49	1, 5, 15, 25	Compared cohorts assessed at 1, 5, 15, 25 y post SCI; mean PHQ-9 scores are significantly lower for 15 and 25 y post SCI (M = 3.8, 3.5, respectively) compared with 1 and 5 y post SCI (M = 5.4, 4.7, respectively)
Hitzig et al,[30] 2008	781	51	14	Cross-sectional study with about 33% indicating on a single item that they experienced depression in the past year; odds of depression decreased as years post SCI increased

Abbreviations: BDI, Beck Depression Inventory; CESD, Centers for Epidemiologic Studies Depression Scale; GDS, Geriatric Depression Scale; IDA, Irritability Depression Anxiety Scale; OAHMQ, Older Adult Health and Mood Questionnaire; PHQ-9, Patient Health Questionnaire-9.

SCI and depression studies generally.[23] Only 1 study examined the relationship of depression to chronologic age at the time of assessment and found a weakly positive relationship.[28] With regard to age at the time of injury, 2 studies found that an older cohort was less likely to be depressed compared with a younger cohort.[23,29] The most consistent finding in cross-sectional studies was an inverse relationship between depression and time since injury.[27,30,31] Krause and colleagues[28] reported a similar pattern with those 1 to 5 years post SCI having higher rates of probable major depression compared with those 6 to 25 years after injury. However, the oldest group, those living with SCI for 26 years or more, was also more likely to be depressed compared with those 6 to 25 years post injury. In contrast, the only longitudinal study of depression found that there was a nonsignificant trend toward increased depression over 6 years.[32] A parallel longitudinal study of quality of life suggested that declines in quality of life preceded increased depression.[33] Only 1 study examined depression as related to historical trends finding that depression rates were higher in the 1990s compared with the previous decades.[29] Few studies reported on more than one age-related factor (see **Table 1**).

The research on depression and aging in SCI leaves many questions unanswered. Studies of people with SCI are generally consistent with research in the nondisabled population in that depression is less pronounced in older than in younger cohorts. However, it may also be that depressive symptoms follow a U-shape in terms of severity, with increasing report of depressive symptoms in mid-life.[23,35] Studies are needed that explicitly examine the relationship of multiple age-related factors to depression. These studies should include suspected moderators of age-related effects on depression such as education, life cycle events, changes in health, and changes in coping. Aging studies with longitudinal designs and studies that examine the health and quality of life correlates of depression at different ages are needed. For example, it has been suggested that the impact of physical health conditions on depression is mediated by restriction of normal activities, and that older adults may find this activity restriction less distressing.[36] However, this has never been tested in an aging population with disability. There are many rich empiric and theoretic concepts from the general aging literature that may be applicable to studies of aging with SCI.

DEPRESSION AND AGING IN PEOPLE WITH MS

A meta-analysis found depression to be more prevalent among people with MS compared with the general population and individuals with other neurologic conditions.[37] In one of the few prospective epidemiologic studies,[38] MDD had a 12-month period prevalence of 15.7% in MS, which is twice the prevalence in the general population. High rates of clinically significant depressive symptoms have been reported in numerous studies of community dwelling individuals with MS.[39] When present, depression adversely affects other domains of functioning, including cognition, fatigue, functioning, and quality of life.[40,41]

To examine relationships between aging and depression in MS, PubMed and PsychLit were searched for papers with the key words such as multiple sclerosis, depression, and age or aging. Study reference lists were also searched for additional papers that included these 3 key words. Given the large volume of studies published on MS and depression, only studies published in 2000 or later were included in the table. **Table 2** displays the subset of studies that analyzed depression and age-related factors in people with MS. Like the SCI studies, cross-study comparisons are difficult because of the diversity of measures.

Similar to the research on depression and aging in SCI, most studies reviewed suggest that younger adults with MS are at a greater risk for depressive symptoms and disorders. Although no study contradicted this pattern, several studies failed to replicate a relationship between depression and age.[42-45] Several MS studies also found that the duration of MS diagnosis was also associated with depression risk; those with a shorter duration of MS were more likely to have a depressive disorder or clinically significant depressive symptoms,[46] although this relationship was not found in other studies.[47] These studies indicate that age is an important factor for further research; however, like SCI, studies are needed that explore in more depth age-related factors that may moderate the influence of age on depression.

AGING, DISABILITY, AND BF/PTG

Although people have myriad reactions to acquiring a physically disabling condition,[48] research has typically focused on negative psychological sequela, such as depression, anxiety, or posttraumatic stress disorder.[49] In recent years, however, researchers have begun to pay attention and systematically investigate the positive shifts in behaviors, beliefs, and emotions that many people report experiencing as a result of living with a disability. In the broader trauma and health literatures, this phenomenon has been given various names (eg, perceived benefits, stress-related growth, adversarial growth, positive by-products),[50] but is perhaps most commonly known as BF[51] or PTG. BF and/or PTG have been investigated in a wide variety of trauma and medical populations such as Oklahoma City bombing residents,[52] individuals with HIV/AIDS,[53] and persons with cancer,[54,55] but few scientific studies of BF/PTG have been conducted in rehabilitation populations. For example, a review of the literature conducted by PubMed and PsycINFO revealed only 20 studies that either qualitatively or quantitatively investigated the nature, scope, and/or correlates of BF/PTG in 5 different disability groups (SCI, amputation, MS, stroke/traumatic brain injury, and burns), whereas literally hundreds of studies have explored these relationships in cancer populations. Despite this, it seems that reports of BF/PTG are fairly common in people with disabilities (eg, 79% of participants with SCI and 83% of participants with an amputation reported growth).[56,57] Among people with disabilities, rates of BF/PTG are comparable to, or even greater than, those reported in other trauma populations, including persons who have experienced sexual assault or abuse (20%–80%),[58,59] witnesses of September 11th (30%),[60] and survivors of tornadoes (90%–95%).[61]

The types of benefit or growth endorsed most frequently can be organized into three categories: (1) enhanced personal relationships (eg, valuing friends and family more, a heightened sense of altruism or compassion for others), (2) a changed view of oneself (eg, a greater awareness of one's strengths and vulnerabilities), and (3) a change in life philosophy (eg, an increased appreciation for each day, renegotiating priorities).[62] Given the dearth of rehabilitation-specific BF/PTG research, however, little to nothing is known about how disability, the aging process, and BF/PTG may interact with one another. Only 3 of the aforementioned 20 studies, reported a significant relationship between BF/PTG and age.[63-65] Until more research is conducted, only tentative conclusions can be drawn regarding how aging may influence, and be influenced by, acquired disability and BF/PTG.

Perhaps one of the more consistent findings in the general BF/PTG literature is that among adults, younger age tends to be associated with increased reports of BF/PTG.[66-69] In a sample of 167 persons with MS, younger age was associated with higher scores on the Benefit-Finding Scale of the Illness Cognitions

Table 2
Depression and age-related factors in MS

Author, Year	Number	Mean Age	Mean Years Since MS Diagnosis	Results
Patten et al,[71] 2000	136	47	9	Cross-sectional population-based Canadian clinic sample; Using the CIDI-A, 23% met DMS-IV criteria for lifetime major depression; 4% had current major depression; 13% reported single episodes of major depression, and 10% reported recurrent episodes. Younger age (<35) associated with greater risk for lifetime major depression (OR = 4.6)
Chwastiak et al,[72] 2002	730	49	13	Cross-sectional study of community dwelling adults; mean CESD score for sample = 16.0; 45% had CESD score ≥ 16; 29% score ≥ 21 on CESD suggestive of probably major depression; younger age was associated with greater risk for depression (≥ 16 on CESD)
Patten et al,[38] 2003	115,071, 332 with MS	NR	NR	Cross-sectional national survey (Canadians); Using the CIDI, the annual prevalence of major depression in MS was 16% compared with 7% in adults without MS; major depression was more prevalent in those <45 y of age (26%) compared with those 45 y or older (8%)
Galeazzi et al,[45] 2005	50	35	10	Cross-sectional; age and duration of MS were not associated with presence of a DSM-IV depressive disorder (based on SCID)
Williams et al,[46] 2005	451	55	18	Cross-sectional survey of US veterans; 22% had current major depressive episode on the PHQ-9; 32% met criteria for a major or minor depressive episode on PHQ. Younger age was a significant risk factor for a current major depressive episode (OR = 0.97). Shorter duration of MS was associated with greater risk for depression

Study				Findings
Arnett & Randolph,[42] 2006	53	47	7	3-y longitudinal study; examined the course and reliable change of different depressive symptom clusters and association with interferon β treatment/coping; mood symptoms more variable over time than neurovegetative or negative evaluative symptoms; age was not associated with the findings; investigators did not report % depressed
Beal et al,[47] 2007	607	51	13	Longitudinal study at 7 y; younger age and longer duration of MS were associated with greater depressive symptoms at time 1 y but did not predict changes in depressive symptoms over time. Greater functional limitations were associated with greater depressive symptoms at all time points
Tsivgoulis et al,[44] 2007	86	39	6	Cross-sectional sample; age and duration of MS were not associated with depression symptom severity as measured on BDI
Bamer et al,[43] 2008	530	52	15	Cross-sectional study of community dwelling adults in a more rural community; 51% had CESD score ≥ 16, 34% score ≥21 on CESD, suggestive of probably major depression; age was not associated with depression
Beiske et al,[73] 2008	140	NR	19	Cross-sectional study; 31% had depression on HSCL-25; younger age at onset of MS was related to presence of depression
Phillips & Stuifbergen,[74] 2008	443	56	19	Cross-sectional; lower age was associated with greater depressive symptoms

Abbreviations: CESD, Centers for Epidemiologic Studies Depression Scale; CIDI-A, Composite International Diagnostic Interview (WHO); GDS, Geriatric Depression Scale; HSCL-25, Hopkins Symptom Checklist; IDA, Irritability Depression Anxiety Scale; NR, not reported; PHQ-9, Patient Health Questionnaire-9.

Questionnaire.[63] The lower bound of this age effect is unclear, but the cognitive processing underlying PTG seems to require some degree of developmental maturity.

A few theories have been put forth to explain the inverse relationship between age and BF/PTG. According to BF/PTG theorists such as Calhoun and Tedeschi,[70] BF/PTG is more likely to occur when a trauma or adverse event shatters a person's pre-existing schemas about how the world works and his or her place in it. The event, therefore, must be of sufficient severity or pose a significant amount of threat to an individual's health and well-being to cause this shattering to occur. Hence, a physical disability that is acquired at a younger age when most individuals are embarking on careers and starting families, that is, when people have their whole life ahead of them, may represent a greater threat to personal integrity, compared with a disabling condition that is acquired at a later age. Similarly, older adults may be more likely to see new physical symptoms and limitations in activity as normative,[75] and therefore new onset disability in old age may not pose a significant threat to pre-existing schemas. However, the relationship between age and BF/PTG in adults aging with long-standing disabilities has not been described. Although the authors are unaware of any rehabilitation-specific studies that have explored the role of threat in the development of BF/PTG, some studies have investigated injury severity or level of functioning and their relationship to BF/PTG. Lower level SCI and greater motor functioning were associated with greater self-efficacy, which is one aspect of PTG/BF.[56] People with relapsing-remitting type of MS reported greater BF compared with other disease variants.[76]

Closer proximity to death has also been cited as a reason for lower rates of reported BF/PTG in older populations. Thoughts and concerns about one's impending mortality may leave little room for continued psychological growth.[67,77] In contrast, younger individuals who acquire a disability may have many years to think about how they will cope with the sequela of this event and go about reaching their desired goals.[63,78]

Notwithstanding the theory and evidence supporting an inverse association between age and BF/PTG, there are studies that have found the opposite. Studies of people with traumatic brain injury[64] and burn injury[65] reported higher rates of BF/PTG among older individuals. The reasons for these inconsistent findings remain unclear.

Few studies have examined BF/PTG over time or how these processes may influence behaviors such as coping styles. Pollard and Kennedy[79] found that depression, mental disengagement and active coping at 12 weeks post SCI predicted PTG at 10 years post injury. However, PTG was only assessed at year 10 and not at 12 weeks. Moreover, they did not report whether depression, mental disengagement, and active coping assessed at year 10 were correlated with PTG at year 10. In a nondisabled sample, Park and colleagues[80] found from elders' reports of PTG that their most traumatic life experiences were positively related to acceptance of death and use of adaptive coping strategies in dealing with a current stressor. However, an average of 32 years had passed since the trauma, PTG was not assessed at the time of the trauma, and PTG was based on retrospective recall of growth that occurred using the Stress-Related Growth Scale.[80,81]

SUMMARY AND FUTURE DIRECTIONS

The literature reviewed in this article suggests that, to date, much of the research on psychological aspects of aging has tended to operationalize age as a unidimensional construct, and this in part may explain variable findings. Most of the studies of aging after acquired disability have looked at 2 factors: chronologic age and disability duration. Although not conclusive, the available research suggests that, like studies of aging in the general population, younger age is associated with a greater risk of depression in people with disabilities. Furthermore, most studies suggest that depression is more common among those who were more recently disabled. However, when major depression does occur in older adults with disabilities, the consequences to long-term health are hypothesized to be greater. The broader aging literature would also suggest that other aspects such as cohort and life cycle events are important and warrant study in disability populations. Cross-sectional and longitudinal studies specifically examining the multidimensional aspects of aging and psychological health in the context of disability are needed.

A notable gap is the lack of theoretically driven conceptualizations of how aging influences psychological functioning and well-being within disability. For example, theoretic models for understanding depression in the context of aging exist in the broader aging literature[82] and could be extended to and tested in disability samples. Several methods may be useful in building theoretic models for understanding aging and psychological functioning, including the use of qualitative research designs,[83] narrative form research,[84] and mixed methods.[85]

An important limitation of the existing literature is that most investigations of age, depression, and BF/PTG have been cross-sectional in nature. Few studies have been longitudinal in design or have taken a life span developmental perspective.[78] To understand depression and BF/PTG in rehabilitation populations, longitudinal research is needed. Such research should be theoretically driven and assesses a broad range of psychological outcomes that include not only psychological distress but also other psychological outcomes such as anxiety, resilience (for a discussion on resilience after traumatic disability),[86] BF, and PTG as they relate to aging with a disability. Application of recent statistical advances, such as structural equation modeling[87] and multilevel modeling,[88] to such longitudinal data could provide analytic approaches for theory development and testing.

In conducting future longitudinal research, several factors seem important to consider. First, several studies (from the general literature and rehabilitation-specific studies) indicate that time since disability onset is associated with psychological outcomes. For example, time since trauma is positively associated with reports of BF/PTG.[63,89,90] As Linley and Joseph[67] caution, however, it may not be time per se that influences development of BF/PTG, but intervening events and processes. These processes, therefore (eg, cognitive processing of the event, attainment of social support), should be measured as possible mediators or moderators, but should also be chosen or based upon relevant biopsychosocial theory. Second, because exposure to trauma that results in a disability may prompt individuals to confront their own vulnerabilities and mortality sooner than they typically would, it may disrupt the normal progression of developmental stages.[91] For example, in a sample of 81 adult cancer survivors, Bellizzi[92] found no significant age difference in the expression of generative concern (ie, concerns that reflect providing and caring for the next generation, thought to emerge in middle-age). The researcher did find that younger adults engaged in a greater number of generative behaviors compared with the older adult cancer survivors in the sample. He also found that across the whole sample, generative concern was positively correlated with PTG. Therefore, future studies may want to investigate specifically how this developmental shift may influence the onset and maintenance of BF/PTG, and other psychological aspects of aging in rehabilitation populations.

Finally, little is understood about the positive psychological outcomes associated with disability.[48,93] For example, little is know about how BF/PTG may result in positive psychological outcomes over time, and how these processes may influence other outcomes or behaviors.

CLINICAL IMPLICATIONS

The modal response to disability and aging is not depression but resilience. Nevertheless, in people with disabilities such as SCI and MS, rates of depression are substantially higher than among the general aging population. Moreover, from the general aging literature there is the specter of under-recognition of clinically significant depressive conditions. In older adults, depression seems to present differently, with milder symptoms or with more prominent somatic symptoms, making it more difficult to distinguish depression from symptoms related to age or physical disability. Further complicating assessment of depression is the fact that MDD is often under-detected and inadequately treated in persons with disabilities such as MS.[94,95] Therefore, one of the greatest challenges is to develop depression screening and assessment procedures that distinguish pathologic syndromes from normal age and disability related symptoms.

This review of the literature also implies that prevention and treatment of depression in people aging with disabilities is likely to be complex. A host of aging related factors may contribute to depressive symptoms. Loss events, poorer health, accelerated functional decline, and economic uncertainties are only some of the factors that may contribute to depression onset, maintenance, and response to treatment. Older adults may not respond as well to standard depression treatments such as antidepressant medication,[96] but a variety of psychosocial interventions such as cognitive behavior therapy[97] or problem solving therapy[98] may be useful alternatives or adjuncts, partly because they target unique mediators of depression in older adults. Developmental or translational research is needed to address the mediators of response to treatment in people aging with disabilities.

Currently the relationship between BF/PTG and psychological distress such as depression is equivocal.[70] More research on these constructs and their relationships, if any, to distress is needed to inform clinical practice. In the broader BF/PTG literature it has been suggested that it is premature to conduct interventions to facilitate BF or PTG, as much remains to be learned about growth, including whether growth is a psychologically and/or physically beneficial outcome for survivors of traumatic or adverse events.[66,99] Furthermore, given the current literature, a lack of BF/PTG in older adults with disabilities should not be viewed as a failure of the individual, the therapist, or the rehabilitation team, given it is not known whether BF/PTG is a psychologically and/or physically beneficial outcome or goal for individuals with disabilities. Like depression assessment and treatment, research in the area of growth is needed to inform clinical practice.

REFERENCES

1. National Institute of Health NIH Consensus Development Conference: diagnosis and treatment of depression in late life. JAMA 1992;268:1018–29.
2. Diagnostic and statistical manual of mental disorders. 4th edition. Washington, DC: American Psychiatric Association; 1994.
3. First MB, Gibbons M, Spitzer R, et al. Structured clinical interview for DSM-IV axis I disorders, clinician version (SCID-CV). Washington, DC: American Psychiatric Press, Inc; 1996.
4. Kalpakjian CZ, Bombardier CH, Schomer K, et al. Measuring depression in persons with spinal cord injury: a systematic review. J Spinal Cord Med 2009; 32(1):6–24.
5. Yang Y. Is old age depressing? Growth trajectories and cohort variations in late-life depression. J Health Soc Behav 2007;48(1):16–32.

6. Carstensen LL, Isaacowitz DM, Charles ST. Taking time seriously. A theory of socioemotional selectivity. Am Psychol 1999;54(3):165–81.
7. Charlifue SW, Weitzenkamp DA, Whiteneck GG. Longitudinal outcomes in spinal cord injury: aging, secondary conditions, and well-being. Arch Phys Med Rehabil 1999;80(11):1429–34.
8. Kemp BJ, Krause JS. Depression and life satisfaction among people ageing with post-polio and spinal cord injury. Disabil Rehabil 1999;21(5–6):241–9.
9. Diener E, Suh ME. Subjective well-being and age: an international analysis. In: Schaie KW, Lawton MP, editors. Annual review of gerontology and geriatrics. New York: Springer; 1997.
10. Kasl-Godley JE, Gatz M, Fiske A. Depression and depressive symptoms in old age. In: Nordhus IH, et al, editors. Clinical geropsychology. Washington, DC: American Psychological Association; 1998. p. 211–7.
11. Wilhelm K, Mitchell P, Slade T, et al. Prevalence and correlates of DSM-IV major depression in an Australian national survey. J Affect Disord 2003;75(2):155–62.
12. Bland RC, Newman SC, Orn H. Period prevalence of psychiatric disorders in Edmonton. Acta Psychiatr Scand Suppl 1988;338:33–42.
13. Cole MG, Yaffe MJ. Pathway to psychiatric care of the elderly with depression. Int J Geriatr Psychiatry 1996;11:157–61.
14. van Marwijk H, Hoeksema HL, Hermans J, et al. Prevalence of depressive symptoms and depressive disorder in primary care patients over 65 years of age. Fam Pract 1994;11(1):80–4.
15. Fiske A, Kasl-Godley JE, Gatz M. Mood disorders in late life. In: Bellack AS, Hersen M, editors. Comprehensive clinical psychology. Oxford (UK): Elsevier Science; 1998. p. 193–229.
16. Caine ED, Lyness JM, King DA, et al. Clinical and etiological heterogeneity of mood disorders in elderly patients. In: Schneider LS, et al, editors. Diagnosis and treatment of depression in late life. Washington, DC: American Psychiatric Press; 1994. p. 21–53.
17. Newman JP, Engel RJ, Jensen JE. Changes in depressive-symptom experiences among older women. Psychol Aging 1991;6:212–22.
18. Cole MG, Bellavance F, Mansour A. Prognosis of depression in elderly community and primary care populations: a systematic review and meta analysis. Am J Psychiatry 1999;156:1182–9.
19. Wells KB, Burnam MA. Caring for depression in America: lessons learned from early findings of the medical outcomes study. Psychiatry Med 1991;9(4):503–19.
20. Benyamini Y, Idler EL. Community studies reporting association between self-rated health and mortality. Res Aging 1999;21:392–401.
21. Idler EL. Discussion: gender differences in self-rated health, in mortality, and in the relationship between the two. Gerontologist 2003;43:372–5.
22. Elliott TR, Frank RG. Depression following spinal cord injury. Arch Phys Med Rehabil 1996;77(8):816–23.
23. Bombardier CH, Richards JS, Krause JS, et al. Symptoms of major depression in people with spinal cord injury: implications for screening. Arch Phys Med Rehabil 2004;85(11):1749–56.
24. Kishi Y, Robinson RG, Kosier JT. Suicidal ideation among patients with acute life-threatening physical illness: patients with stroke, traumatic brain injury, myocardial infarction, and spinal cord injury. Psychosomatics 2001;42(5):382–90.
25. Krause JS, Carter RE, Pickelsimer EE, et al. A prospective study of health and risk of mortality after spinal cord injury. Arch Phys Med Rehabil 2008;89(8):1482–91.

26. Tate D, Forchheimer M, Maynard F, et al. Predicting depression and psychological distress in persons with spinal cord injury based on indicators of handicap. Am J Phys Med Rehabil 1994;73(3):175–8.

27. Glass CA, Jackson HF, Dutton J, et al. Estimating social adjustment following spinal trauma–II: population trends and effects of compensation on adjustment. Spinal Cord 1997;35(6):349–57.

28. Krause JS, Kemp B, Coker J. Depression after spinal cord injury: relation to gender, ethnicity, aging, and socioeconomic indicators. Arch Phys Med Rehabil 2000;81(8):1099–109.

29. Saikkonen J, Karppi P, Huusko TM, et al. Life situation of spinal cord-injured persons in Central Finland. Spinal Cord 2004;42(8):459–65.

30. Hitzig SL, Tonack M, Campbell KA, et al. Secondary health complications in an aging Canadian spinal cord injury sample. Am J Phys Med Rehabil 2008;87(7): 545–55.

31. Richardson EJ, Richards JS. Factor structure of the PHQ-9 screen for depression across time since injury among persons with spinal cord injury. Rehabil Psychol 2008;53(2):243–9.

32. Charlifue S, Gerhart K. Changing psychosocial morbidity in people aging with spinal cord injury. NeuroRehabilitation 2004;19(1):15–23.

33. Charlifue S, Lammertse DP, Adkins RH. Aging with spinal cord injury: changes in selected health indices and life satisfaction. Arch Phys Med Rehabil 2004;85(11): 1848–53.

34. Shulz R, Decker S. Long-term adjustment to physical disability: the role of social support, perceived control and self blame. J Pers Soc Psychol 1985;48(5): 1162–72.

35. Holicky R, Charlifue S. Ageing with spinal cord injury: the impact of spousal support. Disabil Rehabil 1999;21(5–6):250–7.

36. Williamson GM, Schulz R. Activity restriction mediates the association between pain and depressed affect: a study of younger and older adult cancer patients. Psychol Aging 1995;10(3):369–78.

37. Dalton EJ, Heinrichs RW. Depression in multiple sclerosis: a quantitative review of the evidence. Neuropsychology 2005;19(2):152–8.

38. Patten SB, Beck CA, Williams JV, et al. Major depression in multiple sclerosis: a population-based perspective. Neurology 2003;61(11):1524–7.

39. Chwastiak LA, Ehde DM. Psychiatric issues in multiple sclerosis. Psychiatr Clin North Am 2007;30(4):803.

40. Goldman Consensus Group. The Goldman Consensus statement on depression in multiple sclerosis. Mult Scler 2005;11(3):328–37.

41. Ehde DM, Bombardier CH. Depression in persons with multiple sclerosis. Phys Med Rehabil Clin N Am 2005;16(2):437–48, ix.

42. Arnett PA, Randolph JJ. Longitudinal course of depression symptoms in multiple sclerosis. J Neurol Neurosurg Psychiatr 2006;77(5):606–10.

43. Bamer AM, Cetin K, Johnson KL, et al. Validation study of prevalence and correlates of depressive symptomatology in multiple sclerosis. Gen Hosp Psychiatry 2008;30(4):311–7.

44. Tsivgoulis G, Triantafyllou H, Papageorgiou C, et al. Associations of the expanded disability status scale with anxiety and depression in multiple sclerosis outpatients. Acta Neurol Scand 2007;115(1):67–72.

45. Galeazzi GM, Ferrari S, Giaroli G, et al. Psychiatric disorders and depression in multiple sclerosis outpatients: impact of disability and interferon beta therapy. Neurol Sci 2005;26(4):255–62.

46. Williams RM, Turner AP, Hatzakis M, et al. Prevalence and correlates of depression among veterans with multiple sclerosis. Neurology 2005;64(1):75–80.
47. Beal CC, Stuifbergen AK, Brown A. Depression in multiple sclerosis: a longitudinal analysis. Arch Psychiatr Nurs 2007;21(4):181–91.
48. Elliott TR, Kurylo M, Rivera P. Positive growth following acquired physical disability. In: Synder CR, Lopez S, editors. Handbook of positive psychology. New York: Oxford University Press; 2002. p. 687–98.
49. Ehde DM, Williams RM. Adjustment to trauma. In: Robinson LR, editor. Trauma rehabilitation. Philadelphia: Lippincott Williams & Wilkins; 2006. p. 245–72.
50. Tedeschi RG, Calhoun LG. Posttraumatic growth: conceptual foundations and empirical evidence. Psychol Inq 2004;15(1):1–18.
51. Tennen H, Affleck G. Benefit-finding and benefit-reminding. In: Synder CR, Lopez S, editors. Handbook of positive psychology. New York: Oxford University Press; 2002. p. 584–97.
52. Pargament KI, Smith BW, Koenig HG, et al. Patterns of positive and negative religious coping with major life stressors. J Sci Study Relig 1998;37:710–24.
53. Siegel K, Schrimshaw EW. Perceiving benefits in adversity: stress-related growth in women living with HIV/AIDS. Soc Sci Med 2000;51(10):1543–54.
54. Cordova MJ, Cunningham LL, Carlson CR, et al. Posttraumatic growth following breast cancer: a controlled comparison study. Health Psychol 2001;20(3): 176–85.
55. Weiss T. Posttraumatic growth in women with breast cancer and their husbands: an intersubjective validation study. J Psychosoc Oncol 2002;20:65–80.
56. McMillen JC, Cook CL. The positive by-products of spinal cord injury and their correlates. Rehabil Psychol 2003;48:77–85.
57. Oaksford K, Frude N, Cuddihy R. Positive coping and stress-related psychological growth following lower limb amputation. Rehabil Psychol 2005;50(3):266–77.
58. Frazier P, Conlon A, Glaser T. Positive and negative life changes following sexual assault. J Consult Clin Psychol 2001;69(6):1048–55.
59. McMillen C, Zuravin S, Rideout G. Perceived benefit from child sexual abuse. J Consult Clin Psychol 1995;63(6):1037–43.
60. Milam J, Ritt-Olson A, Tan S, et al. The September 11th 2001 terrorist attacks and reports of posttraumatic growth among a multi-ethnic sample of adolescents. Traumatol 2005;11:233–46.
61. McMillen C, Smith EM, Fisher RH. Perceived benefit and mental health after three types of disaster. J Consult Clin Psychol 1997;65(5):733–9.
62. Joseph S, Linley PA. Growth following adversity: theoretical perspectives and implications for clinical practice. Clin Psychol Rev 2006;26(8):1041–53.
63. Evers AW, Kraaimaat FW, van Lankveld W, et al. Beyond unfavorable thinking: the illness Cognition Questionnaire for chronic diseases. J Consult Clin Psychol 2001; 69(6):1026–36.
64. Hawley CA, Joseph S. Predictors of positive growth after traumatic brain injury: a longitudinal study. Brain Inj 2008;22(5):427–35.
65. Rosenbach C, Renneberg B. Positive change after severe burn injuries. J Burn Care Res 2008;29(4):638–43.
66. Helgeson VS, Reynolds KA, Tomich PL. A meta-analytic review of benefit finding and growth. J Consult Clin Psychol 2006;74(5):797–816.
67. Linley PA, Joseph S. Positive change following trauma and adversity: a review. J Trauma Stress 2004;17(1):11–21.
68. Milam JE, Ritt-Olson A, Unger JB. Posttraumatic growth among adolescents. J Res Adolesc 2004;19(2):192–204.

69. Powell S, Rosner R, Butollo W, et al. Posttraumatic growth after war: a study with former refugees and displaced people in Sarajevo. J Clin Psychol 2003;59(1): 71–83.

70. Calhoun LG, Tedeschi RG. Posttraumatic growth: future directions. In: Tedeschi RG, Park CL, Calhoun LG, editors. Posttraumatic growth: positive change in the aftermath of crisis. Mahwah (NJ): Lawrence Erlbaum Associates, Inc; 1998.

71. Patten SB, Metz LM, Reimer MA. Biopsychosocial correlates of lifetime major depression in a multiple sclerosis population. Mult Scler 2000;6:115–20.

72. Chwastiak L, Ehde DM, Gibbons LE, et al. Depressive symptoms and severity of illness in multiple sclerosis: epidemiologic study of a large community sample. Am J Psychiatry 2002;159:1862–8.

73. Beiske AG, Svensson E, Sandanger I, et al. Depression and anxiety amongst multiple sclerosis patients. Eur J Neurol 2008;15:239–45.

74. Phillips LJ, Stuifbergen AK. The influence of positive experiences on depression and quality of life in persons with multiple sclerosis. J Holist Nurs 2008;26:41–8.

75. Prohaska TR, Keller ML, Leventhal EA, et al. Impact of symptoms and aging attribution on emotions and coping. Health Psychol 1987;6(6):495–514.

76. Pakenham KI. Benefit finding in multiple sclerosis and associations with positive and negative outcomes. Health Psychol 2005;24(2):123–32.

77. Davis CG, Nolen-Hoeksema S, Larson J. Making sense of loss and benefiting from the experience: two construals of meaning. J Pers Soc Psychol 1998; 75(2):561–74.

78. Bellizzi KM. Expressions of generativity and posttraumatic growth in adult cancer survivors. Int J Aging Hum Dev 2004;58(4):267–87.

79. Pollard C, Kennedy P. A longitudinal analysis of emotional impact, coping strategies and post-traumatic psychological growth following spinal cord injury: a 10-year review. Br J Health Psychol 2007;12(Pt 3):347–62.

80. Park CL, Mills-Baxter MA, Fenster JR. Post-traumatic growth from life's most traumatic event: Influences on elders' current coping and adjustment. Traumatol 2005;11:297–306.

81. Park CL, Cohen LH, Murch RL. Assessment and prediction of stress-related growth. J Pers 1996;64(1):71–105.

82. Schroots JJ. Theoretical developments in the psychology of aging. Gerontologist 1996;36(6):742–8.

83. Chwalisz K, Shah SR, Hand KM. Facilitating rigorous qualitative research in rehabilitation psychology. Rehabil Psychol 2008;53:387–99.

84. Albright KJ, Duggan CH, Epstein MJ. Analyzing trauma narratives: introducing the narrative form index and matrix. Rehabil Psychol 2008;53:400–11.

85. Teddlie C, Tashakkori A. Foundations of mixed methods research: integrating quantitative and qualitative approaches in the social and behavioral sciences. Thousand Oaks (CA): Sage; 2009.

86. White B, Driver S, Waren A. Considering resilience in the rehabilitation of people with traumatic disabilities. Rehabil Psychol 2008;53:9–17.

87. Weston R, Gore PA Jr, Chan F, et al. An introduction to using structural equation models in rehabilitation psychology. Rehabil Psychol 2008;53:340–56.

88. Kwok OM, Underhill AT, Berry JW, et al. Analyzing longitudinal data with multilevel models: an example with individuals living with lower extremity intra-articular fractures. Rehabil Psychol 2008;53(3):370–86.

89. McGrath JC, Linley PA. Post-traumatic growth in acquired brain injury: a preliminary small scale study. Brain Inj 2006;20(7):767–73.

90. Powell T, Ekin-Wood A, Collin C. Post-traumatic growth after head injury: a long-term follow-up. Brain Inj 2007;21(1):31–8.
91. Lyons JA. Using a life span model to promote recovery and growth in traumatized veterans. In: Joseph S, Linley PA, editors. Trauma, recovery, and growth. Hoboken (NJ): John Wiley & Sons; 2008. p. 233–57.
92. Bellizzi KM. Expressions of generativity and posttraumatic growth in adult cancer survivors. Int J Aging Hum Dev 2004;58(4):267–87.
93. Ehde DM. Application of positive psychology to rehabilitation psychology. In: Frank RG, Caplan R, Rosenthal M, editors. Handbook of rehabilitation psychology. 2nd edition. Washington, DC: American Psychological Association Books; 2009. p. 417–24.
94. Cetin K, Johnson KL, Edhe DM, et al. Antidepressant use in multiple sclerosis: epidemiologic study of a large community sample. Mult Scler 2007;13(8): 1046–53.
95. Mohr DC, Goodkin DE, Likosky W, et al. Screening for depression among patients with multiple sclerosis: two questions may be enough. Mult Scler 2007;13(2): 215–9.
96. Lenze EJ, Sheffrin M, Driscoll HC, et al. Incomplete response in late-life depression: getting to remission. Dialogues Clin Neurosci 2008;10(4):419–30.
97. Laidlaw K, Davidson K, Toner H, et al. A randomized controlled trial of cognitive behaviour therapy vs treatment as usual in the treatment of mild to moderate late life depression. Int J Geriatr Psychiatry 2008;23(8):843–50.
98. Alexopoulos GS, Raue PJ, Kanellopoulos D, et al. Problem solving therapy for the depression-executive dysfunction syndrome of late life. Int J Geriatr Psychiatry 2008;23(8):782–8.
99. Lechner SC, Stoelb BL, Antoni MH. Group-based therapies for benefit finding in cancer. In: Joseph S, Linley PA, editors. Trauma, recovery, and growth: positive psychological perspectives on posttraumatic stress. Hoboken (NJ): John Wiley & Sons Inc; 2008. p. 207–31.

Physical Activity, Disability, and Quality of Life in Older Adults

Robert W. Motl, PhD*, Edward McAuley, PhD

KEYWORDS

• Older adults • Aging • Function • Exercise • Well-being

The United States is undergoing a transformative shift in the demographic composition of adults. Indeed, there is an emergent and staggering rate of growth in the percentage of adults aged 65 years or older and this has been termed the Graying of America. The proportion of the population aged 65 years or older is projected to increase from 12.4% in 2000 to 19.6% in 2030.[1] This reflects a twofold increase in the number of persons aged 65 years or older from nearly 35 million in 2000 to an estimated 71 million in 2030.[1] One of the fastest growing segments of the United States population is those aged 80 years or older. The number of persons in this age group is expected to more than double from 9.3 million in 2000 to 19.5 million in 2030.[1]

The growing percentage and number of older adults is expected to be accompanied by a considerable burden on the public health system, and the medical and social services.[1] This burden is associated with a disproportionate rate of chronic disease conditions among older adults (eg, cancers, diabetes, and stroke) that will represent a primary source of health care services and costs. Of further importance, aging and chronic disease conditions are primary correlates of disablement and compromised quality of life (QOL), and this underscores the importance of identifying factors that might promote healthy aging (ie, optimal mental and physical well-being and function in older adults).

This research was supported, in part, by a grant from the Department of Education, National Institute on Disability and Rehabilitation Research (H133B080024). The contents of this article do not necessarily represent the policy of the Department of Education and the reader should not assume endorsement by the Federal Government.

This article represents an expression of the first author's training under the mentorship of the second author. Robert W. Motl is responsible for the drafting of the article and Edward McAuley is responsible for the critical review of its content along with the revision of the article.

Department of Kinesiology and Community Health, University of Illinois at Urbana-Champaign, 350 Freer Hall, Urbana, IL 61801, USA

* Corresponding author.

E-mail address: robmotl@uiuc.edu.

Physical activity behavior is associated with reduced risks of chronic disease conditions (obesity, heart disease, hypertension, diabetes, depression, and certain cancers) and premature mortality, and might be positively associated with functional limitations, disability, and QOL in older adults.[2–5] This article provides a brief and focused overview of physical activity behavior and its association with functional limitations, disability, and QOL in older adults.

PHYSICAL ACTIVITY BEHAVIOR IN ADULTS: TRENDS FOR AGING AND DISABILITY

There is an abundance of evidence describing the rates of physical activity and inactivity among adults in the United States, and, although the rates vary based on the source of data and nature of the survey questions, the evidence is suggestive of a potential public health problem. The National Center for Health Statistics (NCHS) analyzed data on national estimates of physical activity (usual daily activity and leisure-time physical activity) among adults using the 2000 and 2005 National Health Interview Surveys (NHIS).[6] One important observation was that of little change in the percentage of adults who reported engaging in usual daily activity and leisure-time physical activity between 2000 and 2005. The percentage of adults who reported spending most of the day sitting increased from 36.8% in 2000 to 39.9% in 2005, and the percentage of adults who engaged in no leisure-time physical activity increased from 38.5% in 2000 to 40.0% in 2005.[6] The percentage of adults who engaged in regular leisure-time physical activity decreased from 31.2% in 2000 to 29.7% in 2005, and the percentage of adults who were never active increased from 9.4% in 2000 to 10.3% in 2005.[6] The rates of physical activity/inactivity among adults are not much different based on an analysis by the Center for Disease Control (CDC) of Behavioral Risk Factor Surveillance System (BRFSS) data regarding the prevalence of regular, leisure-time, physical activity between 2001 and 2005.[7] Regular physical activity was defined based on the Healthy People 2010 Objectives as 30 minutes or more per day of moderate-intensity activity on 5 days or more per week, or 20 minutes or more per day of vigorous-intensity activity on 3 days or more per week. The data indicated that between 2001 and 2005 the prevalence of regular physical activity increased 3.5% overall among men (from 48.0% to 49.7%) and 8.6% overall among women (from 43.0% to 46.7%).[7] Nevertheless, fewer than 50% of adults in the United States reported engaging in recommended levels of physical activity,[7] and the overall implication from the NCHS and CDC reports is one of a high rate of physical inactivity and low rate of regular physical activity among adults in the United States.

One noteworthy trend in the NHIS[6] and BRFSS[8] data sets is that of an association between age and the rates of physical activity and inactivity among adults in the United States. Both data sets document that physical activity levels reliably decrease and inactivity levels reliably increase as a function of increasing age. The NCHS reported that the percentage of adults who reported spending most of the day sitting in 2000 was 46.5% for those 65 years and older, whereas it was 38.4%, 33.3%, and 31.2% for those aged 45 to 64 years, 25 to 44 years, and 18 to 24 years.[6] The percentage of adults who engaged in no leisure-time physical activity in 2000 was 51.8% for those 65 years and more, whereas it was 40.8%, 33.7%, and 30.6% for those aged 45 to 64 years, 25 to 44 years, and 18 to 24 years.[6] Finally, the percentage of adults who were never active in 2000 was 22.2% for those aged 65 years and more, whereas it was 9.9%, 5.3%, and 4.3% for those aged 45 to 64 years, 25 to 44 years, and 18 to 24 years.[6] The rates of physical activity/inactivity among older adults are not much different based on BRFSS data regarding the prevalence of no leisure-time physical activity between 1994 and 2004.[8] No leisure-time physical activity was defined based on a "no" response to the question "During the past month, other than your regular job, did you participate in any physical activities or exercise, such as running, calisthenics, golf, gardening, or walking for exercise?" The data indicated that from 1994 to 2004 the prevalence of leisure-time physical inactivity decreased from 29.8% to 23.7% overall, but the rate of leisure-time physical inactivity was consistently higher in men and women aged 70 years or older.[8] The overall implication from both data sets is one of a strong trend for late-life declines in physical activity and associated increases in the rate of physical inactivity.

Another important trend in the BRFSS data set is that of an association between disability and the rates of physical activity and inactivity among older adults in the United States. Indeed, the CDC analyzed data from the 2005 BRFSS on prevalence of physical activity and inactivity among adults with and without a disability.[9] The percentage of adults with a disability who met national recommendations for physical activity in 2005 was 37.7%, whereas the percentage was 49.4% for adults without a disability. The percentage of adults with a disability who were physically inactive in 2005 was 25.6%, whereas the percentage was 12.8% for adults without a disability. The CDC further analyzed data from the 2003 BRFSS on prevalence of physical activity among adults with and without a disability who were 65 years of age and older.[10] The percentage of older adults with a disability who reported engaging in recommended levels of physical activity in 2003 was 14.7%, whereas the percentage was 26.2% for older adults without a disability. Work from the authors' laboratory further supports an inverse association between advancing age and physical activity as measured by a pedometer in persons with multiple sclerosis.[11] Such data support the observation that there is an alarming rate of physical inactivity among adults who are aging with a disability and supports the importance of promoting physical activity among adults who are aging with a disability.

Overall, the age-related trends in the rates of physical activity and inactivity among adults with and without a disability are alarming considering that physical activity is associated with reduced risks of many chronic disease conditions and premature mortality. Physical activity might be associated with beneficial effects on functional limitations, disability, and QOL in older adults,[2–5] and represents a primary component of healthy and successful aging. The following sections focus on the role of physical activity in mitigating the progression of functional limitations and disability and improving QOL among adults who are progressing through advanced years of age.

FUNCTIONAL LIMITATIONS, DISABILITY, AND PHYSICAL ACTIVITY AMONG OLDER ADULTS

As previously noted, there is an unprecedented growth in the older adult population of the United States, and the additional years of life are likely to be associated with chronic disease conditions and the onset of functional limitations and disability. There is considerable evidence that the aging process is associated with declines in function that result in increased risk of disablement.[12] For example, the prevalence of mobility disability was 18.8% and 13.3% for women and men, respectively, aged 65 to 69 years, and the prevalence was 83.3% and 63.4% for women and men, respectively, aged 90 to 95 years.[13] Furthermore, 51.8% of adults more than 65 years of age reported limitations in one or more domains of functioning such as walking, grasping, carrying, or pushing[14] and the prevalence of disability doubled in successive age groups.[14] One final observation is that nearly one-fifth of adults aged 65 years or older reported limitations with basic activities of daily living such as dressing and bathing.[14] The prevalence of functional limitations and disability among older adults supports an examination of factors such as physical activity behavior within the process of disablement.

Theoretically, the process of disablement with advancing age and the role of physical activity can be understood by considering Nagi's[15] Disablement Model. The authors acknowledge the value and innovation offered by the World Health Organization's International Classification of Functioning, Disability, and Health, but opt against this model in favor of Nagi's model for several reasons as recently articulated by Guralnik and Ferrucci.[16] The Disablement Model includes 4 interrelated components. The first component is active pathology. Active pathology describes the interruption of normal cellular processes based on degenerative disease processes, injury/trauma, and infection. The second component of the model is impairment and this involves structural abnormalities and dysfunction in specific body systems. The third component is functional limitations. Functional limitations describe restrictions in basic physical and mental actions (eg, walking 1 mile). Disability is the fourth component and involves the expression of physical or mental limitations in a social context (eg, difficulty doing activities of daily living that are required for one's employment, personal care, and recreation). The 4 aspects of the Disablement Model are interrelated such that activity pathology results in impairment, impairment results in functional limitations, and functional limitations lead to disability. Those basic components have been extended to include personal (eg, lifestyle behaviors and psychosocial attributes) and sociocultural (eg, physical and social environments) variables as core influences of the disablement process.[17,18] Physical activity has been identified as a biobehavioral, intraindividual determinant of disablement in older adults[2,19,20] and is considered a primary determinant of functional limitations.[2,19] To that end, physical activity is a behavior that has a distinct entry point in the process of disablement through its influence on functional limitations in older adults. The authors direct readers to a series of articles on physical activity and disablement in older adults based on Nagi's Disablement Model that are published in a supplement of the *American Journal of Preventive Medicine*.[21]

There is emerging evidence regarding physical activity and its association with functional limitations and disability in older adults. Physical inactivity or sedentary behavior seemingly exacerbates the impairments in physiologic and structural systems that occur with the aging process.[21] Those impairments in physiologic and structural systems will likely result in the accumulation of functional limitations and disability over time. By extension, interventions that promote or maintain physical activity behavior among older adults might represent an effective strategy for attenuating functional decline and reducing the risk of disability in older adults.

Many individual studies have examined physical activity and its association with impairment, function, and disability outcomes in older adults and this literature has been summarized in 2 extensive literature reviews.[2,3] Keysor and Jette[3] performed a literature review of research examining physical activity behavior as a means of improving function and preventing or decreasing disability in older adults. The review included 31 studies published between 1985 and 2000 that examined the effects of aerobic and resistance exercise interventions using experimental and quasi-experimental designs on impairment, function, and disability outcomes in older adults. The effects of exercise on impairment and functional outcomes were reported in 97% and 81% of the studies, respectively, whereas only 50% of the studies reported effects on physical, social, emotional, or overall disability. The most consistent observation was that more than half of the studies reported improvements in strength, aerobic capacity, flexibility, standing balance, and walking after exercise training in older adults. The effects of exercise on physical, social, emotional, and overall disability were less clear with most studies reporting no improvement, and the 5 studies that reported reduced physical disability yielded variable effect sizes ranging between 0.23 and 0.88. Such findings result in ambiguous conclusions regarding physical activity effects on disability in later life, but this might be linked with methodological shortcomings that include variable sample characteristics and exercise parameters, small sample sizes and low power, and inadequate measures of disability as noted by Keysor and Jette.[3] An additional observation of this review was that few studies have actually targeted disability as a primary outcome of physical activity. This literature review and its findings were consistent with those of earlier reviews, including one by Chandler and Hadley.[22]

Keysor[2] later provided another excellent review of the scientific evidence underlying physical activity as an important component for preventing and minimizing functional limitations and disability among older adults. This review used a best-evidence framework and included meta-analyses and systematic reviews of randomized controlled trails (RCTs), individual RCTs, and longitudinal observational studies. The synthesis of the scientific literature clearly supported that exercise, particularly walking, was associated with improvements in strength, aerobic capacity, and function. By comparison, there was again conflicting evidence regarding physical activity and disability outcomes, with minimal evidence that exercise or physical activity prevents or minimizes physical disability from RCTs but stronger evidence from prospective studies of an inverse association between physical activity and disability. One major recommendation of this review for strengthening the scientific evidence on physical activity, function, and disability was a focus on understanding the mechanisms of action.[2] The improved understanding of how physical activity and exercise result in beneficial effects on function and disability would seemingly result in the design of more effective interventions. Such interventions could target exercise behavior plus the presumed mediator variables as a means of maximizing beneficial effects on function and disability in older adults.

To that end, one group of researchers has adopted a social cognitive perspective for examining self-efficacy and physical function performance as possible mediators in the association between physical activity and functional limitations among older adults.[23,24] The first study included a sample of older Black and White women who completed measures of physical activity, self-efficacy, physical function performance, and functional limitations as part of the baseline assessment of an ongoing longitudinal, observational study.[23] The analyses indicated that physical activity was associated with self-efficacy for exercise, efficacy for gait and balance, and physical function performance; measures of self-efficacy and physical functional performance were associated with functional limitations. Those relationships were independent of demographic and health status variables. Such findings support that physical activity, self-efficacy, and physical functional may all be associated with reducing functional limitations, and perhaps disability, in older adults. The findings further suggest that self-efficacy might be an important mediator of physical activity and its association with functional limitations.

This same group of researchers later examined the possibility that changes in self-efficacy and physical functional performance mediated the relationship between changes in physical activity and functional limitations over time.[24] This study used a prospective observational design whereby community-dwelling, older Black and White women completed measures of self-reported physical activity, self-efficacy for exercise and balance, and functional limitations and underwent 4 measures of physical function performance on 2 occasions that were separated by 24 months. The results indicated that a change in physical activity over time was associated with residual changes in exercise and balance self-efficacy. Changes in exercise and balance self-efficacy were, in turn, associated with residual change in physical function performance. Most importantly, changes in self-efficacy for exercise and balance and physical function performance were associated with residual change in functional limitations. This supports that self-efficacy and physical function performance mediated the association between physical activity and functional limitations. The findings further support self-efficacy and physical function performance as possible mediators in the relationship between changes in physical activity and functional limitations in older women.

Overall, there has been an increased interest in the study of physical activity and its role in the process of disablement among older adults. The available evidence supports that exercise is associated with improvements in strength, aerobic capacity, and function, but there is less clear, and perhaps conflicting, evidence regarding physical activity and disability outcomes. Recent work has highlighted the role of self-efficacy in the pathway between physical activity and functional limitations, and such findings suggest that researchers integrate strategies for promoting change in self-efficacy along with physical activity interventions for maximizing improvements in disability outcomes among older adults. Indeed, self-efficacy is a modifiable factor and should be a central component of physical activity programs designed for preventing and minimizing functional limitations and disability in older adults.

QOL AND PHYSICAL ACTIVITY AMONG OLDER ADULTS

We are witnessing a dramatic prolongation of life expectancy, but of central important is maintaining high life quality with increasing age. Indeed, an important goal of healthy aging is living a longer and a better life. This reflects the motto of the Gerontological Society of America, "Adding life to years, not just more years to life." QOL has become a central theme in understanding the effect of chronic disease conditions and monitoring the general well-being of older adults. Indeed, many older adults who develop chronic disease suffer from poor QOL, and seemingly would prefer better QOL over longevity.[5]

Any discussion of QOL would benefit from a definition of terminology. QOL is derived from the behavioral and social sciences for describing subjective well-being or judgments regarding overall satisfaction with life. QOL is considered a global psychological construct that accounts for the weighting or importance of particular areas within an individual's life.[25,26] This conceptualization of QOL differs from that of health-related quality of life (HRQOL). HRQOL is derived from the behavioral medicine and biomedical sciences for considering physical and mental health as 2 related aspects of HRQOL.[27,28] To that end, QOL and HRQOL are related, but not isomorphic constructs,[29,30] and there is evidence of a hierarchical model whereby proximal HRQOL constructs predict distal QOL constructs.[31,32]

Many individual studies have examined physical activity and its association with QOL outcomes in older adults and this literature has been summarized in literature reviews and a meta-analysis. Rejeski and Mihalko[5] undertook a critical review of research on physical activity and QOL in older adults, and focused on QOL as a psychological construct represented by satisfaction with life versus QOL as a clinical or geriatric outcome represented by core dimensions of health status or HRQOL. The investigators located 12 studies on physical activity and QOL, and 6 were RCTs, 1 was a quasi-experimental trial, and 5 were cross-sectional. Of the RCTs, 3 studies reported improvements in QOL after physical activity, whereas the other 3 failed to support such benefits. This presents a confusing picture regarding the effects of physical activity on QOL in older adults, but the equivocal findings are partially explained by activity prescriptions and QOL measures, as noted by Rejeski and Mihalko.[5] The investigators further located 18 studies on physical activity and HRQOL, published since 1996, and nearly two-thirds were RCTs. The review of those studies indicated that physical activity had positive effects on physical function and mental health status as domains of HRQOL among older adults. This pattern is generally consistent with the major conclusion of a previous review of physical activity and HRQOL in older adults by the same lead author.[33]

Netz and colleagues[4] recently conducted a meta-analysis of physical activity and psychological well-being (eg, emotional well-being, self-perceptions, bodily well-being, and global perceptions such as life satisfaction) in advanced age. The meta-analysis included 36 studies of physical activity and well-being in older adults without clinical disorders. The weighted mean-change effect size for the treatment and control groups were 0.24 and 0.09, respectively, indicating that physical activity had a nearly 3 times greater effect on psychological well-being than did the control. Physical activity had its strongest affects on anxiety, overall well-being, self-efficacy, view of the self, and physical symptoms, but had the least effect on life satisfaction compared with the control samples. This pattern of results would support the proximal/distal effects of physical activity and QOL outcomes in older adults[29] and further support the observation that physical activity has its strongest effects on constructs aligned with HRQOL (anxiety, overall well-being, self-efficacy, view of the self, and physical symptoms) than QOL (satisfaction with life).

An important observation of the aforementioned literature and meta-analysis is that of identifying mechanisms or mediators in the pathway between physical activity and QOL in older adults. To this end, one group of researchers has adopted a social cognitive approach for identifying the role of self-efficacy in the relationship between physical activity QOL in older adults[29,34,35] and this model has been further tested and confirmed among persons with multiple sclerosis.[36] Those studies further examined the nature of the relationships among physical activity, HRQOL (ie, health status), and QOL consistent with the conceptual basis offered by Stewart and King.[32] The first study examined the roles played by self-efficacy and health status in the association between physical activity and global QOL in a sample of older Black and White women.[29] The participants completed measures of physical activity, self-efficacy, health status (HRQOL), and QOL as part of the baseline assessment of a 24-month prospective trial. Analyses indicated that relationship between physical activity and QOL was indirect and accounted for by self-efficacy, and physical and mental aspects of HRQOL. Physical activity influenced self-efficacy; self-efficacy influenced physical and mental health status HRQOL; and physical and mental HRQOL, in turn, influenced global QOL. Those findings support the application of a social cognitive model for describing the relationship between physical activity and QOL in older adults.

The subsequent study prospectively examined the roles played by self-efficacy and physical and mental HRQOL in the physical activity and QOL relationship in older women.[34] Older women completed measures of physical activity, self-efficacy relative to balance, mental and physical health status (ie, HRQOL), and global QOL on 2 occasions separated by 24 months. The analysis indicated that change in physical activity over time was associated with residual change in self-efficacy; change in self-efficacy was significantly associated with residual changes in physical and mental aspects of HRQOL; and only changes in mental aspects of HRQOL were significantly related to residual changes in global QOL. Results from this study further support the role of self-efficacy in the relationship between physical activity and QOL.

One final study has recently replicated the observation that physical activity influences global QOL through self-efficacy and physical and mental aspects of HRQOL (ie, health status) in older, community-dwelling men and women.[35] The participants completed measures of physical activity, self-efficacy, physical self-esteem (mental aspect of HRQOL), disability limitations (physical aspect of HRQOL), and global QOL. Analyses indicated that the association between physical activity and global QOL was indirect by way of self-efficacy and then physical self-esteem and disability limitations. The findings provide a replication of self-efficacy's role in the association between physical activity and QOL among older adults.

Overall, there is an important interplay between living longer and living better among older adults, and physical activity has been associated with improvements in longevity and aspects of HRQOL and QOL. This suggests that physical activity should become a central agent in the promotion of healthy aging as a behavioral approach for maximizing the likelihood of quality years along with longevity. Additional research has highlighted the role of self-efficacy within the physical activity and QOL relationship, and this suggests that future researchers should include strategies to enhance self-efficacy as a more effective approach for maximizing QOL outcomes among older adults. As noted previously, self-efficacy is a modifiable construct and should be a central component of physical activity programs designed for maximizing improvements in HRQOL and QOL of older adults.

SUMMARY

This article provided an overview of physical activity and its association with function, disability, and QOL outcomes among older adults. The rationale for this overview is embedded in the Graying of America and the associated onset of chronic disease conditions that erode function, participation, and QOL. The authors provide 3 general observations based on the literature reviewed: (1) an alarming rate of physical inactivity among older adults, particularly those aging with a disability, that supports a critical focus on developing strategies for behavioral change in this demographic segment of society; (2) strong evidence for physical activity exerting positive effects on impairment, function, and HRQOL in older adults, but less conclusive evidence for effects on disability and QOL; and (3) preliminary support for self-efficacy in mediating the association between physical activity and disability and QOL outcomes in older adults.

The authors' review identified obvious directions for future research that will aid in the application of physical activity among older adults. The most obvious direction for future research involves a focus on physical activity and function, disability, and QOL outcomes among persons who are aging with conditions such as multiple sclerosis, spinal cord injury, or muscular dystrophy. This recommendation is based on the limited body of research on adults who are aging with a chronic disabling condition. Another research direction involves the design and testing of programs that incorporate strategies for enhancing self-efficacy along with the promotion of physical activity as a means of mitigating functional declines and disability and improving QOL among older adults and those aging with a chronic disabling condition.

The generation of an expanded body of knowledge will help to identify practical approaches for improving the later years of life and is critical because the number of people affected directly or indirectly by the aging of adults is increasing in the United States. Such work can assist physiatrists who work directly with older adults who have chronic disabling conditions. Physiatrists are on the frontline for the promotion and application of physical activity among adults who are aging with a disability, but are limited by the scope of work on physical activity in older adults with conditions such as multiple sclerosis, spinal cord injury, or muscular dystrophy. Overall, the promotion of physical activity among all persons, particularly those with chronic, disabling conditions, is a central agent in healthy aging of adults in the United States.

REFERENCES

1. Goulding MR, Rogers ME, Smith SM. Public health and aging: trends in aging – United States and worldwide. Morb Mortal Wkly Rep 2003;52(06):101–6.
2. Keysor JJ. Does late-life physical activity or exercise prevent or minimize disability? A critical review of the scientific literature. Am J Prev Med 2003; 25(3Sii):129–36.
3. Keysor JJ, Jette AM. Have we oversold the benefit of late-life exercise? J Gerontol A Biol Sci Med Sci 2001;56(7):M412–23.
4. Netz Y, Wu M-J, Becker BJ, et al. Physical activity and psychological well-being in advanced age: a meta-analysis of intervention studies. Psychol Aging 2005; 20(2):272–84.
5. Rejeski WJ, Mihalko SL. Physical activity and quality of life in older adults. J Gerontol A Biol Sci Med Sci 2001;56(Special Issue II):23–35.
6. Barnes P. Physical activity among adults: United States, 2000 and 2005. Hyattsville (MD): US Department of Health and Human Services, CDC; 2007.
7. Kruger J, Kohl HW. Prevalence of regular physical activity among adults – United States, 2001 and 2005. Morb Mortal Wkly Rep 2007;56(46):1209–12.
8. Kruger J, Ham SA, Kohl HW. Trends in leisure-time physical inactivity by age, sex, race/ethnicity – United States, 1994–2004. MMWR Morb Mortal Wkly Rep 2005; 54(39):991–4.
9. Rimmer JH, Wolf LA, Armour BS, et al. Physical activity among adults with a disability – United States, 2005. MMWR Morb Mortal Wkly Rep 2007;56(39):1021–4.
10. McGuire LC, Strine TW, Okoro CA, et al. Healthy lifestyle behaviors among older adults with and without disabilities, Behavioral Risk Factor Surveillance System, 2003. Prev Chronic Dis 2007;4(1):1–11.
11. Motl RW, Snook EM, McAuley E, et al. Demographic correlates of physical activity in individuals with multiple sclerosis. Disabil Rehabil 2006;29(16):1301–4.
12. Tas Ü, Verhagen AP, Bierma-Zeinstra SMA, et al. Prognostic factors of disability in older people: a systematic review. Br J Gen Pract 2007;57(537):319–23.
13. Leveille SG, Penninx BW, Melzer D, et al. Sex differences in the prevalence of mobility disability in old age: the dynamics of incidence, recovery, and mortality. J Gerontol B Psychol Sci Soc Sci 2000;55(1):S41–50.
14. Brault MW, Hootman J, Helmick CG, et al. Prevalence and most common causes of disability among adults – United States, 2005. MMWR Morb Mortal Wkly Rep 2009;58(16):421–6.
15. Nagi SZ. An epidemiology of disability among adults in the United States. Milbank Mem Fund Q Health Soc 1976;54(4):439–67.
16. Guralnik JM, Ferrucci L. The challenge of understanding the disablement process in older persons. Commentary responding to Jette AM. Toward a common language of disablement. J Gerontol A Biol Sci Med Sci 2009;64(11):1169–71.
17. Jette AM. Toward a common language for function, disability, and health. Phys Ther 2006;86(5):726–34.
18. Verbrugge LM, Jette AM. The disablement process. Soc Sci Med 1994;38(1): 1–14.

19. Jette AM, Keysor JJ. Disability models: implications for arthritis exercise and physical activity interventions. Arthritis Rheum 2003;49:114–20.
20. Stewart AL. Conceptual challenges in linking physical activity and disability research. Am J Prev Med 2003;25(3Sii):137–40.
21. Rejeski WJ, Brawley LR, Haskell WL. Physical activity: preventing physical disablement in older adults. Am J Prev Med 2003;25(3Sii):107–217.
22. Chandler JM, Hadley EC. Exercise to improve physiologic and functional performance in old age. Clin Geriatr Med 1996;12(4):761–84.
23. McAuley E, Konopack JF, Morris KS, et al. Physical activity and functional limitations in older women: influence of self-efficacy. J Gerontol B Psychol Sci Soc Sci 2006;61(5):P270–7.
24. McAuley E, Morris KS, Doerksen SE, et al. Effects of change in physical activity on physical function limitations in older women: mediating roles of physical function performance and self-efficacy. J Am Geriatr Soc 2007;55(12):1967–73.
25. Diener E, Emmons R, Larsen J, et al. The satisfaction with life scale. J Pers Assess 1985;49(1):71–5.
26. Pavot W, Diener E. Review of the satisfaction with life scale. Psychol Assess 1993; 5:164–72.
27. Ware JF. SF-36 Health survey: manual interpretation guide. Boston: The Health Institute; 1993.
28. Ware J, Sherbourne C. The MOS 36 item short-form health survey (SF-36). I. Conceptual framework and item selection. Med Care 1992;36(6):473–83.
29. McAuley E, Konopack JF, Motl RW, et al. Physical activity and quality of life in older adults: influence of health status and self-efficacy. Ann Behav Med 2006;31(1): 99–103.
30. Motl RW, McAuley E, Snook EM, et al. Does the relationship between physical activity and quality of life differ based on generic versus disease-targeted instruments? Ann Behav Med 2008;36(1):93–9.
31. Elavsky S, McAuley E, Motl RW, et al. Physical activity enhances long-term quality of life in older adults: efficacy, esteem, and affective influences. Ann Behav Med 2005;30(2):138–45.
32. Stewart AL, King AC. Evaluating the efficacy of physical activity for influencing quality-of-life outcomes in older adults. Ann Behav Med 1991;13:108–16.
33. Rejeski WJ, Brawley LR, Shumaker SA. Physical activity and health-related quality of life. Exerc Sport Sci Rev 1996;24:71–108.
34. McAuley E, Doerksen SE, Morris KS, et al. Pathways from physical activity to quality of life in older women. Ann Behav Med 2008;36(1):13–20.
35. White SB, Wojcicki TR, McAuley E. Physical activity and quality of life in community dwelling older adults. Health Qual Life Outcomes 2009;7:10.
36. Motl RW, Snook EM. Physical activity, self-efficacy, and quality of life in multiple sclerosis. Ann Behav Med 2008;35:111–5.

Communication and Aging

Kathryn M. Yorkston, PhD[a],*, Michelle S. Bourgeois, PhD[b],
Carolyn R. Baylor, PhD, BC-NCD[a]

KEYWORDS

- Communication disorders • Aging • Dysarthria • Aphasia
- Dual sensory impairment

Interpersonal communication has been described as a critical tool for life adjustment, linking people to their environment.[1] When communication disorders are present these links can be easily broken. Communication disorders form a diverse group of conditions that vary in terms of type, severity, and co-occurrence with other symptoms that limit mobility, vision, endurance, or cognition. Although communication disorders affect people of all ages, the prevalence and complexity of these conditions increase with age, and may be characterized by a stable, recovering or degenerative course. Disabilities associated with communication disorders may best be viewed as a dynamic process that varies over time instead of as a single static event that remains constant. Two broad trajectories of disability and aging have been described[2] and can be applied to those with communication disorders. The disability with aging group includes people who live most of their lives without disability and either experience the subtle communication problems associated with age or the onset of conditions such as stroke that occur most commonly in old age. The aging with disability group includes people who either have lifelong or early onset communication disorders as a result of cerebral palsy or multiple sclerosis (MS) and age in the context of the already-existing disability. Regardless of the trajectory, the burden of communication disorder is cumulative; it grows with age and has important implications for health care providers. This article describes various communication disabilities associated with aging and how these disabilities affect important functions such as access to health care and maintenance of social roles. Suggestions that preserve and enhance communication function in older adults are also provided in this article.

This research was supported, in part, by a grant from the Department of Education, National Institute on Disability and Rehabilitation Research (H133B080024). The contents of this article do not necessarily represent the policy of the Department of Education and the reader should not assume endorsement by the Federal Government.

[a] Division of Speech Pathology, Department of Rehabilitation Medicine, University of Washington, Box 356490, Seattle, WA 98195-6490, USA

[b] Department of Speech and Hearing Science, The Ohio State University, 1070 Carmack Road, Columbus, OH 43210, USA

* Corresponding author.

E-mail address: yorkston@u.washington.edu

COMMUNICATION DISABILITIES

Communication changes are commonly reported by older people. In a large survey of more than 12,000 Medicare beneficiaries aged 65 years or more, 42% reported hearing problems, 26% had writing problems, and 7% had problems using the telephone.[3] Using statistical procedures (sampling weights) to make inferences about the entire Medicare population, more than 16 million Medicare beneficiaries are estimated to experience communication changes. The severity of communication disabilities is based on a health-disease continuum.[4] At one end of the spectrum are the well elderly who wish to prevent disabling communication conditions. In the middle are the worried well or frail elders who struggle to maintain independent function, and at the other end are people with well-defined communication disabilities such as dysarthria, aphasia, and hearing loss.

Communication Changes with Typical Aging

With typical aging, communication skills change subtly at least in part because of changes in physical health, depression, and cognitive decline. Aging is responsible for physiologic changes in hearing, voice, and speech processes.[5,6] A person's age can be predicted with fair accuracy by speech characteristics including voice tremor, pitch, speaking rate, loudness, and fluency.[7] Some language skills remain intact, whereas others tend to decline. For example, vocabulary, grammatical judgment, and repetition ability are relatively stable with age; comprehension of complex utterances and naming may decline.[8] Although changes in communication skills such as voice may be subtle and gradual, they have clear life consequences such as avoidance of social situations.[9]

Aging with a Preexisting Communication Disorder

Conditions that are associated with preexisting, long-term communication disorders may compound the challenges faced by people as they age. MS, which is one such condition, is discussed in this article. MS is a chronic, progressive, neurologic condition, frequently with an onset in mid-life. Multiple lesions in the central nervous system result in a complex constellation of symptoms, including changes in communication especially changes in speech and cognition. Communication problems are common, and occur in approximately half of the people with MS.[10] They typically do not occur in isolation, but rather as part of a collection of other physical and sensory changes. Fatigue and depression are commonly referred to as invisible symptoms of MS and are particularly distressing and disruptive.[11] Even when relatively mild, communication problems have an important effect on the ability to take part in valued life situations partially because of their interaction with other symptoms of MS.[12] People aging with MS report that they need more assistance and have less freedom than their peers of the same age.[13] In a study that followed people with MS over a period of 9 years, 1 of the important changes was a narrowing of participants' social and geographic arenas. People aging with MS stayed closer to home, dropped activities, and restricted the number of people with whom they stayed in close contact.[14] Often social contacts were maintained via telephone. Thus, for those aging with a long-standing disability, the effects are cumulative reflecting normal aging processes and the potentially increasing burden of the long-standing disability.

Onset of New Communication Disorders in Old Age

In addition to changes in communication resulting from the normal aging process and those from long-standing chronic conditions, many neurologic conditions associated with communication disabilities have their onset in old age. These conditions may affect anyone regardless of disability status and are common in aging. For example, hearing loss is ranked as the third most prevalent chronic condition in older adults.[15] Nearly half of adults older than 75 years have some hearing loss. Parkinson disease, which is estimated to occur in about 1% of people more than 60 years old, is commonly associated with dysarthria.[16] One million people in the United States are estimated to have aphasia, commonly as a result of stroke.[17] Adult onset of neurologic conditions adds to the existing burden of changes with aging. When examining changes in participation and social roles after a stroke, Desrosiers and colleagues[18] found that changes could not be attributed entirely to the stroke itself but also to the process of normal aging.

In the 2008 study of Aging, Demographics, and Memory, the prevalence of dementia in persons older than 71 years is estimated to be 14% of the population, with 3.4 million women and 1 million men affected by the most common form of dementia, Alzheimer disease.[19] Dementia is the general term used to describe the continuum of degenerative brain diseases characterized by cognitive impairment across multiple domains. Alzheimer disease, Pick disease, Huntington disease, Parkinson disease, multi-infarct or vascular dementia, and Lewy body disease are some of the presentations of dementia that have their own unique features but have 1 common characteristic: the presence of memory impairment, particularly impairment in the ability to learn new information.[20] Dementia affects communication and eventually limits social roles, because of the gradual deterioration of cognitive skills, including memory, attention, perception, executive functions, and problem solving. The degenerative course of dementing illnesses contributes to an ever-changing presentation of symptoms. In the early stages, individuals experience mild forgetfulness for names and objects, mild word finding, abstract reasoning, attention, language, and spatial cognition difficulties.[21] As the disease progresses, moderately severe impairments in memory, language, judgment, and activities of daily living are apparent, thus increasing the need for assistance and surveillance by caregivers. Late stage patients exhibit loss of language (ie, incoherent babbling or muteness) and decreased recognition of family and self, delusions, hallucinations, repetitive, and bizarre behaviors.[20] Individuals with dementia experience a gradual transformation from an independent, fully functioning participant in their own life, to total dependence on others, oblivious to the world around them.

IMPORTANT FUNCTIONS OF COMMUNICATION

People use communication to perform many functions in their day-to-day activities, including employment, social and leisure activities, community involvement, personal relationships, and meeting needs for daily living. Many of these functions change with typical aging. People retire from careers. Their social circles and personal relationships may change as they adjust their life roles and change their activity patterns. They may require more services such as health care services or in-home help to meet their daily needs. With these changing roles, the effects of communication disorders also change. One important way to understand the roles played by older adults is to study the tasks that occupy their time. Community-dwelling older adults who were receiving some kind of occupational therapy spent most of their time at home and alone.[22] Almost half of their time was spent in tasks involving instrumental activities of daily living. When asked to rate the importance of these activities, tasks involving communication were rated among the highest with using the telephone rated as the most important activity.

The psychosocial consequences of communication disorders in older adults have not been studied thoroughly. However, the following sections provide some examples of research that illustrate the effect of communication disorders on social roles in populations with various trajectories of disability, including cerebral palsy where people experience lifelong disability, MS where people experience the onset of disability in mid-life, and dual sensory impairment and aphasia where onset occurs in old age. This is followed by a specific discussion on the role of communication disorders and aging in an individual's access to and management of their health care.

Maintaining Social Roles

Communication is not just about transactions such as exchanging information and transferring messages; it also serves an important role in establishing and maintaining social affiliation. Lubinski[8] proposed that communication serves several critical roles in the lives of older adults, including maintaining a sense of identity, and relieving loneliness, depression, or anxiety. Communication also allows older adults to exert influence and to help others by listening, reflecting, and offering advice. If communication is compromised, social life is affected.

Cerebral palsy

People aging with cerebral palsy have lived their lives with a disability that may have increased with age, see the article by Strax and colleagues elsewhere in this issue for exploration of this topic. Problems with communication may result in loneliness and difficulties in developing and maintaining social relationships.[23,24] Ballin and Balandin[25] conducted in-depth interviews with adults with cerebral palsy (>40 years of age) focusing on issues of loneliness. The investigators believe that loneliness and social isolation are not the same. Loneliness is a subjective experience that correlates only weakly with objective characteristics, such as social network size or frequency of contact with friends. Analyses of these interviews suggested that these participants experienced loneliness for some of the same reasons as older adults without lifelong disability, including being without a partner or feeling of reduced person control. Communication disorders appear to put an additional burden on people aging with cerebral palsy at least in part due to unsuccessful communication with unfamiliar conversational partners, insufficient time for satisfactory communication, and unacceptable telephone communication.

MS

MS is a progressive neurologic condition that is typically diagnosed in mid-life when people are engaged in many preexisting roles, such as parent, spouse, friend, employee, or homemaker. An important challenge is the premature transition out of valued roles that were expected to continue into older age. For example, they may need to retire long before their nondisabled peers. Analysis of a series of in-depth interviews of people with MS who were experiencing mild communication problems suggests that participation in important roles changed markedly, not only because of the communication problems but also because of issues related to fatigue, cognitive changes, and mobility limitations commonly associated with MS.[12] People who retired early spoke of the need to construct roles that did not require flawless speech for participation. Others expressed frustration in relinquishing their valued roles. For example, a former teacher described retirement as a major loss because "education was my life." Participants also felt the loss of friendship that had developed in the workplace. Thus, many of the life transitions made by people with MS occur before the expected time. When these transitions are rapid or undesirable, psychosocial stress may occur.[26]

Sensory loss

Dual sensory loss (decreased vision and hearing acuity) is increasingly common especially in the very old and those in institutional settings. In a survey of people with dual sensory loss, more than two-thirds reported frequent difficulty in conversation especially in noisy situations or with groups.[27,28] Poor hearing is often the cause of misunderstandings and negative reactions by communication partners, yet fewer than 24% of people who could benefit from hearing aids actually purchase them.[29]

Aphasia

Aphasia is a language impairment commonly associated with left hemisphere stroke. Davidson and colleagues[30] observed older people with aphasia in everyday communication situations. They found that people with aphasia engaged in similar activities as older people without disability. For example, conversation was the most common activity for both groups. However, differences were evident in the frequency of communication activities and in specific activities such as making telephone calls, reading, writing, and business activities such as making appointments or completing forms. Thus, communication activities that were rated as important by older community-dwelling adults were more limited in those with communication disorders. Older adults with aphasia also had fewer communication partners and took part in fewer social situations than peers without aphasia. These differences were viewed as documentation of losses in relationships and social networks experienced by people with aphasia. The differences may reflect a lack of connectedness reported by older adults with aphasia.[31]

Access to Health Care

Although maintaining social roles is important to people as they age, another significant concern is the ability to access services that they perhaps have not needed in the past, or that they now need to a greater degree. Health care is a primary example of these types of services. The ability to communicate successfully, including speaking, listening, reading, and writing, is a critical factor in obtaining health care. The importance of communication is reflected in Ruben's[32] suggestion that in the 21st century a person's fitness for survival will be defined in terms of his or her ability to communicate effectively. Communication disabilities are especially common in the hospital setting. Although they are estimated to occur in 5% to 10% of the general population, this rate is higher in people who are hospitalized. Ebert and Heckerling[33] found that approximately 16% of patients on general inpatient services had 1 or more severe disabilities affecting communication. These patients were more likely to be older men. The presence of a communication problem was significantly associated with an increased risk of experiencing a preventable adverse event.[34] Patients with communication problems were 3 times more likely to experience adverse events than those without such problems.

Limitations in communication also have an undesirable affect on outpatient health care, where time is increasingly limited for patient visits and health care relies more on communication via written information, telephone, and computer (eg, e-mail). Research focused on the Medicare population suggests a significant relationship between the presence of communication problems and dissatisfaction with health care including overall quality, accessibility, and receipt of information.[3] Iezzoni and colleagues[35] also found that older people with hearing or vision problems affecting communication were more likely to be dissatisfied with physicians' understanding of their conditions and with the time spent discussing their problem and answering questions.

In their review of empiric studies examining the physician-older patient interaction, Adelman and colleagues[36] found that several dimensions were better with younger rather than older patients. These included physician responsiveness (eg, the quality of questions), agreement in setting major goals, and joint decision making. Another issue that distinguished physician visits in the geriatric population is the frequent presence of a third party. As much as half of the time, the older patient is accompanied to the visit by someone else who may play the role of advocate, passive participant or antagonist.[36] The third party may play an important role in decision making and be a conduit for education. The term ageism has been used to describe an important barrier to good communication between health care providers and older patients.[37] This type of bias may lead to communication that is characterized by stereotyped expectations rather than the recognition of highly variable individual characteristics of older patients. It is also associated with interaction patterns in which the physician dominates.

CLINICAL IMPLICATIONS

Although people aging with communication disabilities are certainly a heterogeneous group, some issues with important clinical implications are common to all. First, research suggests that quality of life in older adults is related to more than health status. Social contacts may be as valued as health status in quality of life.[38] Although people with communication disabilities may experience more challenges developing and maintaining social contacts, factors they report as important to quality of life may be similar to those reported by people aging without communication disorders. After interviewing people living with aphasia, Cruice and colleagues[39] found several factors related to quality of life including having affirming experiences in sharing one's life with others, having control over one's life, taking part in personally rewarding leisure activities, coping with loss and change, and continuing to grow personally.

Second, the burden of disability is cumulative with the added conditions associated with aging. Because the burden of disability increases with aging, adaptive resources may be insufficient to accommodate the cumulative effects of these sources of disablement. Finally, the presence of communication problems is especially taxing in areas in which older adults are experiencing increasing needs, such as accessing health care. Communication disabilities hinder the implementation of strategies to compensate for many aspects of disablement. Therefore, health care providers should be aware of potential communication disabilities and make provisions for these problems when interacting with older adults. The final section provides a review of issues and suggestions for enhancing communication in health care settings and in everyday social interaction.

Communication in Heath Care Settings

Health literacy, defined as the ability to understand the basic health information and services necessary for making appropriate decisions about health services, is becoming an increasingly critical factor in health care communication. It has been estimated that one-third of people older than 65 years have inadequate or marginal health literacy.[40] This proportion is no doubt much higher in those with communication disabilities. Although accommodations such as wheelchair ramps to allow physical access to health care and other facilities are now taken for granted, similar accommodations to improve access to health care settings for those with health literacy issues are often not acknowledged as part of standard clinical practice.[41]

Iezzoni and colleagues[35] suggest that 3 types of accommodations in health care settings are needed to improve access to health care for people with communication disorders. These include brick and mortar (eg, a quiet room with furniture that allows eye to eye contact), tools (eg, reading material appropriate for people with aphasia), and policy changes (eg, longer appointments). A list of general suggestions for communicating with older adults with communication disabilities is provided in **Box 1**. Excellent resources are also available to guide patients in talking with doctors.[42] Other guidelines are being developed and effective written materials are available.[43,44] For example, Hoffman and Worral[44] suggest that key stakeholders pretest and give feedback about educational material for people with communication disorders, particularly disorders affecting language comprehension or cognitive function. Their recommendations for effective written material focus on content (eg, inclusion of a clear purpose statement), language (eg, aim for 5th to 6th reading grade level), organization (eg, use subheadings and bulleted lists), layout (eg, use large print), and illustrations (eg, use simple line drawings).

In addition to these types of accommodations, it is important to identify the roster of decision makers who will be involved in the care of each individual patient. This set of decision makers may be large, diverse, and changing, and may include those who accompany the older person to the health care visit and those who do not, for example, distant adult children.[45] Once the set of decision makers has been identified it is important that educational materials are provided to all and that a partnership is formed between health care providers and decision makers. The goals of this partnership include identification of the problems, potential option or options and expectations, and the pros and cons of each option. The health care provider should determine the patient's preferred format for receiving information (written, verbal, Internet), explore the concerns, and identify the preferred level of involvement in decision making. The health care provider should also check the patient's understanding of the information and provide ample opportunity for questions. Arrangement should be made for future review of the decisions.

Enhancing Everyday Communication

By definition, communication involves an exchange between people. Thus, the focus of intervention to address communication disabilities must be on the person with the disorder and the communication partner. Research suggests that training communication partners such as nursing assistants in residential facilities can bring about

---

Box 1
Suggestions for communicating with older adults with communication disability

- Know the patient's communication strengths and weaknesses
- Make sure that sensory aids (eg, eye glasses, hearing aids, communication devices, memory aids) are available and used
- Take extra time for communication
- Make sure the environment is communication friendly, that is, quiet, well lit, furniture arranged for face-to-face interactions
- Use living room language not medical terminology
- Speak slowly and simplify your sentences
- Supplement verbal descriptions with pictures and writing
- Confirm understanding with teach-back approaches
- Limit the information given in one session
- Provide take-home educational material in the preferred format and at the appropriate reading level

encouraging changes such as more positive communication without increasing care-giving time.[46] Several programs for enhancing everyday communication are available. Some of these programs provide a general framework for enhancing communication, including approaches to enrich communication opportunities (eg, modifying the physical and social environment in resident care facilities) or enhancing communication effectiveness through identification of communication strategies for the person with the communication disorder and frequent communication partners. These strategies may involve manipulating the environment by decreasing background noise, distractions, and distance between speakers.[4,47–49] Other programs involve training in specific techniques, such as use of memory books and other written and graphic cues for people with dementia.[50]

SUMMARY

People who age with communication disabilities face many challenges in areas such as maintaining social roles and identity and accessing needed services such as health care. Although research in this area is as yet limited, preliminary evidence suggests that many of the challenges of aging with a communication disorder are common across different types of communication disorders and different times of onset. Because of the complex and chronic nature of many of the communication disorders experienced by older adults, intervention efforts must include strategies to reduce overall disability even in the context of persistent communication disorders. These strategies may include working with the person with the disability and with people in that person's environment and broader social institutions to maximize accessibility to a wide range of settings and situations for people with communication disabilities. Because of the increasing need for health care in older adults, and the higher prevalence of communication disorders in older adults, health care providers need to be well versed in the appropriate strategies for communicating effectively with these populations. Their medical institutions will need to support health care providers with the tools and training to serve these populations most efficaciously. Further research is needed to better understand the experiences and implications of aging with communication disorders, and to learn how to best minimize the disability associated with those disorders. In summary, older people with communication disabilities form a diverse group in which the burden of disability increases over time. Because these disabilities may interfere with access to health and maintenance of valued social interaction, identification and management is critical.

REFERENCES

1. Kaakinen J. Talking among elderly nursing home residents. Top Lang Disord 1995;15:36–46.
2. Verbrugge LM, Yang L-S. Aging with disability and disability with aging. J Disabil Pol Stud 2002;12(4):253.
3. Hoffman JM, Yorkston KM, Shumway-Cook A, et al. Effects of communication disability on satisfaction with health care: a survey of Medicare beneficiaries. Am J Speech Lang Pathol 2005;14(3):221–8.
4. Worrall LE, Hickson LM. Communication disability in aging: from prevention to intervention. Clifton Park (NY): Delmar Learning; 2003.
5. Caruso AJ, Mueller PB, Shadden BB. Effects of aging on speech and voice. Phys Occup Ther Geriatr 1995;13(1–2):63–79.

6. Zraick RI, Gregg BA, Whitehouse EL. Speech and voice characteristics of geriatric speakers: a review of the literature and a call for research and training. J Med Speech Lang Pathol 2006;14(3):133–42.

7. Ryan EB. Normal aging and language. In: Lubinski R, editor. Dementia and communication. San Diego (CA): Singular Publishing Co; 1996. p. 84–97.

8. Lubinski R, editor. Dementia and communication. San Diego (CA): Singular Publishing Group; 1995. p. 147.

9. Verdonck-de Leeuw IM, Mahieu HF. Vocal aging and the impact on daily life: a longitudinal study. J Voice 2004;18(2):193–202.

10. Yorkston KM, Klasner ER, Bowen J, et al. Characteristics of multiple sclerosis as a function of the severity of speech disorders. J Med Speech Lang Pathol 2003; 11(2):73–85.

11. White CP, White MB, Russell CS. Invisible and visible symptoms of multiple sclerosis: which are more predictive of health distress? J Neurosci Nurs 2008;40(2): 85–95, 102.

12. Yorkston KM, Klasner ER, Swanson KM. Communication in context: a qualitative study of the experiences of individuals with multiple sclerosis. Am J Speech Lang Pathol 2001;10(2):126–37.

13. Finlayson M, Van Denend T, Hudson E. Aging with multiple sclerosis. J Neurosci Nurs 2004;36(5):245–51.

14. Bringfelt P, Hartelius L, Runmarker B. Communication problems in multiple sclerosis: 9-year follow-up. Int J MS Care 2006;8:130–40.

15. Aging America. Trends and projections. Washington, DC: Department of Health and Human Services; 1991.

16. Samii A, Nutt JG, Ranson BR. Parkinson's disease. Lancet 2004;363(9423): 1783–93.

17. National Institute of deafness and other communication disorders. Aphasia. Available at: http://www.nidcd.nih.gov/health/voice/aphasia.htm. Accessed February 18, 2009.

18. Desrosiers J, Bourbonnais D, Noreau L, et al. Participation after stroke compared to normal aging. J Rehabil Med 2005;37(6):353–7.

19. Plassiman BL, Langer KM, Fisher GG, et al. Prevalence of dementia in the United States: the aging, demographics and memory study. Neuroepidemiology 2007; 29(1–2):125–32.

20. Brandt J, Rich JB. Memory disorders in the dementias. In: Baddeley AD, Wilson BA, Watts FN, editors. Handbook of memory disorders. Chichester (UK): Wiley; 1995. p. 243–70.

21. Grady CL, Haxby JV, Horwitz B, et al. Longitudinal study of the early neuropsychological and cerebral metabolic changes in dementia of the Alzheimer type. J Clin Neurophysiol 1988;10:576–96.

22. Fricke J, Unsworth C. Time use and importance of instrumental activities of daily living. Aust Occup Ther J 2001;48:118–31.

23. Higginbotham DJ, Wilkins DP. Slipping through the timestream: social issues of time and timing in augmented interactions. In: Duchan J, Kovarsky D, Maxwell M, editors. The social construction of language incompetence. Mahwah (NJ): Lawrence Erlbaum; 1999. p. 49–82.

24. Balandin S, Berg N, Waller A. Assessing the loneliness of older people with cerebral palsy. Disabil Rehabil 2006;28(8):469–79.

25. Ballin L, Balandin S. An exploration of loneliness: communication and the social networks of older people with cerebral palsy. J Intellect Dev Disabil 2007;32(4): 315–27.

26. Starks H, Morris M, Yorkston K, et al. Being in- or out-of-sync: a qualitative study of couples' adaptation to change in multiple sclerosis. Disabil Rehabil 2010;32(3):196–206.
27. Heine C, Erber NP, Osborn R, et al. Communication perceptions of older adults with sensory loss and their communication partners: implications for intervention. Disabil Rehabil 2002;24(7):356–63.
28. Heine C, Browning CJ. Communication and psychosocial consequences of sensory loss in older adults: overview and rehabilitation directions. Disabil Rehabil 2002;24(15):763–73.
29. Garstecki DC, Erler S. Hearing in older adults. In: Shadden BB, Toner MA, editors. Aging and communication. Austin (TX): ProEd; 1997. p. 97–116.
30. Davidson B, Worrall L, Hickson L. Identifying the communication activities of older people with aphasia: evidence from naturalistic observation. Aphasiology 2003;17(3):243–64.
31. Davidson B, Worrall L, Hickson L. Social communication in older age: lessons from people with aphasia. Top Stroke Rehabil 2006;13(1):1–13.
32. Ruben RJ. Redefining the survival of the fittest: communication disorders in the 21st century. Laryngoscope 2000;10:241–5.
33. Ebert DA, Heckerling P. Communication disabilities among medical inpatients. N Engl J Med 1998;339:271–3.
34. Bartlett G, Blais T, Tamblyn R, et al. Impact of patient communication problems on the risk of preventable adverse events in acute care settings. Can Med Assoc J 2008;178(12):1555–62.
35. Iezzoni LI, Davis RB, Soukup J, et al. Quality dimensions that most concern people with physical and sensory disabilities. Arch Intern Med 2003;163:2085–92.
36. Adelman RD, Greene MG, Ory MG. Communication between older patients and their physicians. Clin Geriatr Med 2000;16(1):1–24.
37. Ryan EB, Butler RN. Communication, aging and health: toward understanding health provider relationships with older clients. Health Commun 1996;8(3):191–8.
38. Farquhar M. Elderly people's definitions of quality of life. Soc Sci Med 1995;41(10):1439–46.
39. Cruice M, Worrall L, Hickson L. Perspectives of quality of life by people with aphasia and their family: suggestions for successful living. Top Stroke Rehabil 2006;13(1):14–24.
40. Williams MV, Davis T, Parker RM, et al. The role of health literacy in patient-physician communication. Fam Med 2002;34(5):383–9.
41. Kagan A, LeBlanc K. Motivating for infrastructure change: toward a communicatively accessible, participation-based stroke care system for all those affected by aphasia. J Commun Dis 2002;35(2):153–69.
42. U.S. Department of Health and Human Services. 2005. Talking with your doctor. In NIH Publication No. 05-3452 Available at: http://www.nia.nih.gov/HealthInformation/Publications/TalkingWithYourDoctor/. Accessed February 18, 2009.
43. Billek-Sawhney B, Reicherter EA. Literacy and the older adult: educational considerations for health professionals. Top Geriatr Rehabil 2005;21(4):275–81.
44. Hoffmn T, Worrall L. Designing effective written health education materials: considerations for health professionals. Disabil Rehabil 2004;26(19):1166–73.
45. Beukelman DR, Yorkston KM, Garrett KL. AAC decision-making teams: achieving change and maintaining social support. In: Beukelman DR, Garrett KL,

Yorkston KM, editors. AAC intervention for adults in medical settings: integrated assessment and treatment protocols. Baltimore (MD): Brookes Publishing; 2007. p. 369–90.

46. Bourgeois MS, Camp C, Rose M, et al. A comparison of training strategies to enhance use of external aids by persons with dementia. J Commun Dis 2003; 36:361–78.

47. Lubinski R, Organe JB. A framework for the assessment and treatment of functional communication in dementia. In: Worral LE, Frattali CM, editors. Neurogenic communication disorders: a functional approach. New York: Thieme; 2000. p. 220–47.

48. Beukelman DR, Garrett KL, Yorkston KM, editors. Augmentative communication strategies for adults with acute and chronic medical conditions. Baltimore (MD): Brookes Publications; 2007. p. 369–90.

49. Bourgeois MS, Hickey EM. Dementia: from diagnosis to management - a functional approach. Oxford (UK): Taylor & Francis; 2009.

50. Bourgeois MS, Mason LA. Memory wallet interventions in an adult day care setting. Behav Interv 1996;11(1):3–18.

Aging with a Disability: Physical Impairment, Pain, and Fatigue

Eva Widerström-Noga, DDS, PhD[a,b,c,d],*,
Marcia L. Finlayson, OT, PhD, OTR/L[e]

KEYWORDS

• Aging • Disability • Physical impairment • Pain • Fatigue

Central nervous system trauma (eg, spinal cord injury, traumatic brain injury, stroke), diseases of the nervous system (eg, multiple sclerosis, post-polio syndrome, Parkinson's disease), and degenerative muscle diseases (eg, muscular dystrophy) can result in significant physical impairments and alterations in functional abilities. People living and aging with these underlying medical conditions often experience pain and fatigue secondary to their primary impairments that may worsen over time and negatively influence health-related quality of life.[1–3]

A broad array of biologic and psychosocial factors may contribute to the development and impact of these secondary conditions, including general medical status, underlying pathophysiological mechanisms, emotional and psychosocial factors, intrinsic and personal characteristics, and interactions with the broader physical and social environment.[2,4] Alone or in combination, the extent and consequences of common secondary conditions among people aging with physical impairments associated with trauma or disease are staggering and may further increase physical disability and depression.

When these individuals age, the frequency and severity of persistent pain, fatigue, or sleep disorders can be expected to increase because of the reduced biologic,

[a] Miami Project to Cure Paralysis, University of Miami Miller School of Medicine, Lois Pope Life Center (R-48), 1095 NW 14th Terrace, Miami, FL 33136, USA
[b] VA Medical Center, 1201 NW 16th Street, Miami, FL 33125, USA
[c] Department of Neurological Surgery, University of Miami Miller School of Medicine, Lois Pope Life Center (R-48), 1095 NW 14th Terrace, Miami, FL 33136, USA
[d] Department of Rehabilitation Medicine, University of Miami Miller School of Medicine, PO Box 016960, Miami, FL 33101, USA
[e] Department of Occupational Therapy, University of Illinois at Chicago, 327 Applied Health Sciences Building, 1919 West Taylor, Chicago, IL 60612, USA
* Corresponding author. Miami Project to Cure Paralysis, University of Miami Miller School of Medicine, Lois Pope Life Center (R-48), 1095 NW 14th Terrace, Miami, FL 33136.
E-mail address: ewiderstrom-noga@med.miami.edu

Phys Med Rehabil Clin N Am 21 (2010) 321–337
doi:10.1016/j.pmr.2009.12.010
1047-9651/10/$ – see front matter. Published by Elsevier Inc.

psychological, and social reserves associated with aging.[5] Therefore, in aging persons who have physical impairments, long-term secondary conditions may result in significantly increased levels of disability and depression.

With this background, the critical need to understand what is currently known about the nature, extent, and impact of pain and fatigue among people living and aging with physical impairments becomes apparent. Understanding the epidemiology, assessment procedures, and treatment options for these secondary conditions can help guide practitioners to make informed decisions during interactions with their patients. This article provides a brief summary of this information, with a specific focus on people who have trauma or disease of the nervous and muscular systems. The specific objectives are to:

1. Offer definitions, descriptions and classifications of pain and fatigue;
2. Describe the implications of these secondary conditions on the health and functioning of people who experience them;
3. Highlight key issues with respect to multidisciplinary assessment and treatment options; and
4. Identify critical gaps in knowledge regarding these conditions and their interactions, and describe directions for future research.

DEFINITIONS, DESCRIPTIONS, AND CLASSIFICATIONS
Pain

Pain is defined by the International Association for the Study of Pain as "an unpleasant sensory and emotional experience associated with actual or potential tissue damage, or described in terms of such damage."[6] Although pain is a sensation in the body, it is always unpleasant and therefore can be considered an emotional experience. Based on this definition, activity induced in the nociceptor per se is clearly not pain, because the nociceptive signal must be processed in the brain and consciously appreciated before it can be called pain. This fact must be taken into account when translating basic pain research findings into clinical applications. For example, a discrepancy exists between basic and clinical research in that most basic research studies use evoked pain or reflex behaviors as their primary outcome measures, although usually the spontaneous pain is the primary problem in the clinical situation.

The rates of persistent pain in people who have multiple sclerosis range from 43% to 79%.[7–10] Among people who have spinal cord injuries, the reported prevalence of pain is similar and ranges between 26% to 96%[11]; however, many large-scale studies report frequencies around two thirds.[12–17] Similarly, pain and fatigue have been reported by most people experiencing post-polio syndrome.[18–20]

Pain can be divided into two general categories regardless of the underlying medical condition: nociceptive, which is pain caused by activation of specific pain receptors (ie, nociceptors), and neuropathic, which is pain initiated or caused by a primary lesion or dysfunction in the nervous system. Nociceptive pain is usually experienced as being located in a region of sensory preservation and may be described as dull, aching, and cramping. In contrast, neuropathic pain is usually located in a region of sensory dysfunction and may be described as sharp, shooting, electric, or burning.[21] Neuropathic pain is often associated with sensory deficits and abnormal sensory phenomena, such as allodynia or hyperalgesia.[22,23] Allodynia is pain that is evoked by a normally innocuous (nonpainful) stimulus, such as touch, cooling, or warmth. Hyperalgesia is pain that is felt as abnormally intense when evoked by a mild to moderately intense nociceptive stimulus. Both hyperalgesia and allodynia can be evoked by thermal or mechanical stimuli.

The classification of pain into specific pain types is based on a combination of pain characteristics (eg, pain locations and various pain descriptors) and injury character-istics, if applicable (eg, level of injury). Recently, Treede and colleagues[24] suggested revising the definition of neuropathic pain to "pain, arising as a direct consequence of a lesion or disease affecting the somatosensory system." Because the diagnosis of neuropathic pain is not always straightforward, they also suggested including a grading system of "definite," "probable," and "possible" neuropathic pain with specific criteria, including the presence of symptoms such as hyperalgesia and allodynia.

Fatigue

For healthy people, the experience of fatigue can be a positive one, reflecting a normal response to a busy day or period of exercise. This type of fatigue can be remediated with rest.[25] However, for people who are aging with a physical impairment or have a chronic health condition, fatigue is often a multidimensional, disabling, and negative symptom that significantly disrupts everyday life. Fatigue is a common problem among several groups of people who may experience aging and physical disability concurrently, such as people who have multiple sclerosis,[26–30] late-effects polio,[31–35] spinal cord injury,[36–39] muscular dystrophy,[31,40–45] and stroke.[46,47]

Fatigue has many definitions, ranging from broad, subjective ones (eg, over-whelming sense of tiredness, subjective lack of physical or mental energy)[29,48] to others that are narrow, objective, and physiologically based (eg, exercise-induced reduction in maximal voluntary muscle force).[44] Fatigue has also been described as a common, protective response to reduce the likelihood of individuals engaging in an activity beyond their functional reserve,[49] either physically or mentally.[34] Ultimately, fatigue "may be best characterized as the absence of energy and the mind-body response to that absence."[50]

Among some populations, fatigue may be one of the major presenting symptoms of the disease process. When fatigue can be directly attributed to the disease state, it is labeled primary fatigue. In multiple sclerosis, primary fatigue may be related to lesion load, immune activation, neuroendocrine involvement, and/or peripheral abnormali-ties.[26,28] Among people who have late-effects polio, primary fatigue is believed to be a function of the extra demands and resulting overload placed on surviving motor neuron units.[34,35] The extent of injury (ie, full or partial) may be a factor in the primary fatigue of people who have spinal cord injury, with partial injury contributing to greater fatigue.[36]

Many other factors, not directly related to the disease process itself, may also contribute to fatigue. This secondary fatigue is associated with inefficient movement patterns or cardiorespiratory functions, deconditioning, sleep problems, medication side effects, depression, pain, nutritional deficiencies, or chronic infections.[28,34,36,43] Because many secondary factors can contribute to fatigue, health care providers must conduct comprehensive assessments to identify and remediate as many of them as possible.[51]

The distinction between primary and secondary fatigue is only one way to concep-tualize fatigue. Other conceptualizations include acute versus chronic, experienced versus physiologic, and physical versus cognitive. Acute fatigue has a recent onset and a short duration, and is usually produced by physical activity. It can typically be remediated through appropriate rest.[31]

Generally, acute fatigue is not considered disabling, whereas chronic fatigue is disabling. It is often unrelated to physical activity, is not fully resolved with rest, and tends to be more generalized (physical, cognitive, and emotional components).[48,51] The point at which fatigue is considered chronic varies according to diagnosis. Among people who have multiple sclerosis, fatigue lasting more than 6 weeks is considered chronic.[48] However, in people who have many other potentially disabling diagnoses, such as congestive heart failure, diabetes, sleep apnea, rheumatoid arthritis, depression,[51] and late-effects polio, fatigue lasting more than 6 months is considered chronic.[34]

Experienced fatigue reflects the subjective experience, such as severity and impact on daily life. Prevalence of severe fatigue as measured by an average score of 4 or greater on the Fatigue Severity Scale was reported in 74% of people who had multiple sclerosis (N = 9205).[27] In much smaller studies of people who had spinal cord injury (N = 76), muscular dystrophy (N = 200), and stroke (N = 40), rates of severe fatigue using this same scale were reported as 57%, 62%, and 30%, respectively.[36,41,52]

In comparison to the subjective nature of experienced fatigue, physiologic fatigue captures exercise-induced muscle weakness or fatigability, and reflects reduction in maximal voluntary muscle force. It has both central and peripheral components, and is common in people who have neuromuscular disorders.[44] Central fatigue is also linked to subjective feelings of exhaustion, and difficulties with alertness and arousal.[53]

EFFECTS ON HEALTH AND FUNCTIONING
Pain

Aging is associated with several common comorbidities that in combination may decrease physical function and increase disability. For example, a large-scale study in persons aged 85 to 105 years showed that the presence of persistent pain was predictive of functional limitations, fatigue, sleeping problems, depressed mood, and a decreased quality of life.[54] Similarly, lower scores on the physical subscale of the Medical Outcomes Study 36-item Short Form Survey[55] were significantly associated with increased frequencies of common diseases, such as congestive heart failure, chronic lung disease, and arthritis, however, the associations were more pronounced between the physical function scores and common symptoms such as muscle weakness, pain, and shortness of breath in older adults.[56]

Another large-scale study in older individuals showed that approximately 50% experience pain that interferes with physical and psychological functioning, and that the severity and chronicity of pain are the primary determinants for this interference.[57] Similarly, a study in women showed that sleep problems, pain, and visual and hearing impairments increased significantly with age.[58] Studies also suggest that the effects of pain on distress and disability may be less pronounced in older adults than in younger cohorts,[59,60] possibly because older adults either underreport pain or see it as part of the aging process,[61–63] or because they have acquired better pain coping skills.[64]

Emotional distress, such as depression, anxiety and anger, is intimately linked to the experience of chronic pain in various heterogeneous populations.[65,66] Thus, in people with physical impairments, persistent pain is yet another significant burden that contributes to increased psychological distress and disability.[67–71] Although it may be difficult to interpret the influence of pain on emotional functioning in a person who has a physical impairment,[72] this domain must be evaluated because it is central to individuals' assessment of their well-being and satisfaction with life.[73]

The term pain interference refers to the extent that pain hinders or interferes with common activities of daily life. Persistent pain naturally increases disability through limiting a person's ability to perform and participate in daily activities.[74,75] For example, pain interfering with the performance of daily activities can result in decreased independence, ultimately leading to affective distress.[76,77] In fact, high levels of pain interference assessed by the spinal cord injury (SCI) version of the Multi-dimensional Pain Inventory,[78] rather than the severity of pain, were predictive of decreased life satisfaction in 161 persons who had SCI and chronic pain.[68] The extent to which chronic pain specifically (distinct from physical impairments) hinders or inter-feres with activities of daily life may be more important than general physical function in populations experiencing physical impairment. Furthermore, when an individual is aging, the capacity to deal with added physical and emotional stress imposed by persistent pain and an underlying disease is reduced and may result in additional disability.[5]

Up to 60% of people who have multiple sclerosis, SCI, and post-polio syndrome experience fatigue severe enough to interfere with daily activities.[34,36,70,79,80] Research shows that pain and fatigue are common comorbidities in diseases affecting the nervous and muscular systems, such as post-polio syndrome,[81] muscular dystrophy,[82] and cancer,[83] and in older people.[84] The combination of pain and fatigue was associated with an increased degree of disability in older individuals who had experienced a stroke.[85]

The relationship between sleep problems and disability in persons who have persis-tent pain is not straightforward. Although poor quality of sleep has been shown to be significantly related to pain-related disability and depression, these relationships may be primarily mediated by the severity of pain and by depression.[86] Additionally, although sleep problems are often considered a consequence of chronic pain, some studies suggest that the relationship between pain and sleep may be bidirectional.[87]

Fatigue

Although acute fatigue can typically be remedied by a short rest or a good night's sleep, chronic fatigue typically does not resolve with these strategies alone. For this reason, individuals who have chronic fatigue often stop performing important and valued activities in their everyday lives, including instrumental activities of daily living (eg, shopping, home management responsibilities), employment, socializing, and other leisure interests, which often contributes to reductions in quality of life and over-all life satisfaction.[32,38,41] Among people who have multiple sclerosis[88,89] and muscular dystrophy,[41] fatigue has been identified as a major factor in the inability to maintain employment.

In a mixed sample of 961 adults with a mean age of 43.6 years (SD = 10.2), 25 different adjectives were used to describe fatigue. Using principal components anal-ysis, the authors identified four factors: frustrating, exhausting, pleasant, and fright-ening, which explained 24%, 9%, 6%, and 5% of the variance, respectively. Healthy controls and individuals who did not report fatigue were significantly more likely to report fatigue as pleasant than those who reported fatigue caused by chronic fatigue syndrome, neuromuscular disorders, pancreatitis, or cancer. People who had unexplained fatigue were more likely to report fatigue as frightening than those who had chronic disease.[25]

These descriptions are consistent with findings from qualitative research involving people who had multiple sclerosis,[88–91] muscular dystrophy,[40]and SCI.[92] Among people who had multiple sclerosis, fatigue has been described as frustrating, overwhelming, and disabling.[91] People who had SCI used similar descriptors for their fatigue and also identified it as stressful.[92] People who had muscular dystrophy linked fatigue to feebleness and lack of initiative.[40]

For people who have multiple sclerosis, fatigue contributes to redefinitions of work and the need to prioritize everyday tasks, find and use resources, plan in advance, and develop and evaluate strategies to change how tasks get completed.[89] However, making change is not easy, because it requires disclosure to others who often do not understand the fatigue experience, or requires simply deciding that some tasks will not get done.[90] Similarly, people who have SCI have described how fatigue leads to prioritization of tasks and the need to reduce or eliminate recreational, leisure, and other pleasant activities from their daily life because of lack of energy. Curtailing pleasant activities contributes to stress, depression, and increased fatigue, creating a vicious cycle.[92]

The findings of two recent longitudinal studies of fatigue among patients who had multiple sclerosis indicate the complexity and variability of this symptom over time, and raise questions about how its impact may also vary over time. Both studies used the Fatigue Severity Scale for assessment; one used it every 6 months for 2 years[93] and the other every year for 3 years.[94] Across the two studies, one fifth to one quarter of participants were nonfatigued throughout the study period, but 25% to 38% experienced persistent fatigue. Factors associated with increased fatigue over time included depressive symptoms, weak/moderate sense of coherence, living with a partner, and not working.[93] Factors associated with persistent or sporadic fatigue over time included depression, heat sensitivity, and physical impairment.[94] Together with literature about how fatigue influences everyday life, these longitudinal studies indicate the need for more nuanced investigations of fatigue and its impact on health and functioning.

ASSESSMENT
Pain

Because pain is a subjective and conscious experience, the individual experience of pain and its perceived impact on daily life are integral parts of the pain evaluation.[95] This concept was recognized by The Initiative on Methods, Measurement, and Pain Assessment in Clinical Trials (IMMPACT) group,[96] which recommends that investigators consider including a standard core set of outcome domains in clinical pain trials regardless of pain population. Complete relief of pain problems that have persisted over a long time is unlikely, either spontaneously or as a result of treatment, especially in persons who have experienced neurologic injury or disease and who have developed neuropathic pain.[20,97–100] Therefore, domains such as pain severity and physical and emotional function that reflect Health-Related Quality of Life are of particular interest for the multidimensional evaluation of pain.[96]

However, in populations of individuals who have physical impairments, a decrease in physical function may be more dependent on physical impairments than on pain.[101] Therefore, a decrease in function specifically because of pain (ie, pain interference) should be assessed.

Standardized pain assessments in physically impaired populations are needed, and recent efforts have been made to this end. For instance, in the SCI pain field, the International Spinal Cord Injury Pain Data Set (ISCIPDS) committee developed a basic pain dataset (ISCIBPDS) that contains a basic amount of clinically relevant information concerning pain.[102] The ISCIBPDS is consistent with the recommendations made by the IMMPACT group and includes questions about pain severity and physical and emotional function. Several other international workgroups in this field also have made important contributions toward the standardization of SCI pain measures.[103,104]

Ratings of pain intensity or severity using Numerical Rating or Visual Analog Scales are common primary outcome measures in most clinical pain trials.[105] However, additional information regarding location, quality, and temporal pattern of pain is usually evaluated in the pain history,[95] and this information provides information important for diagnosing pain. The pain evaluation in individuals who have experienced neurologic trauma or disease is particularly complicated, because these individuals frequently experience different types of pain that may have different underlying origins.[106] Thus, different pain types are important to evaluate separately to determine treatment effect.[102]

In neuropathic pain conditions, an evaluation of neurologic dysfunction is often performed to quantify and determine sensory, motor, or autonomic function.[23] Bedside clinical examination of sensory function and the more time-consuming quantitative sensory testing (QST) assess decreased function of specific spinal pathways, such as the dorsal column and the spinothalamocortical tract, and stimulus-evoked pain.[22,107] Although QST may potentially be a useful diagnostic and outcome measure in clinical settings and trials, further research is needed to establish validity and reliability in physically impaired populations.[108]

In summary, the assessment domains recommended by the IMMPACT group are appropriate for diverse chronic pain populations, including persons who have nervous system trauma (eg, spinal cord injury, traumatic brain injury, stroke), diseases of the nervous system (eg, multiple sclerosis, post-polio syndrome, Parkinson's disease), and degenerative muscle diseases (eg, muscular dystrophy). When people experiencing chronic pain also have varying degrees of physical impairments, specific assessment of pain-related interference with physical and emotional functioning is more useful than general measures of physical and emotional function. A set of core outcome measures in combination with more disease-specific measures would be useful for comparing clinical outcomes and trials in these populations. When selecting specific instruments to be used as core outcome measures, not only validity and reliability but also whether the instrument can be used in pain populations associated with underlying disease or trauma must be considered.

Fatigue

Although fatigue can be experienced and physiologic, its measurement among people who have chronic illness is largely based on self-report.[30] Many instruments are available, but no gold standard currently exists.[109] Several review papers have been published recently that identify methods of fatigue assessment among people who have chronic illness[109] or critically examine specific self-report fatigue assessment scales.[110–113] In one study, 252 different ways to measure fatigue were identified across 2285 papers published between 1975 and 2004. Only 152 of these methods were used more than once.[109] Overall, the authors found that single-item questions, retrospective chart review, and ad hoc scales were the most frequently used methods for assessing fatigue. Among fatigue specific scales, 71 multidimensional ones were identified, primarily for assessing cancer-related fatigue.[109]

Across the reviews by Dittner and colleagues,[110] Kos and colleagues,[111] Mota and Pimenta,[112] and Taylor and colleageus,[113] a total of 34 fatigue-specific instruments are described and critiqued. Individuals interested in fatigue assessment are strongly encouraged to read these papers because the instruments described include both unidimensional (eg, Brief Fatigue Inventory, Fatigue Severity Scale [FSS]) and multidimensional measures (eg, Fatigue Impact Scale, Fatigue Assessment Instrument), identify the populations for which the tool was developed and have been validated, and offer a detailed critique of psychometric properties and overall usefulness.

According to Hjollund and colleagues,[109] the most frequently used fatigue-specific assessment instruments include the FSS,[114] the Fatigue Questionnaire (FQ; also called the *Fatigue Rating Scale* or the *Chalder Fatigue Scale*),[115] and the Multidimensional Fatigue Inventory (MFI).[116] Although the instruments are used widely, they were originally developed for chronic medical patients (FSS), individuals who have chronic fatigue syndrome (FQ), and general medical patients (MFI).[110] Each instrument uses Likert-scale response options for its items (9, 11, and 20, respectively), has good internal consistency documented across several studies, and has some documentation of different aspects of validity and reliability.[110] Despite the strong psychometric properties reported on the FSS, a recent evaluation of this instrument using Rasch analysis has raised some questions about the 9-item structure of the tool, which will require further examination given its common use.[117]

Because of the wide range of fatigue assessment instruments that are available, clinicians and researchers must be focused and deliberate in choosing a tool for use in their setting. Considerations must include availability, ease of administration, level of measurement, applicability to the specific patient population, and psychometric properties (reliability, validity, and sensitivity to change as a result of intervention).[111] In addition, consideration must be given to the definition of fatigue used in the setting and the extent to which an instrument provides a suitable match. In clinical settings, a comprehensive history will also be needed to identify potential sources of secondary fatigue so that they can be addressed through appropriate referrals and intervention.[51]

In the future, self-reported assessment of fatigue may become more consistent because of the Patient-Reported Outcomes Measurement System (PROMIS) initiative, established in 2004 by the National Institutes of Health. The focus of PROMIS is on developing "efficient, consistent, well-validated" ways to measure patient-reported symptoms that are known to be difficult to measure (eg, fatigue). The preliminary item bank on fatigue contains 95 items, with 55 addressing the fatigue experience and 40 addressing fatigue impact. Testing and calibration continues, and eventually these instruments will be possible to access publicly through computerized adaptive tests (http://www.nihpromis.org/default.aspx).

TREATMENTS
Pain

Some of the pain conditions that occur after neurologic trauma or disease and degenerative muscle diseases are complex and often resistant to available treatments.[98,99] Similar to younger persons, older persons who have these conditions may experience pain of various origins, including neuropathic pains, which are inadequately relieved through prescribed or self-initiated treatments. However, persistent pain in older adults is associated with multiple factors that may differ from those in a younger population, and these factors must be considered in the management of pain.

Aging is associated with gradual changes in areas such as cognitive ability, physiologic responses to pharmacologic treatments, emotional and physical function, and social support, and these factors all play a role in the treatment response and person's ability to adapt to the added stress of pain.[5] Because aging is associated with cognitive decline, the pros and cons of specific pharmacologic interventions that may further worsen cognitive deficits may need particular consideration in this population. For example, although severe pain is associated with negative effects on cognition (eg, mental flexibility[118]), some available medications also may be associated with this unwanted effect.[119]

According to the biopsychosocial perspective, a dynamic interaction exists among biologic factors, psychological status, and social factors. Although biologic mechanisms may initiate, maintain, and modulate pain, psychological factors may influence the appraisal and perception of pain, and social factors may modulate the individual's behavior in response to these perceptions.[120] Thus, adaptation to persistent pain not only is dependent on psychosocial factors but also involves adapting to specific types of pain, some of which may have characteristics that are more difficult to deal with and adapt to than other pain types.[121]

As in younger persons, treatments targeting the pathophysiologic mechanisms of the pain condition in combination with treatments aimed at reducing psychosocial distress and disability may be more effective than a single type of therapy in reducing pain severity and impact in older persons.[122–125] A mechanisms-based approach to classifying and managing pain is of high priority in the pain field,[126–128] because it may help identify appropriate and effective treatments that specifically address the causative mechanisms underlying a specific type of pain.

The treatment of persistent pain varies depending on several factors, including the diagnosis of pain, contributing psychosocial factors, and the preferences of the patient and health care professional. Pain is a prevalent problem in populations that have sustained trauma or disease of the nervous system and degenerative muscle diseases, and one that can significantly affect quality of life. Therefore, diagnosis, assessment, and management of pain should be integral parts of the care of older persons who have neurologic trauma or disease and degenerative muscle diseases, and interdisciplinary approaches to pain management should be applied.

Fatigue

Interventions to reduce the impact of fatigue on everyday life include (1) identification and remediation of factors contributing to secondary fatigue (eg, correcting nutritional deficiencies through diet and supplements, controlling pain, promoting good sleep hygiene, reducing deconditioning through exercise); (2) education to promote self-management of available energy through selection and application of energy management strategies; (3) cognitive behavioral therapy to enhance adaptive functioning with fatigue; and (4) use of pharmaceuticals. The extent to which these approaches have been evaluated and found effective across different populations varies. The literature on fatigue management interventions for people who have multiple sclerosis is more plentiful than for those who have SCI, late-effects polio, and muscular dystrophy. Excluding pharmacologic investigations, exercise and energy management education predominate this literature.

A recent meta-analysis examining the impact of exercise on quality of life among people who had multiple sclerosis[129] identified 25 studies and reviewed 13 (both nonexperimental and experimental) that included a total of 484 people. Eight of the studies used fatigue as a quality of life outcome measure; seven of these provided an aerobic exercise intervention, whereas the other one used a nonaerobic intervention. Average effect sizes for these eight studies ranged from a low of 0.04 to a high of 1.51. The authors concluded that exercise training was associated with a small but significant improvement in quality of life among people who had multiple sclerosis and is worthy of further investigation.[129]

Energy management education involves teaching people to identify and develop modifications to their daily activities to reduce fatigue,[48] and has been examined extensively in multiple sclerosis.[90,130–137] Energy management education focuses on teaching people who experience fatigue to evaluate their energy expenditures for daily activities, determine ways to modify their activities, evaluate their rest–activity ratios, and examine their use of adaptive equipment and community resources for fatigue management. It also teaches people how to use their bodies to perform various tasks efficiently, to prioritize their work, and to plan ahead to manage their fatigue.[138] Although some variability is present across studies, overall findings indicate that energy management education can reduce fatigue severity and impact among people who have multiple sclerosis. One randomized controlled trial found that effects on quality of life could be maintained for up to 1 year in people who had multiple sclerosis.[130]

GAPS AND FUTURE DIRECTIONS

Important areas for future research on pain and fatigue in persons who have preexisting physical impairments include the identification of conditions that require age-specific considerations. Currently, the role age and aging play in the experience of pain and fatigue, or in the interaction between pain and fatigue among people who have physical impairment, is unclear. Without this knowledge, ensuring that clinical practice is adequately addressing age-related issues when diagnosing and managing pain and fatigue will be difficult.

Another important area for future research is the identification of symptom clusters (eg, pain, fatigue, depression) and how they evolve over time as people simultaneously cope with physical impairments and aging-specific issues. Understanding the interaction among these symptoms may facilitate the development of comprehensive yet targeted assessment tools and interdisciplinary intervention protocols. These tools and protocols must be standardized, valid, and reliable, and most likely specific to populations that have an underlying physical impairment.

Intervention protocols, whether pain- or fatigue-specific, and targeting of symptom clusters will need to address type of pain or fatigue, relevant psychosocial factors, and age-specific considerations (eg, comorbidities, cognitive function, physiologic response to treatment, social support, retirement).

Both pain and fatigue are complex conditions, with many contributing factors and important life consequences. Because of this complexity, addressing these conditions requires the input of many individuals, including members of the interdisciplinary team, family members, and most important, the persons who are living with these conditions.

REFERENCES

1. Cruz-Almeida Y, Martinez-Arizala A, Widerstrom-Noga EG. Chronicity of pain associated with spinal cord injury: a longitudinal analysis. J Rehabil Res Dev 2005;42:585–94.
2. Nosek MA, Hughes RB, Petersen NJ, et al. Secondary conditions in a community-based sample of women with physical disabilities over a 1-year period. Arch Phys Med Rehabil 2006;87:320–7.
3. Hagell P, Brundin L. Towards an understanding of fatigue in Parkinson disease. J Neurol Neurosurg Psychiatr 2009;80:489–92.
4. World Health Organization. International classification of functioning, disability and health. World Health Organization; 2001. Available at: http://www.who.int/classifications/icf/wha-en.pdf. Accessed July 19, 2009.
5. Karp JF, Shega JW, Morone NE, et al. Advances in understanding the mechanisms and management of persistent pain in older adults. Br J Anaesth 2008; 101:111–20.

6. Merskey H. Classification of chronic pain, description of chronic pain syndromes and definitions of pain terms. Seattle (WA): IASP Press; 1994.
7. Solaro C, Brichetto G, Amato MP, et al. The prevalence of pain in multiple sclerosis: a multicenter cross-sectional study. Neurology 2004;63:919–21.
8. Khan F, Pallant J. Chronic pain in multiple sclerosis: prevalence, characteristics, and impact on quality of life in an Australian community cohort. J Pain 2007;8: 614–23.
9. O'Connor AB, Schwid SR, Herrmann DN, et al. Pain associated with multiple sclerosis: systematic review and proposed classification. Pain 2008;137:96–111.
10. Svendsen KB, Jensen TS, Overvad K, et al. Pain in patients with multiple sclerosis: a population-based study. Arch Neurol 2003;60:1089–94.
11. Dijkers M, Bryce T, Zanca J. Prevalence of chronic pain after traumatic spinal cord injury: a systematic review. J Rehabil Res Dev 2009;46:13–29.
12. Wollaars MM, Post MW, Brand N. Spinal cord injury pain: the influence of psychologic factors and impact on quality of life. Clin J Pain 2007;23: 383–91.
13. Widerstrom-Noga EG, Felipe-Cuervo E, Broton JG, et al. Perceived difficulty in dealing with consequences of spinal cord injury. Arch Phys Med Rehabil 1999; 80:580–6.
14. Turner JA, Cardenas DD. Chronic pain problems in individuals with spinal cord injuries. Semin Clin Neuropsychiatry 1999;4:186–94.
15. Rintala DH, Loubser PG, Castro J, et al. Chronic pain in a community-based sample of men with spinal cord injury: prevalence, severity, and relationship with impairment, disability, handicap, and subjective well-being. Arch Phys Med Rehabil 1998;79:604–14.
16. Siddall PJ, Taylor DA, McClelland JM, et al. Pain report and the relationship of pain to physical factors in the first 6 months following spinal cord injury. Pain 1999;81:187–97.
17. Finnerup NB, Johannesen IL, Sindrup SH, et al. Pain and dysesthesia in patients with spinal cord injury: a postal survey. Spinal Cord 2001;39:256–62.
18. Wekre LL, Stanghelle JK, Lobben B, et al. The Norwegian Polio Study 1994: a nation-wide survey of problems in long-standing poliomyelitis. Spinal Cord 1998;36:280–4.
19. Halstead LS, Rossi CD. New problems in old polio patients: results of a survey of 539 polio survivors. Orthopedics 1985;8:845–50.
20. Stoelb BL, Carter GT, Abresch RT, et al. Pain in persons with post-polio syndrome: frequency, intensity, and impact. Arch Phys Med Rehabil 2008;89: 1933–40.
21. Loeser JD, Treede RD. The Kyoto protocol of IASP basic pain terminology. Pain 2008;137:473–7.
22. Lindblom U. Analysis of abnormal touch, pain, and temperature sensation in patients. In: Hansson P, Lindblom U, editors. Touch, temperature, and pain in health and disease: mechanisms and assessments. Progress in pain research and management. Seattle (WA): IASP Press; 1994. p. 63–84.
23. Cruccu G, Anand P, Attal N, et al. EFNS guidelines on neuropathic pain assessment. Eur J Neurol 2004;11:153–62.
24. Treede RD, Jensen TS, Campbell JN, et al. Neuropathic pain: redefinition and a grading system for clinical and research purposes. Neurology 2008;70:1630–5.
25. Gielissen MF, Knoop H, Servaes P, et al. Differences in the experience of fatigue in patients and healthy controls: patients' descriptions. Health Qual Life Outcomes 2007;5:36.

26. Bakshi R. Fatigue associated with multiple sclerosis: diagnosis, impact and management. Mult Scler 2003;9:219–27.
27. Hadjimichael O, Vollmer T, Oleen-Burkey M, et al. Fatigue characteristics in multiple sclerosis: the North American Research Committee on Multiple Sclerosis (NARCOMS) survey. Health Qual Life Outcomes 2008;6:100.
28. Kos D, Kerckhofs E, Nagels G, et al. Origin of fatigue in multiple sclerosis: review of the literature. Neurorehabil Neural Repair 2008;22:91–100.
29. Krupp LB, Christodoulou C. Fatigue in multiple sclerosis. Curr Neurol Neurosci Rep 2001;1:294–8.
30. MacAllister WS, Krupp LB. Multiple sclerosis-related fatigue. Phys Med Rehabil Clin N Am 2005;16:483–502.
31. Feasson L, Camdessanche JP, El ML, et al. Fatigue and neuromuscular diseases. Ann Readapt Med Phys 2006;49:375–84.
32. On AY, Oncu J, Atamaz F, et al. Impact of post-polio-related fatigue on quality of life. J Rehabil Med 2006;38:329–32.
33. Schanke AK, Stanghelle JK, Andersson S, et al. Mild versus severe fatigue in polio survivors: special characteristics. J Rehabil Med 2002;34:134–40.
34. Schanke AK, Stanghelle JK. Fatigue in polio survivors. Spinal Cord 2001;39: 243–51.
35. Trojan DA, Cashman NR. Post-poliomyelitis syndrome. Muscle Nerve 2005;31: 6–19.
36. Fawkes-Kirby TM, Wheeler MA, Anton HA, et al. Clinical correlates of fatigue in spinal cord injury. Spinal Cord 2008;46:21–5.
37. Liem NR, McColl MA, King W, et al. Aging with a spinal cord injury: factors associated with the need for more help with activities of daily living. Arch Phys Med Rehabil 2004;85:1567–77.
38. McColl MA, Arnold R, Charlifue S, et al. Aging, spinal cord injury, and quality of life: structural relationships. Arch Phys Med Rehabil 2003;84:1137–44.
39. McColl MA, Charlifue S, Glass C, et al. Aging, gender, and spinal cord injury. Arch Phys Med Rehabil 2004;85:363–7.
40. Bostrom K, Ahlstrom G. Living with a chronic deteriorating disease: the trajectory with muscular dystrophy over ten years. Disabil Rehabil 2004;26: 1388–98.
41. Gagnon C, Mathieu J, Jean S, et al. Predictors of disrupted social participation in myotonic dystrophy type 1. Arch Phys Med Rehabil 2008;89:1246–55.
42. Kalkman JS, Schillings ML, van der Werf SP, et al. Experienced fatigue in facioscapulohumeral dystrophy, myotonic dystrophy, and HMSN-I. J Neurol Neurosurg Psychiatr 2005;76:1406–9.
43. Kalkman JS, Schillings ML, Zwarts MJ, et al. The development of a model of fatigue in neuromuscular disorders: a longitudinal study. J Psychosom Res 2007;62:571–9.
44. Kalkman JS, Zwarts MJ, Schillings ML, et al. Different types of fatigue in patients with facioscapulohumeral dystrophy, myotonic dystrophy and HMSN-I. Experienced fatigue and physiological fatigue. Neurol Sci 2008;29(Suppl 40): S238–40.
45. Schillings ML, Kalkman JS, Janssen HM, et al. Experienced and physiological fatigue in neuromuscular disorders. Clin Neurophysiol 2007;118:292–300.
46. Annoni JM, Staub F, Bogousslavsky J, et al. Frequency, characterisation and therapies of fatigue after stroke. Neurol Sci 2008;29(Suppl 2):S244–6.
47. Colle F, Bonan I, Gellez Leman MC, et al. Fatigue after stroke. Ann Readapt Med Phys 2006;49:272–6.

48. Multiple Sclerosis Council for Clinical Practice Guidelines. Fatigue and multiple sclerosis: Evidence-based management strategies for fatigue in multiple sclerosis. Washington, DC: Paralyzed Veterans of America; 1998.

49. Tralongo P, Respini D, Ferra F. Fatigue and aging. Crit Rev Oncol Hematol 2003; 48:S57–64.

50. National Institute on Aging. Unexplained fatigue in the elderly. Available at: http://www.nia.nih.gov/ResearchInformation/ConferencesAndMeetings/Unexplained Fatigue.htm. Accessed July 19, 2009.

51. Rosenthal TC, Majeroni BA, Pretorius R, et al. Fatigue: an overview. Am Fam Physician 2008;78:1173–9.

52. Park JY, Chun MH, Kang SH, et al. Functional outcome in poststroke patients with or without fatigue. Am J Phys Med Rehabil 2009;88:554–8.

53. Shah A. Fatigue in multiple sclerosis. Phys Med Rehabil Clin N Am 2009;20:363–72.

54. Jakobsson U, Hallberg IR, Westergren A. Overall and health related quality of life among the oldest old in pain. Qual Life Res 2004;13:125–36.

55. Ware JE Jr, Sherbourne CD. The MOS 36-item short-form health survey (SF-36). I. Conceptual framework and item selection. Med Care 1992;30:473–83.

56. Whitson HE, Sanders LL, Pieper CF, et al. Correlation between symptoms and function in older adults with comorbidity. J Am Geriatr Soc 2009;57:676–82.

57. Scudds RJ, Ostbye T. Pain and pain-related interference with function in older Canadians: the Canadian Study of Health and Aging. Disabil Rehabil 2001; 23:654–64.

58. Bardel A, Wallander MA, Wedel H, et al. Age-specific symptom prevalence in women 35–64 years old: a population-based study. BMC Public Health 2009; 9:37.

59. Riley JL, Wade JB. The stages of pain processing across the adult lifespan. J Pain 2000;1:162–70.

60. Rustoen T, Wahl AK, Hanestad BR, et al. Age and the experience of chronic pain: differences in health and quality of life among younger, middle-aged, and older adults. Clin J Pain 2005;21:513–23.

61. LaChapelle DL, Hadjistavropoulos T. Age-related differences among adults coping with pain: evaluation of a developmental life-context model. Can J Behav Sci 2005;37:123–37.

62. Parmelee PA, Smith B, Katz IR. Pain complaints and cognitive status among elderly institution residents. J Am Geriatr Soc 1993;41:517–22.

63. Williamson GM, Schulz R. Activity restriction mediates the association between pain and depressed affect: a study of younger and older adult cancer patients. Psychol Aging 1995;10:369–78.

64. Molton IR, Jensen MP, Ehde DM, et al. Coping with chronic pain among younger, middle-aged, and older adults living with neurological injury and disease. J Aging Health 2008;20:972–96.

65. Ohayon MM. Specific characteristics of the pain/depression association in the general population. J Clin Psychiatry 2004;65(Suppl 12):5–9.

66. Banks SM, Kerns RD. Explaining high rates of depression in chronic pain: a diathesis-stress framework. Psychol Bull 1996;119:95–110.

67. Hirsh AT, Turner AP, Ehde DM, et al. Prevalence and impact of pain in multiple sclerosis: physical and psychologic contributors. Arch Phys Med Rehabil 2009; 90:646–51.

68. Widerstrom-Noga EG, Cruz-Almeida Y, Martinez-Arizala A, et al. Internal consistency, stability, and validity of the spinal cord injury version of the multidimensional pain inventory. Arch Phys Med Rehabil 2006;87:516–23.

69. Kennedy P, Frankel H, Gardner B, et al. Factors associated with acute and chronic pain following traumatic spinal cord injuries. Spinal Cord 1997;35: 814–7.

70. Ostlund G, Wahlin A, Sunnerhagen KS, et al. Vitality among Swedish patients with post-polio: a physiological phenomenon. J Rehabil Med 2008;40:709–14.

71. Padua L, Aprile I, Frusciante R, et al. Quality of life and pain in patients with facioscapulohumeral muscular dystrophy. Muscle Nerve 2009;40:200–5.

72. Jacob KS, Zachariah K, Bhattacharji S. Depression in individuals with spinal cord injury: methodological issues. Paraplegia 1995;33:377–80.

73. Strine TW, Kroenke K, Dhingra S, et al. The associations between depression, health-related quality of life, social support, life satisfaction, and disability in community-dwelling US adults. J Nerv Ment Dis 2009;197:61–4.

74. Widerstrom-Noga EG, Felipe-Cuervo E, Yezierski RP. Chronic pain after spinal injury: interference with sleep and daily activities. Arch Phys Med Rehabil 2001;82:1571–7.

75. Douglas C, Wollin JA, Windsor C. Illness and demographic correlates of chronic pain among a community-based sample of people with multiple sclerosis. Arch Phys Med Rehabil 2008;89:1923–32.

76. Turk DC, Rudy TE. Toward an empirically derived taxonomy of chronic pain patients: integration of psychological assessment data. J Consult Clin Psychol 1988;56:233–8.

77. Kishi Y, Robinson RG, Forrester AW. Prospective longitudinal study of depression following spinal cord injury. J Neuropsychiatry Clin Neurosci 1994;6:237–44.

78. Kerns RD, Turk DC, Rudy TE. The West Haven-Yale Multidimensional Pain Inventory (WHYMPI). Pain 1985;23:345–56.

79. Anton HA, Miller WC, Townson AF. Measuring fatigue in persons with spinal cord injury. Arch Phys Med Rehabil 2008;89:538–42.

80. Fisk JD, Pontefract A, Ritvo PG, et al. The impact of fatigue on patients with multiple sclerosis. Can J Neurol Sci 1994;21:9–14.

81. Hansson B, Ahlstrom G. Coping with chronic illness: a qualitative study of coping with postpolio syndrome. Int J Nurs Stud 1999;36:255–62.

82. van der Kooi EL, Kalkman JS, Lindeman E, et al. Effects of training and albuterol on pain and fatigue in facioscapulohumeral muscular dystrophy. J Neurol 2007; 254:931–40.

83. Hoffman AJ, Given BA, von EA, et al. Relationships among pain, fatigue, insomnia, and gender in persons with lung cancer. Oncol Nurs Forum 2007; 34:785–92.

84. Wolkove N, Elkholy O, Baltzan M, et al. Sleep and aging: 2. Management of sleep disorders in older people. CMAJ 2007;176:1449–54.

85. Appelros P. Prevalence and predictors of pain and fatigue after stroke: a population-based study. Int J Rehabil Res 2006;29:329–33.

86. Naughton F, Ashworth P, Skevington SM. Does sleep quality predict pain-related disability in chronic pain patients? The mediating roles of depression and pain severity. Pain 2007;127:243–52.

87. McCracken LM, Iverson GL. Disrupted sleep patterns and daily functioning in patients with chronic pain. Pain Res Manag 2002;7:75–9.

88. Johnson KL, Yorkston KM, Klasner ER, et al. The cost and benefits of employment: a qualitative study of experiences of persons with multiple sclerosis. Arch Phys Med Rehabil 2004;85:201–9.

89. Yorkston KM, Johnson K, Klasner ER, et al. Getting the work done: a qualitative study of individuals with multiple sclerosis. Disabil Rehabil 2003;25:369–79.

90. Holberg C, Finlayson M. Factors influencing the use of energy conservation strategies by persons with multiple sclerosis. Am J Occup Ther 2007;61:96–107.
91. McLaughlin J, Zeeberg I. Self-care and multiple sclerosis: a view from two cultures. Soc Sci Med 1993;37:315–29.
92. Hammell KW, Miller WC, Forwell SJ, et al. Fatigue and spinal cord injury: a qualitative analysis. Spinal Cord 2009;47:44–9.
93. Johansson S, Ytterberg C, Hillert J, et al. A longitudinal study of variations in and predictors of fatigue in multiple sclerosis. J Neurol Neurosurg Psychiatr 2008;79:454–7.
94. Lerdal A, Celius EG, Krupp L, et al. A prospective study of patterns of fatigue in multiple sclerosis. Eur J Neurol 2007;14:1338–43.
95. Wincent A, Liden Y, Arner S. Pain questionnaires in the analysis of long lasting (chronic) pain conditions. Eur J Pain 2003;7:311–21.
96. Turk DC, Dworkin RH, Allen RR, et al. Core outcome domains for chronic pain clinical trials: IMMPACT recommendations. Pain 2003;106:337–45.
97. Bowsher D. Central pain following spinal and supraspinal lesions. Spinal Cord 1999;37:235–8.
98. Warms CA, Turner JA, Marshall HM, et al. Treatments for chronic pain associated with spinal cord injuries: many are tried, few are helpful. Clin J Pain 2002;18:154–63.
99. Widerstrom-Noga EG, Turk DC. Types and effectiveness of treatments used by people with chronic pain associated with spinal cord injuries: influence of pain and psychosocial characteristics. Spinal Cord 2003;41:600–9.
100. Finnerup NB. A review of central neuropathic pain states. Curr Opin Anaesthesiol 2008;21:586–9.
101. Cruz-Almeida Y, Alameda G, Widerstrom-Noga EG. Differentiation between pain-related interference and interference caused by the functional impairments of spinal cord injury. Spinal Cord 2009;47:390–5.
102. Widerstrom-Noga E, Biering-Sorensen F, Bryce T, et al. The international spinal cord injury pain basic data set. Spinal Cord 2008;46:818–23.
103. Bryce TN, Budh CN, Cardenas DD, et al. Pain after spinal cord injury: an evidence-based review for clinical practice and research. Report of the National Institute on Disability and Rehabilitation Research Spinal Cord Injury Measures meeting. J Spinal Cord Med 2007;30:421–40.
104. Sawatzky B, Bishop CM, Miller WC. Classification and measurement of pain in the spinal cord-injured population. Spinal Cord 2008;46:2–10.
105. Farrar JT, Young JP Jr, Lamoreaux L, et al. Clinical importance of changes in chronic pain intensity measured on an 11-point numerical pain rating scale. Pain 2001;94:149–58.
106. Felix ER, Cruz-Almeida Y, Widerstrom-Noga EG. Chronic pain after spinal cord injury: What characteristics make some pains more disturbing than others? J Rehabil Res Dev 2007;44:703–16.
107. Hansson P, Backonja M, Bouhassira D. Usefulness and limitations of quantitative sensory testing: clinical and research application in neuropathic pain states. Pain 2007;129:256–9.
108. Felix ER, Widerstrom-Noga EG. Reliability and validity of quantitative sensory testing in persons with spinal cord injury and neuropathic pain. J Rehabil Res Dev 2009;46:69–83.
109. Hjollund NH, Andersen JH, Bech P. Assessment of fatigue in chronic disease: a bibliographic study of fatigue measurement scales. Health Qual Life Outcomes 2007;5:12.

110. Dittner AJ, Wessely SC, Brown RG. The assessment of fatigue: a practical guide for clinicians and researchers. J Psychosom Res 2004;56:157–70.
111. Kos D, Kerckhofs E, Ketelaer P, et al. Self-report assessment of fatigue in multiple sclerosis: a critical evaluation. Occup Ther Health Care 2003;17:45–62.
112. Mota DC, Pimenta CA. Self-report instruments for fatigue assessment: a systematic review. Res Theory Nurs Pract 2006;20:49–78.
113. Taylor R, Jason L, Torres A. Fatigue rating scales: an empirical comparison. Psychol Med 2000;30:849–56.
114. Krupp LB, LaRocca NG, Muir-Nash J, et al. The fatigue severity scale. Application to patients with multiple sclerosis and systemic lupus erythematosus. Arch Neurol 1989;46:1121–3.
115. Chalder T, Berelowitz G, Pawlikowska T, et al. Development of a fatigue scale. J Psychosom Res 1993;37:147–53.
116. Smets EM, Garssen B, Bonke B, et al. The Multidimensional Fatigue Inventory (MFI) psychometric qualities of an instrument to assess fatigue. J Psychosom Res 1995;39:315–25.
117. Mills R, Young C, Nicholas R, et al. Rasch analysis of the fatigue severity scale in multiple sclerosis. Mult Scler 2009;15:81–7.
118. Karp JF, Reynolds CF III, Butters MA, et al. The relationship between pain and mental flexibility in older adult pain clinic patients. Pain Med 2006;7:444–52.
119. Closs SJ, Barr B, Briggs M. Cognitive status and analgesic provision in nursing home residents. Br J Gen Pract 2004;54:919–21.
120. Turk DC. Biopsychosocial perspective on chronic pain. In: Gatchel R, Turk DC, editors. Psychological approaches to chronic pain management: a clinician's handbook. New York: Guilford Press; 1996. p. 3–33.
121. Widerstrom-Noga EG, Cruz-Almeida Y, Felix ER, et al. Relationship between pain characteristics and pain adaptation type in persons with SCI. J Rehabil Res Dev 2009;46:43–56.
122. Oslund S, Robinson RC, Clark TC, et al. Long-term effectiveness of a comprehensive pain management program: strengthening the case for interdisciplinary care. Proc (Bayl Univ Med Cent) 2009;22:211–4.
123. Molton IR, Graham C, Stoelb BL, et al. Current psychological approaches to the management of chronic pain. Curr Opin Anaesthesiol 2007;20:485–9.
124. Norrbrink BC, Kowalski J, Lundeberg T. A comprehensive pain management programme comprising educational, cognitive and behavioural interventions for neuropathic pain following spinal cord injury. J Rehabil Med 2006;38:172–80.
125. Jensen MP, Turner JA, Romano JM. Changes after multidisciplinary pain treatment in patient pain beliefs and coping are associated with concurrent changes in patient functioning. Pain 2007;131:38–47.
126. Woolf CJ, Bennett GJ, Doherty M, et al. Towards a mechanism-based classification of pain? Pain 1998;77:227–9.
127. Woolf CJ, Salter MW. Neuronal plasticity: increasing the gain in pain. Science 2000;288:1765–9.
128. Hansson P. Neuropathic pain: clinical characteristics and diagnostic workup. Eur J Pain 2002;6(Suppl A):47–50.
129. Motl RW, Gosney JL. Effect of exercise training on quality of life in multiple sclerosis: a meta-analysis. Mult Scler 2008;14:129–35.
130. Mathiowetz VG, Matuska KM, Finlayson ML, et al. One-year follow-up to a randomized controlled trial of an energy conservation course for persons with multiple sclerosis. Int J Rehabil Res 2007;30:305–13.

131. Matuska K, Mathiowetz V, Finlayson M. Use and perceived effectiveness of energy conservation strategies for managing multiple sclerosis fatigue. Am J Occup Ther 2007;61:62–9.

132. Mathiowetz V, Busch ML. Participant evaluation of energy conservation course for people with multiple sclerosis. Int J Ms Care 2006;8:98–106.

133. Lamb AL, Finlayson M, Mathiowetz V, et al. The outcomes of using self-study modules in energy conservation education for people with multiple sclerosis. Clin Rehabil 2005;19(5):475–81.

134. Mathiowetz V, Finlayson M, Matuska K, et al. A randomized trial of energy conservation for persons with multiple sclerosis. Mult Scler 2005;11:592–601.

135. Vanage SM, Gilbertson KK, Mathiowetz V. Effects of an energy conservation course on fatigue impact for persons with progressive multiple sclerosis. Am J Occup Ther 2003;57:315–23.

136. Kos D, Duportail M, D'hooghe M, et al. Multidisciplinary fatigue management programme in multiple sclerosis: a randomized clinical trial. Mult Scler 2007; 13:996–1003.

137. Sauter C, Zebenholzer K, Hisakawa J, et al. A longitudinal study on effects of a six-week course for energy conservation for multiple sclerosis patients. Mult Scler 2008;14:500–5.

138. Packer TL, Brink N, Sauriol A. Managing fatigue: a six-week course for energy conservation. Tucson (AZ): Therapy Skill Builders; 1995.

The Potential of Virtual Reality and Gaming to Assist Successful Aging with Disability

B.S. Lange, PhD, BPhysio[a], P. Requejo, PhD[b,*], S.M. Flynn, PhD, PT[a],
A.A. Rizzo, PhD[a], F.J. Valero-Cuevas, PhD[c],
L. Baker, PhD, PT[d], C. Winstein, PhD, PT, FAPTA[d]

KEYWORDS

- Aging • Disability • Rehabilitation • Technology
- Virtual reality • Games

The probability for acquired disability increases with age.[1] Accordingly, the number of middle-aged and older adults living with disabilities will grow significantly as the United States population ages rapidly.[2] Emerging evidence from social and cognitive neuroscience suggests that new learning, productivity, and social engagement are possible for those aging with and into disability.[3] Although such evidence-based techniques and interventions are currently available, they are seldom used for those who are aging with and into disabilities. Moreover, research indicates that functional motor capacity can be improved, maintained, or recovered via consistent participation in motor exercises and rehabilitation regimens,[4] but independent adherence to such preventative and rehabilitative programming outside the clinic setting is low.[5] Given

This material is based upon work supported by NSF Grants EFRI-COPN 0836042, BES-0237258 and IGERT-0333366, and NIH Grant R21-HD048566 to FVC. Its contents are solely the responsibility of the authors and do not necessarily represent the official views of the NSF or NIH.
[a] VRPSYCH Laboratory, Institute for Creative Technologies, University of Southern California, 13274 Fiji Way, Marina Del Rey, CA 90292, USA
[b] Rancho Los Amigos National Rehabilitation Center, Building 500, Room 64, 7601 East Imperial Highway, Downey, CA 90242, USA
[c] Division of Biokinesiology and Physical Therapy at the School of Dentistry, Department of Biomedical Engineering, University of Southern California, RTH 402, Los Angeles, CA 90089, USA
[d] Division of Biokinesiology and Physical Therapy at the School of Dentistry, University of Southern California, CHP 155, Los Angeles, CA 90089-9006, USA
* Corresponding author.
E-mail address: prequejo@larei.org

the importance and high costs of health care for those aging with disability, the applications of technology that can improve health maintenance and health care, or reduce the associated costs, would be especially valuable. Moreover, the technology needs to be introduced into everyday life well before sensory, sensorimotor, and cognitive impairments have occurred.[6] Such technology should not be centered only on disability and pathology, but should also be geared at promoting successful lifespan development at all ages.[7] It should be a pleasure to use,[8] and some would argue, a status symbol to possess.[9]

Maintaining functional independence is a high priority for those aging with and into disability. Advancements in computer technologies and information systems have the potential to assist in this goal by enhancing sensorimotor and cognitive functions required for day-to-day activities. As technology is rapidly being integrated into most aspects of life and is changing the nature of work, the form and scope of personal communication, education, and health care delivery has been transformed. It is highly likely that older people, specifically those aging with physical disability, will need to interact with some form of computer technology to carry out routine activities. Consequently, technology has the potential to enhance participation in community living and thus enhance the health and functional outcomes for individuals aging with disability because it may augment their ability and capacity to perform a variety of tasks that have traditionally presented a barrier to their daily living.[10,11]

One tangible way to show that virtual reality (VR) and gaming technologies can maximize function and participation for those aging with and into a disability is through the incorporation of outcome measures across the 3 disablement domains described in the framework defined by the International Classification of Functioning, Disability and Health (ICF) (**Fig. 1**).[12] The ICF classification system is an effective organizational framework to allow assessment of outcome interactions that are associated with health-related problems (ie, body function/structure impairments, activity limitations, participation restrictions) and across disease or injury-specific health conditions.[13] The true effect of a reduction in activity limitation on participation in home, work, and community life is of primary importance.

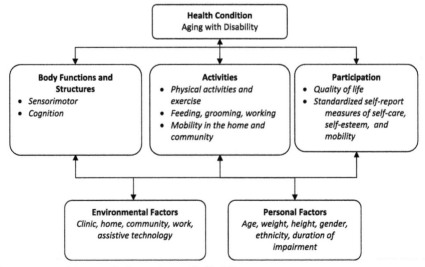

Fig. 1. ICF model as applied to aging with disability.

The application of VR and gaming technology that focuses on research and development of multimodal technology-therapy programs designed to address specific motor activity limitations (ie, posture and balance, dexterous manipulation, and integrated functional behaviors during wheeled mobility) presents an unique opportunity to address the challenges of linking multiple domains of the ICF, particularly in the context of negating the impairment at the body function/structure level (eg, game-based exercise for targeted and progressive strengthening), at the activity level (eg, Improved walking function because of game-based physical exercise), and at the home and community participation level (eg, increased family and social interaction when playing the games). For example, an individual who is recovering from a stroke may begin to play a home-based video game for hand and arm rehabilitation, but may benefit from the social interaction when playing with his or her grandchildren. The use of VR-based games can provide the means to address all the 3 disablement domains because a controllable range of stimuli can be delivered and systematically quantified at each stage of an intervention.[14]

This article presents an approach for maximizing function and participation for those aging with and into a disability by combining task-specific training with advances in VR and gaming technologies to enable positive behavioral modifications for independence in the home and community. This approach is unique, and stands in sharp contrast to the more conventional use of technologies that are primarily assistive, such as a device that can be used as a stand-alone assist for a specific task like walking (eg, a cane or walker). In this article, the authors present the rationale for the clinical application of VR and gaming technology, examples from the authors' work, and a description of some of the applications within their Rehabilitation Engineering Research Center on aging with disability (http://www.usc.edu/agingrerc). In each application, the authors combine the potential offered by immersive game-based VR technology with evidence-based rehabilitation approaches, such as muscle-specific exercises or sophisticated task-specific training protocols that harness the benefits of meaningful task practice for sustained improvements in sensorimotor functions, thereby fostering successful cognitive "unloading" and facilitating activity and social participation in home, work, and community life.

VIRTUAL REALITY AND GAMING TECHNOLOGY FOR SENSORIMOTOR AND COGNITIVE REHABILITATION

The effectiveness of sensorimotor function retraining is influenced by the quantity, duration, and intensity of practice.[15–21] High-intensity exercise programs are often fraught with low compliance and adherence. Exercise adherence is a significant hurdle to overcome, especially in the presence of a long-term chronic illness. Maintaining motivation and engagement are central to long-term functional improvement and success. Self-worth, motivation, and activity enjoyment have been reported to be vital to long-term exercise adherence.[22,23] It has also been suggested that when a client "focuses" on a game than his or her impairment, exercise becomes more enjoyable, motivating, and is more likely to be maintained over the many trials needed to induce plastic changes in the nervous system.[24–26] Providing a treatment that is fun, motivating, and distracting while simultaneously enhancing function would serve to improve exercise adherence and, therefore, effect motor learning and functional outcomes. One method that is showing great potential to meet this need is the use of VR games for rehabilitation.

VR is defined as "an immersive and interactive system that provides users with the illusion of entering a virtual world."[27] Immersion and interactivity suggest a virtual or imaginary world that can be entered and explored. Gobbetti and Scateni[28] 1998 state the "goal of virtual reality is to put the user in the loop of a real-time simulation, immersed in a world that can be both autonomous and responsive to its actions." The user is connected to the VR system as part of the input/output loop, allowing individuals to provide input to the virtual environment (VE) and experience the result of that input. In 2003 Burdea[29] described VR as "a high-end user-computer interface that involves real-time simulation and interactions through multiple sensorial channels." These definitions require that legitimate VR systems provide a computer simulated situation or environment with which the user can interact in real time, giving a sense of actually being in that situation or environment. To place the user within a loop of real-time simulation, VR systems require an output device or visual interface (flat screen or head mounted display) and input devices for interaction (mouse, joystick, data glove) and tracking (tracking device). The software or VE can be viewed through the output device and manipulated or interacted with via the input devices.[29] **Fig. 2** shows the components of a VR system.[29]

VR applications, historically used for the training of motor tasks involving highly complex activities such as surgical techniques,[30] flight simulation,[31] and military exercises[32] allow the user to enter a simulated world through multimodal sensory feedback. With the reduction in cost of computing hardware and software technologies,

VR System Architecture

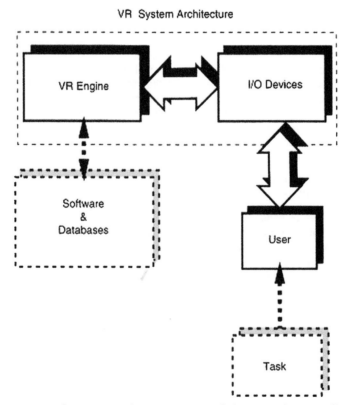

Fig. 2. Components of a VR system (I, input; O, output). (*From* Burdea G, Coiffet P. Virtual reality technology. 2nd edition. New York: Wiley; 1994, copyright 2003. Reprinted with permission of John Wiley & Sons, Inc.)

and the increasing expansion of the video game market, video game consoles and video games can be labeled as VR systems. These VR systems are interactive, immersive, and provide the user with a sense of presence within a VE. The use of video games and VR systems for rehabilitation has expanded rapidly over the past few years. Early research in the area of the use of VR systems to assist people to relearn how to move suggests that VR game-based technology can be used effectively to improve motor skill rehabilitation of a range of functional deficits. VR systems demand focus and attention, but can motivate the user to move, and can provide the user with a sense of achievement even if they cannot perform that task in the "real world."

There is a compelling and ethical motivation to address the needs of individuals who are aging with disabilities by promoting home-based access to low-cost, interactive VR systems designed to engage and motivate individuals to participate with game-driven physical activities and rehabilitation programming. The creation of such systems can serve to enhance, maintain, and rehabilitate the motor processes that underlie the integrated functional behaviors that are needed to maximize independence and quality of life beyond what exists with currently available, labor intensive, underutilized, and more costly approaches. There are fundamental and dramatic advantages inherent in the use of game-based approaches for treating cognitive, motor, and behavioral impairments. VR offers an ideal core technology because it allows for the creation of computer-generated 3-dimensional simulations, within which hierarchical task relevant challenges can be delivered and titrated across a range of difficulty levels.[33] In this way, an individual's treatment plan can be customized to begin at a stimulus challenge level that is attainable and comfortable for them, and then proceed with a gradual progression of challenge that is informed by the individual's performance in real time. Furthermore, VR game-based environments allow for the presentation of more ecologically relevant stimuli that are embedded in meaningful and familiar contexts. By designing VEs that not only "look like" the real world but also actually incorporate challenges that require real-world functional behaviors, the ecological validity of cognitive/motor interventions can be enhanced. Within such simulations, the complexity of stimulus challenges found in naturalistic settings can be delivered while still maintaining the experimental control required for rigorous scientific analysis and replication. Alternatively, it is possible that the use of novel environments and game play can engage and motivate the user to perform activities that they would not normally perform of their own accord. VR technology also supports precise and detailed capture and analysis of complex responses (ie, kinematic assessments of speed, accuracy, timing, consistency).

VR has recently been explored as a therapeutic tool to retrain faulty movement patterns resulting from neurologic dysfunction and to augment rehabilitation of the upper limb of patients in the chronic phase after stroke.[17,34] VR technology using specialized interface devices has been applied to improve motor skill rehabilitation of functional deficits including reaching,[35–37] hand function,[17,20,34,38–40] and walking.[41–43] Substantial effort and expertise have been focused on developing these innovative technology/interventions to exploit the neuroplastic properties associated with the sensorimotor systems in the adult brain. It has been proposed that such VR-based activities can be delivered in the home via a telerehabilitation approach to support these patients' increased access to rehabilitation and preventative exercise programming.[44,45] Moreover, when such VR training is embedded in an interactive game-based context, there is a potential to enhance the engagement and motivation needed to drive neuroplastic changes that underlie motor process maintenance and improvement. However, home-based VR systems need to be affordable, and easy to deploy and maintain, while still providing the interactional fidelity required to produce the meaningful motor activity required to foster rehabilitative aims and promote transfer to real-world activities.

Use of computer-based cognitive fitness and assessment technologies have rapidly expanded over the past 5 years with the introduction of a range of game-based training tools, such as BrainAge (Nintendo of America, Redmond, WA, USA), BrainFitness (PositScience Corporation, San Francisco, CA, USA), and Posit Science (Posit Science Corporation, San Francisco, CA, USA). Sales of cognitive fitness and assessment products in the United States have grown an estimated $100 million to $265 million between the period of 2005 and 2008.[46] Many products offer cognitive fitness games for regular long-term use. These brain-training games are often based on common neuropsychological assessment tools. Common areas of focus for games include long-term and short-term memory, language, executive function, visuospatial orientation, and critical thinking. The Posit Science program has been shown to reduce the effects of age-related cognitive decline through training in areas of memory, concentration, language, executive function, reaction time, and visual attention.[47,48] BrainFitness by Dakim (http://www.dakim.com/dakim) is a touch-screen device that assesses and trains long- and short-term memory, language, computation, visuospatial orientation, and critical thinking. These types of applications may include the neuropsychological tests that are often used for assessment, raising some concern that these tasks are training the user for the test rather than training the cognitive domain itself. Playing casual computer games has also been shown to improve cognitive abilities in older adults. Older adults who play video games have shown improvements in reaction time,[49–51] cognitive functioning,[52] intelligence,[53] visuomotor coordination,[53] attention and concentration,[54] and self-esteem and quality of life.[49,55] The use of physical computer games for improvement of cognitive and functional deficits has to be shown; however, several researchers across the globe are currently exploring the use of video game consoles, such as the Sony Playstation2 EyeToy (Sony Corporation, Minato, Tokyo, Japan) and the Nintendo Wii and WiiFit (Nintendo Co. Ltd, Kyoto, Japan) with groups of individuals who are healthy aged and those aging with a disability.

One of the issues with the use of commercial games and consoles such as the Nintendo Wii, Nintendo WiiFit, and Sony Playstation2 EyeToy is that these applications have been developed and tested for the purpose of entertainment. Commercial video game consoles and games have been tested on a diverse audience; however, they were not designed as medical devices or with a primary focus of a rehabilitation tool. Because these games were initially designed for entertainment, the game-play mechanics are not entirely applicable to those with disabilities. Thus, there is a need to gain a better understanding of the qualities of the commercial games and gaming consoles before these devices can be approved as appropriate rehabilitation tools for people with disabilities. Many of these applications are too difficult to use as a therapy tool by people with disabilities, and cannot be accessed or altered to improve usability.[56] The development of low-cost VR applications for rehabilitation must provide versatile and accurate interaction devices with the ability to track the user's movements and present information about performance to the user and their therapist in an appropriate and user-friendly format. The games and VEs must allow the user to interact in a way that is appropriate for their level of impairment, and must be easily changed to increase the level of challenge as the user improves.

The potential of the use of VR game-based applications, as they pertain to those aging with and into disability, involves the integration of cognitive and physical tasks within an engaging and meaningful environment in which it is safe to (or in some cases the system makes the user unable to) make mistakes and errors. The operating premise is that cognitive demand for daily functional behaviors increases with age-related physical decline. The approach is to enhance physical function in meaningful activities by harnessing advances in science and technology (especially immersive technologies) that increase sensorimotor capacity and unload cognitive demands in those aging with and into disability. By taking advantage of VR technologies for facilitating focused task-specific practice and gaming for enjoyment and adherence, it is anticipated that the core processes at the body function level and activities level as represented in the ICF model will be affected, which can enable active participation and enhance quality of life for the intended beneficiaries. Examples of clinical situations in which the use of VR and gaming technologies can serve to complement and improve on existing assessment and training applications are described in the following sections.

VR REHABILITATION FOR BALANCE IMPAIRMENTS

Balance, defined as the ability to maintain the body's center of gravity over the base of support, requires full integrity of an elegant and complicated system. Postural control is the ability to maintain an upright position (in sitting or standing) when stationary or when performing activities. The postural control system incorporates (1) sensory detection (through the visual, vestibular, and somatosensory systems), (2) integration of sensorimotor information within the central nervous system, and (3) proper coordinated movement patterns and responses.[57–59] When deterioration or damage occurs to one or more of these systems, impairment of balance occurs.[60–62] More specifically, an ability to accurately assess (sense) the position of the center of gravity relative to the base of support will disrupt balance. Second, when automatic movements to maintain balance are triggered too slowly or ineffectively, balance becomes distorted. Impairments affecting balance, such as muscular weakness, proprioceptive deficits, limitations in range of motion, and visual/vestibular deficits, can lead to falls and restrict an individual's normal motor activities, thereby limiting one's sense of independence, and adversely affecting the quality of life. The prevalence of balance disorders in the overall population of the United States is unknown. It is estimated that at least half of the overall population of the United States are affected by a balance or vestibular disorder sometime during their life (http://www.cdc.gov). Thus, there is a high probability that individuals aging with and into disability will experience balance problems sometime in their lifetime. Finding low-cost and safe balance training tools is imperative as the baby boomers continue to age and potentially increase the risk of falls.

The recent release and worldwide acceptance and enjoyment of Nintendo's WiiFit has provided significant evidence for the notion that exercise can be fun, provided it is presented in a manner that is entertaining, motivating, and distracting. The Nintendo WiiFit challenges balance in a variety of ways. By using a low-tech forceplate platform, the player controls the movements of an onscreen avatar by shifting their weight on the platform. When the player shifts right, the avatar shifts right and vice versa. Games such as hoola-hooping, defending a soccer goal, floating down a river, skiing down a mountain, and a variety of yoga positions are used in this device. This type of game challenges balance in a variety of ways. The player must watch, that is, engage the visual system, in a way that he or she can interpret the images presented and decide if movements to the right or to the left would be most successful. Visual feedback is given by, for example, seeing the avatar move between ski flags. Furthermore, knowledge of performance is provided visually as an individual moves into a yoga position, and is challenged to maintain his or her balance as precisely as possible by keeping a small red dot inside a yellow circle. Challenging the player to maintain the center of pressure and center of balance in a precise location while using visual feedback to guide the cursor on the screen tests the player's balance symmetry. The games challenge a person's vestibular system as the person moves through the challenging positions, and the vestibular system is being activated as the player moves into the various positions. If an individual has a deficit in any of these systems (visual, vestibular, or somatosensory) these games become a significant challenge. The Sony Playstation EyeToy has shown promising results as a low-cost tool for balance rehabilitation.[63,64] The EyeToy (Sony Computer Entertainment, Europe) is a projected video capture system that uses a motion-sensitive USB camera to display mirror image of the player into the game, allowing the player to interact with the VE using the entire body. In a feasibility study in 2007, Flynn and colleagues[63] applied the Eye-Toy with an individual with chronic stroke for 20 1-hour sessions. The game's task requirements included target-based motion, dynamic balance, and motor planning. The study showed clinically relevant improvements in the Dynamic Gait Index, and trends toward improvement on the Fugl-Meyer Assessment, Berg Balance Scale, UE Functional Index, Motor Activity Log, and Beck Depression Inventory.

Physical activities, including strengthening exercises, tai chi, dancing, and walking have been shown to improve balance and decrease the risk of falls in older adults.[65] Dancing is a fun filled, physical, and expressive activity open for participation by people of all levels of coordination. Modified dance-based exercises have been shown to improve endurance and balance in older adults.[66–68] Dancing can improve and maintain strength, endurance, balance, and coordination. Dancing can also increase body awareness and kinesthetic awareness, challenge attention, and improve self-esteem and confidence.[66–68] Dance-based training has been shown to be beneficial in improving static balance and reducing the risk of a fall.[67] The effectiveness of physical activity and aerobic exercise in preservation of balance and reduction of falls has been well documented.[65] A systematic review of prevention of falls exercise regimes found that the greatest relative effects of exercise on fall rates were seen in programs that included a combination of a higher total dose of exercise (>50 hours over the trial period) and consisted of challenging balance exercises (exercises conducted while standing in which people aimed to stand with their feet closer together or on one leg, minimize use of their hands to assist, and practice controlled movements of the center of mass).[65] Dancing can be considered a challenging balance exercise, because dancers are required to change their base of support while moving to music, not looking at their feet, and controlling their weight shift between poses or movements. Dancing can increase body awareness, kinesthetic awareness, and improve and maintain flexibility, balance, coordination, endurance, strength, and self-esteem.[69] Hopkins and colleagues[68] found in 1990 that a 12-week low-impact aerobic dance program significantly improved cardiorespiratory endurance, strength/endurance, body agility, flexibility, body fat, and balance in a sample of 53 women older than 65 years. Shigematsu and colleagues[67] in 2002 similarly found that, compared with a control group, a 12-week danced-based exercise class showed significantly greater improvements in balance measures (single leg balance, functional reach, and walking time around obstacles) in 38 women aged 72 to 87 years. Hui and colleagues[66] in 2009 found that a 12-week danced-based exercise program of a sample of 111 older adults significantly improved balance measures (6-minute walk test, flexibility, timed up-and-go test), resting heart rate, endurance, and physical and mental well-being (SF-36) compared with a control group. Most of the dance group felt the intervention improved their health status. These findings show that dancing has physical and psychological benefits, and should be promoted as a form of leisure activity for older adults. Dance games, such as Dance-Dance Revolution, first developed by Konami in 1998, are physically active video games that challenge endurance and dynamic balance. However, the primary function of current dance and music-based video games such as Dance-Dance Revolution is entertainment. These games are beneficial from a rehabilitative perspective because they require skills related to timing, rhythm, balance, endurance, and strength. Using a dance mat with areas that the player must step on in time with cues on the screen, these games have the ability to get the player to perform specific moves in a specific pattern, and have been shown to improve activity and mood as well as reduce weight in children and youth.[70–72] Dance-Dance Revolution has been shown to increase heart rate and motivate adolescents to exercise in an effort to improve motor coordination, self-esteem, and aerobic fitness.[70,72] Dance games are currently being used in schools and a variety of workplaces across the United States to encourage children and adults to become more active. These games have the potential to be used as a part of a balance training prevention program for older adults (with and without disability) in clinics or within the home.

VR REHABILITATION FOR A HOME EXERCISE PROGRAM FOR THE SHOULDER

An estimated 1.5 million people in the United States use a manual wheelchair.[73] The proportion of the population using wheelchairs increases sharply with age. In the population of age 18 to 64 years, 560,000 individuals use a manual wheelchair. This number increases to 864,000 in those 65 years and older. Four-fifths (80.2%) of wheelchair users in all age groups report some degree of difficulty in at least one activity of daily living. Of those aged 64 years and younger, spinal cord injury (SCI) is the most common diagnosis in manual wheelchair users.[73] Approximately 12,000 new survivors of SCI are added each year to the total population of approximately 300,000 persons now living with SCI (http://www.spinalcord.uab.edu, 2008). Improved life expectancy and increasing age at injury have resulted in a population that is increasingly experiencing the impact of aging with a disability.[74] One of the most common secondary complaints in the SCI population is shoulder joint pain that has been attributed to the high demand on the upper limbs during manual wheelchair use, transfers, and raises.[75–78] The incidence of shoulder joint pain after SCI is greater than that in the nondisabled population at every age and increases steadily with time post injury, affecting a full 70% of individuals at 20 years post SCI.[79] A consequence of the current near-normal life expectancy for individuals with SCI is that most of this population will eventually experience significant and function-limiting shoulder pain. Because individuals who use a manual wheelchair are dependent on their upper extremities for mobility and daily activities, shoulder dysfunction and pain can present a devastating loss of independence and decreased quality of life.[80] Although this clinical problem has been documented extensively in the SCI population, individuals with other primary diagnoses that preclude function of the lower extremities (eg, lower extremity amputation, poliomyelitis, myelomeningocele, multiple sclerosis) experience a similar course of shoulder pain with prolonged wheelchair use.[77,81–84]

Rotator cuff strengthening and shoulder joint stretching exercise programs modified for performance from a manual wheelchair have been shown to reduce shoulder pain and improve function in individuals who are dependent on manual wheelchair use for community mobility.[85–87] A randomized control trial confirmed the effectiveness of a home-based, progressive resistive exercise program that was designed to be simple and to require minimal equipment.[84] Participants in this trial had chronic shoulder pain (mean duration of 5 years) from prolonged wheelchair use after SCI (average time since injury 20 years). Shoulder pain, as measured by the Wheelchair User's Shoulder Pain Index (WUSPI),[67] was reduced after the 12-week exercise program in the experimental group from 51 to 15 out of a total possible score of 150. In contrast, WUSPI scores in the attention-control group were unchanged at a score of 45 after 12 weeks.[84] Moreover, participants in the experimental group showed a small but statistically significant improvement overall; subjective quality of life increased from 4.8 to 5.3 out of a total possible score of 7.0 where as quality of life scores were unchanged at 5.0 in the control participants. Thus this simple, low-cost home exercise program is dramatically effective at reducing long-standing, debilitating shoulder pain in individuals who use a manual wheelchair for community mobility.

A vital component to long-term adherence to an exercise program is maintaining the person's interest in the repetitive tasks and ensuring that they complete the training program. A lack of interest or short attention span can also impair the potential effectiveness of the exercise program. The use of rewarding activities and biofeedback has been shown to improve task performance and motivations to practice.[88,89] For instance, an interface (GAME[Wheels]) between a portable roller system and a computer that enables a wheelchair user to play commercially available computer video games during wheelchair propulsion exercise was shown to increase the individual's physiologic response, and allowed the users to reach their exercise training zone faster and maintain it for the entire exercise trial.[90–92] Moreover, of the 15 subjects tested, 87% indicated that having a video game during exercise would help them work out on a regular basis.[91] Similarly, a game-based arm exercise using an interface between an arm ergometer and a computer game (GAME[Cycle]) that allows the user to control game play on the screen as if using a joystick was shown to elicit the same physiologic response and perceived exertion as arm ergometry, but the games made the exercise more exciting and, thus, motivated a person to exercise more or for a longer period of time, yielding increased energy expenditure.[93] A shoulder strengthening and flexibility home exercise program performed to prevent the onset of shoulder pain would require long-term or intermittent commitment for individuals with chronic disability. Therefore, the development of a low-cost game-based application that can be deployed in the home environment is vital for long-term commitment to such a shoulder preservation program.

VR REHABILITATION FOR DEXTEROUS MANIPULATION WITH THE FINGERTIPS

Dexterous fingertip tasks are ubiquitous in daily life (eg, writing, sorting coins, or buttoning a shirt) and differ greatly from static pinch tasks (eg, holding a key or pressing a button) in that the magnitude and direction of fingertip forces need to be dynamically controlled to fulfill the task. The retention and restoration of hand function in aging, in injury, and in disease is the subject of an entire medical field.[94–97] Maintaining and restoring finger dexterity is a gateway to a productive and entertaining lifestyle for the elderly: from feeding and dressing oneself to using a cell phone or computer, to participating in a knitting club or playing cards. Dexterous manipulation with the fingertips is disproportionately impaired by orthopedic (eg, thumb osteoarthritis) and neurologic (eg, stroke, cerebral palsy, Parkinson disease, traumatic brain injury, and SCI) condition and natural aging because it requires a complex balance and interactions among all neuromusculoskeletal elements of the body: from cortical and spinal sensorimotor systems, to musculotendon integrity, to joint and ligament flexibility and stability of the hand.[98,99] The medical and rehabilitation communities are in dire need of effective means to promote the retention or restoration of dexterous manipulation in aging, and especially in aging with a disability.

To address this need, the authors have developed a novel engineering paradigm and technologies that focus on the ability of a person to perform dexterous fingertip tasks at submaximal force levels.[100] The manipulating ability of a multifinger hand is defined by the mechanical effect each fingertip can produce on an object.[101] Effective and dexterous manipulation arises when the coordinated action of the fingertips can generate the desired resultant 3-dimensional force/torque vector at the center of mass of the object being held. The ability with which the magnitude and direction of the fingertip force vectors are dynamically regulated determines the effectiveness of dynamic manipulation. The Strength-Dexterity (S-D) system targets the functional cornerstone of dexterous manipulation in healthy and clinical populations, which is the ability to simultaneously and dynamically regulate the magnitude and direction of fingertip force vectors. The S-D system is based on the principle of buckling of compression springs. When compressed the spring is initially stable, but as the compression increases to a critical point the combined handspring system becomes unstable and relies on the passive anatomic structures and active sensorimotor control of the fingers to dynamically hold that level of compression force. The compression of this device involves low forces (2–3 N), but requires careful collaborative control of finger motions and fingertip force vectors to prevent the spring from buckling. The one parameter that can characterize performance during the production of dexterous manipulation with the fingertips is the maximal compression a person can achieve with a spring that is impossible to compress fully. The maximal compression a person can achieve indicates the limit of sensorimotor integration ability by indicating how much instability the person can control. The S-D system has the potential to be used to quantify impairment and compare treatment outcomes in orthopedic and neurologic afflictions that degrade dynamic manipulation.[100]

The application of VR and a game-based system to rehabilitate hand and finger function in persons with stroke,[38,39,102] cervical level SCI,[103] and cerebral palsy[103] has shown promising outcomes. In 2004 Adamovich and colleagues[38] used a VR-based system for hand rehabilitation using a CyberGlove (Cyber Glove Systems, San Jose, CA, USA) and a Rutgers Master II-ND haptic glove that trained finger range of motion, finger flexion speed, independence of finger motion, and finger strength in 8 individuals with chronic stroke. All participants showed improvements in functional tests that transferred into gains in clinical tests and task completion times.[39] To rehabilitate finger-hand function in patients with SCI and stroke, Szturm and colleagues[103] in 2008 used an interactive computer gaming system, coupled with the manipulation of common objects, as a form of repetitive, task-specific movement therapy for 15 1-hour therapy sessions, 3 sessions a week. Participants could select from 25 different commercial video games (rated "everyone"), each offering different precision levels, speed constraints, visuospatial demands, and either single- or dual-axis movements. The training levels were progressive and emulated the functional properties of objects used daily. This therapy resulted in positive effects on the recovery of finger motion and hand function.

VR REHABILITATION AND STIMULATED ACTIVE SEATING FOR PRESSURE ULCER PREVENTION

Pressure ulcers (PUs) are a significant and frequent problem for those who depend on a wheelchair for mobility. Pressure ulcers are a debilitating pathology resulting from pressure and shear in the soft tissues of immobilized individuals who do not shift their weight.[104] Blood vessels become occluded and the soft tissues they supply become necrotic. PUs are particularly high in incidence in individuals who are insensate but who sit for long periods of time. About 30% of immobile people develop pressure ulcers at some time during their lives.[105] Age- and pathology-matched patient trials have shown that hospital stays increase 3- to 5-fold in patients suffering from PUs, incurring significant hospital expense.[106] Pressure, immobility, and disuse atrophy also contribute to a high incidence of PUs in elderly patients who lose mobility from stroke, dementia, Parkinson disease, and so forth. The cost of treating PUs in the United States was estimated to be more than $55 billion annually in 1994 (average increase in hospital stay of 21.6 days at $2360 per day in almost 1.1 million patients per year).[106] Current treatment of PUs requires prolonged passive tissue load reduction, when individuals are required to be removed from their seating systems, sometimes in bed for long periods of time. In some cases, surgical repair is required. Even when healed, PUs have a high (more than 60%) recurrence rate,[107] with the monetary costs for treatment ranging from $50,000 to $80,000 per incident. A pressure ulcer is devastating on personal well-being, self-esteem, and the ability to contribute to and participate in society in general.[108] Thus, prevention of occurrence or recurrence of PUs are a high priority for aging wheelchair users.

Today's strategies require cognitive awareness to manually or mechanically shift weight several times each hour. When individuals are actively engaged in activities of daily life, this cognitive burden is often lost and can result in pressure breakdown of high-risk sitting areas, such as the ischia, sacrum, and sometimes over the trochanters.[109–111] Stimulated active seating for pressure ulcer prevention (SASyPUP) is designed to allow significant weight relief, especially over the ischia, on a preprogrammed schedule. The SASyPUP uses chronically implanted, wireless microstimulators[112,113] to deliver preprogrammed stimulations to electrically activate the gluteal muscles to shift the paralyzed participant's weight, as well as to build up gluteal muscle volume (padding) and musculocutaneous circulation for exercise, and hamstring muscles as hip extensors. Implanted neuromuscular electrical stimulation has been shown to activate strong muscle contractions and to produce skeletal motion, with associated increases in muscle bulk (hypertrophy), strength, and metabolic capacity, as well as vascularization.[112–115] Thus the stimulation has the potential to counteract the 3 major etiologic factors in PU development: immobility, soft-tissue atrophy, and hypoxia. The individual does not need to generate cognitive strategies for weight shifting, because implanted microstimulators will automatically activate muscles to shift pressure. This will serve the seated individual who lacks sensation much more like the automatic position changes used by seated individuals with intact sensation.

Unlike individuals with normal sensation, who subconsciously automatically shift their seated weight, the SASyPUP system shifts the user, but without the coordinated trunk muscles used to maintain upright balance. Thus there is the potential to shift the seated individual and alter their base of support unexpectedly. In this instance, a unique application of VR and gaming technology helps in enhancing sitting posture and balance to allow individuals to practice and develop automatic strategies to maintain upright seated balance both at rest and while experiencing the periodic stimulated weight shift. Conceptually, the stimulated cycles can use a gradual ramping up of the weight-shifting contraction, and users of the system will be made aware of the impending weight shift so that appropriate and perhaps automatic compensations can be employed. Because the SASyPUP system is engaged during most of the day while participants are in their wheelchair, a wide range of activities and postures may be interrupted by the weight-shifting stimulation. The VR and gaming applications can allow users to develop and practice strategies that will minimize the potential loss of balance regardless of position or activity in which they are engaged when the weight-shifting cycle begins.

SUMMARY

The use of VR technology to design games with a focus on augmenting traditional rehabilitation interventions will likely play a large part in the future of treatment and training of people aging with and into a disability. More research is required in several areas before this technology can be incorporated into daily life and rehabilitation plans, including a systematic analysis of the characteristics of optimal design and use of VR games in the clinic and home environment, increasing the capacity to conduct interdisciplinary research and knowledge translation in the emerging area of VR and gaming applications for those aging with or into disability, and the effective incorporation of VR and games technology into the clinical setting and proper potential incorporation (through commercialization) of low-cost VR technology in the home environment. In addition to translational research, Adamovich and colleagues[116] suggest a need for future research to follow several important paths. There is a need for imaging studies to evaluate the effects of sensory manipulation on brain activation patterns and the effects of various training parameters on long-term changes in brain function. Larger clinical studies are also needed to establish the efficacy of sensorimotor rehabilitation using VR in various clinical populations and, most importantly, to identify VR training parameters that are associated with optimal transfer to real-world functional improvements. Finally, the application of robust outcome measures across the 3 domains of functioning as defined in the ICF, particularly in the participation domain, is vital for the development of evidence-based guidelines regarding the effectiveness of VR and gaming interventions that could have the potential to impact the local and national agenda for the future.

REFERENCES

1. Steinmetz E. American with disabilities: 2002 current population reports. Washington, DC: U.S. Census Bureau; 2006. p. 70.
2. Experience C. Fact sheet on aging in America. Washington, DC: Experience Corps; 2007. p. 1.
3. Ochsner KN, Lieberman MD. The emergence of social cognitive neuroscience. Am Psychol 2001;56:717.
4. Galvin R, Cusack T, Stokes E. A randomised controlled trial evaluating family mediated exercise (FAME) therapy following stroke. BMC Neurol 2008;8:22.
5. Vincent C, Deaudelin I, Robichaud L, et al. Rehabilitation needs for older adults with stroke living at home: perceptions of four populations. BMC Geriatr 2007;7:20.
6. Lindenberger U, Lovden M, Schellenbach M, et al. Psychological principles of successful aging technologies: a mini-review. Gerontology 2008;54:59.
7. Baltes PB, Staudinger UM, Lindenberger U. Lifespan psychology: theory and application to intellectual functioning. Annu Rev Psychol 1999;50:471.
8. Mykityshyn AL, Fisk AD, Rogers WA. Learning to use a home medical device: mediating age-related differences with training. Hum Factors 2002;44:354.
9. Mynatt E, Rogers W. Developing technology to support the functional independence of older adults. Ageing Int 2002;27:24.
10. Pew RW, Van Hemel SB, National Research Council (U.S.). Steering Committee for the Workshop on Technology for Adaptive Aging, et al. Technology for adaptive aging. Washington, DC: National Academies Press; 2004.
11. Helal AA, Mokhtari M, Abdulrazak B. The engineering handbook of smart technology for aging, disability, and independence. Hoboken (NJ): John Wiley; 2008.
12. WHO. International Classification of Functioning, Disability and Health (ICF). New York: World Health Organization (WHO); 2001.

13. Rejeski WJ, Ip EH, Marsh AP, et al. Measuring disability in older adults: the International Classification System of Functioning, Disability and Health (ICF) framework. Geriatr Gerontol Int 2008;8:48.

14. Jung Y, Yeh SC, McLaughlin M, et al. Three-dimensional game environments for recovery from stroke. In: Ritterfeld U, Cody M, Vorderer P, editors. Serious games: mechanisms and effects. New York: Routledge, Taylor and Francis; 2009. p. 413–28.

15. Krakauer JW. Motor learning: its relevance to stroke recovery and neurorehabilitation. Curr Opin Neurol 2006;19:84.

16. Winstein CJ, Merians AS, Sullivan KJ. Motor learning after unilateral brain damage. Neuropsychologia 1999;37:975.

17. Merians AS, Jack D, Boian R, et al. Virtual reality-augmented rehabilitation for patients following stroke. Phys Ther 2002;82:898.

18. Shaw SE, Morris DM, Uswatte G, et al. Constraint-induced movement therapy for recovery of upper-limb function following traumatic brain injury. J Rehabil Res Dev 2005;42:769.

19. Merians AS, Poizner H, Boian R, et al. Sensorimotor training in a virtual reality environment: does it improve functional recovery poststroke? Neurorehabil Neural Repair 2006;20:252.

20. Merians AS, Tunik E, Adamovich SV. Virtual reality to maximize function for hand and arm rehabilitation: exploration of neural mechanisms. Stud Health Technol Inform 2009;145:109.

21. Merians AS, Tunik E, Fluet GG, et al. Innovative approaches to the rehabilitation of upper extremity hemiparesis using virtual environments. Eur J Phys Rehabil Med 2009;45:123.

22. Huberty J, Ransdell L, Sidman C, et al. Explaining long-term exercise adherence in women who complete a structured exercise program. Res Q Exerc Sport 2008;79:374.

23. Huberty JL, Vener J, Sidman C, et al. Women bound to be active: a pilot study to explore the feasibility of an intervention to increase physical activity and self-worth in women. Womens Health 2008;48:83.

24. Bach-y-Rita P. Conceptual issues relevant to present and future neurologic rehabilitation. New York: Oxford University Press; 2000.

25. Ferguson J, Trombly C. The effect of added-purpose and meaningful occupation on motor learning. Am J Occup Ther 1997;51:508.

26. Wood S, Murillo N, Bach-y-Rita P, et al. Motivating, game-based stroke rehabilitation: a brief report. Top Stroke Rehabil 2003;10:134.

27. Heim M. Virtual realism. New York: Oxford University Press; 1998.

28. Gobbetti E, Scateni R. Virtual reality: past, present and future. In: Riva G, Weiderhold BK, Molinari E, editors, Virtual environments in clinical psychology and neuroscience: methods and techniques in advances patient-therapist interaction, vol. 58. Amsterdam: IOS; 1998. p. 3.

29. Burdea GC. Virtual rehabilitation—benefits and challenges. Methods Inf Med 2003;42:519.

30. McCloy R, Stone R. Science, medicine, and the future: virtual reality in surgery. BMJ 2001;323:912.

31. Ungs TJ. Simulator induced syndrome: evidence for long-term aftereffects. Aviat Space Environ Med 1989;60:252.

32. Rizzo A, Pair J, McNerney PJ, et al. Development of a VR therapy application for Iraq war military personnel with PTSD. Stud Health Technol Inform 2005;111:407.

33. Rizzo A, Schultheis M, Kerns K, et al. Analysis of assets for virtual reality applications in neuropsychology. Neuropsychol Rehabil 2004;14:207.
34. Stewart JC, Yeh SC, Jung Y, et al. Intervention to enhance skilled arm and hand movements after stroke: a feasibility study using a new virtual reality system. J Neuroeng Rehabil 2007;4:21.
35. Crosbie JH, Lennon S, McNeill MD, et al. Virtual reality in the rehabilitation of the upper limb after stroke: the user's perspective. Cyberpsychol Behav 2006;9:137.
36. Dvorkin AY, Shahar M, Weiss PL. Reaching within video-capture virtual reality: using virtual reality as a motor control paradigm. Cyberpsychol Behav 2006;9:133.
37. Sanchez RJ, Liu J, Rao S, et al. Automating arm movement training following severe stroke: functional exercises with quantitative feedback in a gravity-reduced environment. IEEE Trans Neural Syst Rehabil Eng 2006;14:378.
38. Adamovich SV, Merians AS, Boian R, et al. A virtual reality based exercise system for hand rehabilitation post-stroke: transfer to function. Conf Proc IEEE Eng Med Biol Soc 2004;7:4936.
39. Boian R, Sharma A, Han C, et al. Virtual reality-based post-stroke hand rehabilitation. Stud Health Technol Inform 2002;85:64.
40. Broeren J, Rydmark M, Sunnerhagen KS. Virtual reality and haptics as a training device for movement rehabilitation after stroke: a single-case study. Arch Phys Med Rehabil 2004;85:1247.
41. Baram Y, Miller A. Virtual reality cues for improvement of gait in patients with multiple sclerosis. Neurology 2006;66:178.
42. Fung J, Malouin F, McFadyen BJ, et al. Locomotor rehabilitation in a complex virtual environment. Conf Proc IEEE Eng Med Biol Soc 2004;7:4859.
43. Riva G. Virtual reality in paraplegia: a VR-enhanced orthopaedic appliance for walking and rehabilitation. Stud Health Technol Inform 1998;58:209.
44. Holden MK. Virtual environments for motor rehabilitation: review. Cyberpsychol Behav 2005;8:187.
45. Lange B, Flynn SM, Rizzo AA. Game-based telerehabilitation. Eur J Phys Rehabil Med 2009;45:143.
46. SharpBrains. The state of the brain fitness software market. San Francisco: SharpBrains; 2009.
47. Mahncke HW, Bronstone A, Merzenich MM. Brain plasticity and functional losses in the aged: scientific bases for a novel intervention. Prog Brain Res 2006;157:81.
48. Mahncke HW, Connor BB, Appelman J, et al. Memory enhancement in healthy older adults using a brain plasticity-based training program: a randomized, controlled study. Proc Natl Acad Sci U S A 2006;103:12523.
49. Goldstein J, Cajko L, Oosterbroek M, et al. Video games and the elderly. Soc Behav Pers 1997;25:345.
50. Dustman RE, Emmerson RY, Steinhaus LA, et al. The effects of videogame playing on neuropsychological performance of elderly individuals. J Gerontol 1992;47:168.
51. Clark JE, Lanphear AK, Riddick CC. The effects of videogame playing on the response selection processing of elderly adults. J Gerontol 1987;42:82.
52. Farris M, Bates R, Resnick H, et al, editors. Evaluation of computer games' impact upon cognitively impaired frail elderly. (Electronic tools for social work practice and education). Haworth (UK): Haworth Press; 1994. p. 219–28.
53. Drew B, Waters J. Video games: utilization of a novel strategy to improve perceptual motor skills and cognitive functioning in the noninstitutionalized elderly. Cognit Rehabil 1986;4:26.

54. Weisman S. Computer games for the frail elderly. Gerontologist 1983;23:361.
55. McGuire FA. Improving the quality of life for residents of long term care facilities through Video games. Activities, Adaptation & Aging 1984;6:1.
56. Lange BS, Flynn SM, Rizzo AR. Initial usability assessment of off-the-shelf video game consoles for clinical game-based motor rehabilitation. Physical therapy reviews: special issue on virtual reality and rehabilitation. Phys Ther Rev 2009; 14(5):355–63.
57. Massion J. Postural control system. Curr Opin Neurobiol 1994;4:877.
58. Massion J. Movement, posture and equilibrium: interaction and coordination. Prog Neurobiol 1992;38:35.
59. Massion J. Postural changes accompanying voluntary movements. Normal and pathological aspects. Hum Neurobiol 1984;2:261.
60. Brauer SG, Woollacott M, Shumway-Cook A. The interacting effects of cognitive demand and recovery of postural stability in balance-impaired elderly persons. J Gerontol A Biol Sci Med Sci 2001;56:M489.
61. Dietz V, Zijlstra W, Assaiante C, et al. Balance control in Parkinson's disease. Gait Posture 1993;1(2):77–84.
62. Woollacott M, Inglin B, Manchester D. Response preparation and posture control. Neuromuscular changes in the older adult. Ann N Y Acad Sci 1988; 515:42.
63. Flynn S, Palma P, Bender A. Feasibility of using the Sony PlayStation 2 gaming platform for an individual poststroke: a case report. J Neurol Phys Ther 2007;31:180.
64. Rand D, Kizony R, Weiss PT. The Sony PlayStation II EyeToy: low-cost virtual reality for use in rehabilitation. J Neurol Phys Ther 2008;32:155.
65. Sherrington C, Whitney JC, Lord SR, et al. Effective exercise for the prevention of falls: a systematic review and meta-analysis. J Am Geriatr Soc 2008;56:2234.
66. Hui E, Chui BT, Woo J. Effects of dance on physical and psychological well-being in older persons. Arch Gerontol Geriatr 2009;49:e45.
67. Shigematsu R, Chang M, Yabushita N, et al. Dance-based aerobic exercise may improve indices of falling risk in older women. Age Ageing 2002;31:261.
68. Hopkins DR, Murrah B, Hoeger WW, et al. Effect of low-impact aerobic dance on the functional fitness of elderly women. Gerontologist 1990;30:189.
69. De Lucia R, Martin-Dominguez E. Biomechanics of the Caribbean dance: a preliminary study. Dance Ther Sport Med 1997;17:7.
70. Hindery R. Japanese video game helps people stay fit and lose weight. New York: Associated Press AP Worldstream; 2005.
71. Tan B, Aziz AR, Chua K, et al. Aerobic demands of the dance simulation game. Int J Sports Med 2002;23:125.
72. Unnithan VB, Houser W, Fernhall B. Evaluation of the energy cost of playing a dance simulation video game in overweight and nonoverweight children and adolescents. Int J Sports Med 2006;27:804.
73. Kaye HS, Kang T, LaPlante MP. Wheelchair use in the United States. Washington, DC: National Institute on Disability and Rehabilitation Research; 2002. p. 1.
74. Kemp B, Thompson L. Aging and spinal cord injury: medical, functional, and psychosocial changes. SCI Nurs 2002;19:51.
75. Bayley JC, Cochran TP, Sledge CB. The weight-bearing shoulder. The impingement syndrome in paraplegics. J Bone Joint Surg Am 1987;69:676.
76. Dalyan M, Cardenas DD, Gerard B. Upper extremity pain after spinal cord injury. Spinal Cord 1999;37:191.
77. Nichols PJ, Norman PA, Ennis JR. Wheelchair user's shoulder? Shoulder pain in patients with spinal cord lesions. Scand J Rehabil Med 1979;11:29.

78. Wing PC, Tredwell SJ. The weightbearing shoulder. Paraplegia 1983;21:107.
79. Sie IH, Waters RL, Adkins RH, et al. Upper extremity pain in the postrehabilitation spinal cord injured patient. Arch Phys Med Rehabil 1992;73:44.
80. Gutierrez DD, Thompson L, Kemp B, et al. The relationship of shoulder pain intensity to quality of life, physical activity, and community participation in persons with paraplegia. J Spinal Cord Med 2007;30:251.
81. Burnham RS, May L, Nelson E, et al. Shoulder pain in wheelchair athletes. The role of muscle imbalance. Am J Sports Med 1993;21:238.
82. Curtis KA, Roach KE, Applegate EB, et al. Reliability and validity of the Wheelchair User's Shoulder Pain Index (WUSPI). Paraplegia 1995;33:595.
83. Curtis KA, Roach KE, Applegate EB, et al. Development of the Wheelchair User's Shoulder Pain Index (WUSPI). Paraplegia 1995;33:290.
84. Mulroy SJ, Farrokhi S, Newsam CJ, et al. Effects of spinal cord injury level on the activity of shoulder muscles during wheelchair propulsion: an electromyographic study. Arch Phys Med Rehabil 2004;85:925–34.
85. Curtis KA, Tyner TM, Zachary L, et al. Effect of a standard exercise protocol on shoulder pain in long-term wheelchair users. Spinal Cord 1999;37:421.
86. Nash MS, van de Ven I, van Elk N, et al. Effects of circuit resistance training on fitness attributes and upper-extremity pain in middle-aged men with paraplegia. Arch Phys Med Rehabil 2007;88:70.
87. Nawoczenski DA, Ritter-Soronen JM, Wilson CM, et al. Clinical trial of exercise for shoulder pain in chronic spinal injury. Phys Ther 2006;86:1604.
88. Cunningham D, Krishack M. Virtual reality: a holistic approach to rehabilitation. Stud Health Technol Inform 1999;62:90.
89. Nelson DL, Konosky K, Fleharty K, et al. The effects of an occupationally embedded exercise on bilaterally assisted supination in persons with hemiplegia. Am J Occup Ther 1996;50:639.
90. O'Connor TJ, Cooper RA, Fitzgerald SG, et al. Evaluation of a manual wheelchair interface to computer games. Neurorehabil Neural Repair 2000;14:21.
91. O'Connor TJ, Fitzgerald SG, Cooper RA, et al. Does computer game play aid in motivation of exercise and increase metabolic activity during wheelchair ergometry? Med Eng Phys 2001;23:267.
92. O'Connor TJ, Fitzgerald SG, Cooper RA, et al. Kinetic and physiological analysis of the GAME(Wheels) system. J Rehabil Res Dev 2002;39:627.
93. Fitzgerald SG, Cooper RA, Thorman T, et al. The GAME(Cycle) exercise system: comparison with standard ergometry. J Spinal Cord Med 2004;27:453.
94. Tubiana R. The hand, vol. 3. Philadelphia: WB Saunders; 1981.
95. McKenzie C, Iberall T, editors. The grasping hand (advances in psychology). Amsterdam: North-Holland; 1994. p. 15–42.
96. Brand P, Hollester A. Clinical mechanics of the hand, vol. 3. St Louis: Mosby Year-book, Inc; 1999. p. 2–6.
97. Green DP, Hotchkiss RN, Pederson WC, et al. Green's operative hand surgery, vol. 1–2. 4th edition. Philadelphia: Churchill Livingstone, 1999.
98. Valero-Cuevas FJ. An integrative approach to the biomechanical function and neuromuscular control of the fingers. J Biomech 2005;38:673–84.
99. Kandel E, Schwartz J, Jessell T. Principles of neural science. New York: McGraw-Hill; 2000.
100. Valero-Cuevas FJ, Smaby N, Venkadesan M, et al. The strength-dexterity test as a measure of dynamic pinch performance. J Biomech 2003;36:265.
101. Murray R, Li Z, Sastry S. A mathematical introduction to robotic manipulation. Boca Raton (FL): CRC; 1994.

102. Brewer BR, Klatzky R, Matsuoka Y. Visual feedback distortion in a robotic environment for hand rehabilitation. Brain Res Bull 2008;75:804.
103. Szturm T, Peters JF, Otto C, et al. Task-specific rehabilitation of finger-hand function using interactive computer gaming. Arch Phys Med Rehabil 2008;89:2213.
104. Yarkony GM. Pressure ulcers: a review. Arch Phys Med Rehabil 1994;75:908.
105. National Pressure Ulcer Advisory Panel Board of Director. Prevalence, incidence and implications for the future: an executive summary of the National Pressure Ulcer Advisory Panel Monograph. Adv Skin Wound Care 2001;14:208–15.
106. National Decubitis Foundation. Cost savings through bedsore avoidance. Aurora (CO): National Decubitus Foundation; 2006.
107. Disa JJ, Carlton JM, Goldberg NH. Efficacy of operative cure in pressure sore patients. Plast Reconstr Surg 1992;89:272.
108. Krause JS. Skin sores after spinal cord injury: relationship to life adjustment. Spinal Cord 1998;36:51.
109. Clark F, Rubayi S, Jackson J, et al. The role of daily activities in pressure ulcer development. Adv Skin Wound Care 2001;14:52.
110. Clark FA, Jackson JM, Scott MD, et al. Data-based models of how pressure ulcers develop in daily-living contexts of adults with spinal cord injury. Arch Phys Med Rehabil 2006;87:1516.
111. Dunn CA, Carlson M, Jackson JM, et al. Response factors surrounding progression of pressure ulcers in community-residing adults with spinal cord injury. Am J Occup Ther 2009;63:301.
112. Baker LL, Eberly V, Rakoski D. Preliminary experience with implanted microstimulators for management of post-stroke impairments. J Neurol Phys Ther 2006;30.
113. Baker LL, Palmer E, Waters RL, et al. Rehabilitation of the arm and hand following stroke—a clinical trial with BIONs. Conf Proc IEEE Eng Med Biol Soc 2004;6:4186.
114. Dupont Salter AC, Bagg S, Creasy J, et al. First clinical experience with BION implants for therapeutic electrical stimulation. Neuromodulation 2004;38:38.
115. Richmond FJR, Baker LL, Winstein C, et al. A modular approach to retraining muscles after stroke. Procceding at the 9th Annual Meeting of the International Functional Electrical Stimulation Society. Bournemouth, UK, September 6–9, 2004.
116. Adamovich SV, Fluet GG, Tunik E, et al. Sensorimotor training in virtual reality: a review. NeuroRehabilitation 2009;25:29.

Falls, Aging, and Disability

Marcia L. Finlayson, OT, PhD, OTR/L*,
Elizabeth W. Peterson, PhD, MPH, OTR/L

KEYWORDS

- Accidental falls • Risk factors • Fall prevention
- Aging • Chronic illness

Falls are a major public health problem. In the United States, falls are the leading cause of injury deaths for adults over age 65 and the most common cause of nonfatal injuries and hospital admissions for traumatic injuries.[1] Nonfatal fall injuries are associated loss of independence[2] as well as significant use of health care services.[3] By 2020, the combined direct and indirect costs of injurious falls among people over the age of 65 are expected to exceed $54.2 billion dollars in the United States.[4]

A fall is an unexpected event during which the individual comes to rest on the ground, floor, or lower level,[5] typically during the performance of basic daily activities (eg, walking, getting up from a chair, bending down).[6,7] To date, most falls-related research has focused on older community-dwelling adults. Only recently have researchers started to study falls among adults and older adults with chronic illness or existing physical disability.

The purposes of this article are to summarize and then compare (1) fall prevalence rates, (2) fall risk factors, (3) consequences of falls, and (4) current knowledge about fall prevention interventions between community-dwelling older adults and people aging with physical disability. In this latter group, the article focuses on individuals with multiple sclerosis (MS), late effects of polio, muscular dystrophies, and spinal cord injuries. These groups have been selected because they are the target populations for the work currently being conducted through the Rehabilitation Research and Training Center on Aging with Physical Disability, based at the University of Washington at Seattle. To locate falls-related information on these populations, a MEDLINE search was conducted using the index term "accidental falls" in combination with one of the following index terms: "multiple sclerosis," "postpoliomyelitis syndrome," "muscular dystrophies," or "spinal cord injuries."

PREVALENCE OF FALLS
Prevalence of Falls Among Community-Dwelling Older Adults

Approximately 30% of community-dwelling adults aged 65 years or older fall each year.[8,9] Among individuals aged over 75 years, the proportion increases to

Department of Occupational Therapy, University of Illinois at Chicago, 1919 West Taylor Street, Mail Code 811, Chicago, IL 60612-7250, USA
* Corresponding author
E-mail address: marciaf@uic.edu

Phys Med Rehabil Clin N Am 21 (2010) 357–373
doi:10.1016/j.pmr.2009.12.003
1047-9651/10/$ – see front matter © 2010 Elsevier Inc. All rights reserved.

pmr.theclinics.com

50%.[10,11] Based on data from the 2006 Behavioral Risk Factor Surveillance System (BRFSS) survey, which was drawn from interviews involving 92,808 persons aged 65 years or older, Stevens and colleagues[12] found that approximately 5.8 million (almost 16%) of people aged 65 years or older reported falling at least once during the preceding 3 months. Recurrent falls are common. For example, in one study conducted over a 48-week period, researchers followed 409 community-dwelling persons aged 65 years or more and found that 11.5% fell two or more times.[13]

Prevalence of Falls Among People Aging with Physical Disability

MS
Rates of falls have been reported in three cross-sectional studies[14–16] and one longitudinal study[7] of people with MS. In one of the cross-sectional studies, an Italian research team found 54% of 50 participants (20 from the community, 30 from an extended care ward) reported at least one fall in the previous 2 months, and 32% of these fallers experienced recurrent falls. The average age of the fallers was 40 years (SD = 11). The other two cross-sectional studies were conducted by a US research team. In one of their studies, the researchers found 52% of 1089 participants aged 45 to 90 years from the Midwest had experienced a fall over the previous six-month period.[16] Using a national US sample, this same research team reported that 64% of 354 study participants, aged 55 to 94 years, reported at least two falls per year. Of these individuals, 30% reported falling once a month or more.[15]

The longitudinal study was conducted in Sweden with 76 participants, ranging in age from 25 to 75 years.[7] Falls data were collected prospectively over 9 months. In this period, 63% (48 of 76) of participants reported at least one fall. Among the fallers, 32 participants fell two times or more, and 11 fell 10 times or more. A total of 2352 near-fall incidents were reported across the study period.[7]

Late effects of polio
Two cross-sectional studies were identified that reported on fall prevalence rates among people with late effects of polio. In the first study, an Australian team reported prevalence of falling among 40 people with prior polio, who had an average age of 50.7 years. Of these individuals, 47.5% reported falling three or more times in the previous year, and an additional 20% reported falling twice. The remaining participants either experienced a single fall or no falls at all (not reported separately).[17] In the second study, a US team reported that 84% of 172 survey respondents experienced a fall over the previous year. Average participant age was not reported, although the median age of post-polio syndrome onset was 48 years.[18]

Muscular dystrophies
Only one study was located that reported fall prevalence rates among adults with a form of muscular dystrophy.[19] In this study, 13 adults with myotonic dystrophy, with a mean age of 46.5 years (SD = 1.68), reported retrospectively on falls and also monitored falls prospectively for 13 weeks. Retrospectively, 5 of 13 (38%) participants reported that they fell and injured themselves more than once in the past 6 months. Over the prospective monitoring period, 10 of 13 (77%) participants experienced a total of 127 stumbles, and 6 of 13 (46%) participants experienced a total of 34 falls. On average, participants experienced a total of 12.2 events over the 13 weeks (falls and stumbles combined).[19]

Spinal cord injuries
Only one study was located that reported the prevalence of falling among people with spinal cord injury. In this retrospective survey study, 75% of 119 individuals with

incomplete spinal cord injury (average age 52.2 years), reported falling in the past year.[20]

Summary and Comparison

Although the time periods considered across the studies reported in this section vary from 2 months to 1 year, findings suggest that the fall rates are considerably higher among people aging with physical disability compared with community-dwelling older adults aged 65 years and over. From the findings reported here, it appears that in some cases, the fall rates of people aging with physical disability may be double that of their community-dwelling older adult peers. Even if one considers only the fall rates among community-dwelling older adults 75 years and older, the rates for people aging with physical disability are still often greater.

FALL RISK FACTORS

Research to identify risk factors for falls has been fairly consistent in showing that most falls result from multiple, interacting factors.[21] Fall risk factors typically are classified as intrinsic (within-subject) or extrinsic.[22] Overall, balanced attention to both intrinsic and extrinsic risk factors is warranted, because the interaction between a person's physical abilities and his or her exposure to environmental stressors appears to influence fall risk.[23]

Fall Risks Among Community-Dwelling Older Adults

To date, epidemiologic research to inform fall prevention efforts among community-dwelling older adults has focused heavily on intrinsic fall risk factors. This research has led to understanding of both modifiable and nonmodifiable fall risk factors, and the realization that the risk of falling increases dramatically as the number of risk factors increases.[8,24] For community-dwelling older adults, nonmodifiable risk factors include being female, having a history of falls, and higher age.[22,25,26] Several cohort studies have identified gait and balance disorders, functional impairment, visual deficits, and cognitive impairment as the most important intrinsic risk factors for falling.[8,27–29] Often, these risk factors are modifiable.

Data from a prospective cohort study of community-dwelling older adults (n = 1285) that was undertaken to construct a fall-risk model suggest that key risk factors for men and women may differ.[27] Findings indicated that previous falls and visual impairment were the strongest predictors for women (area under curve = .66), whereas previous falls, visual impairment, urinary incontinence, functional limitations, and low level of physical activity were the strongest predictors for men (area under curve = .74). Other research has suggested that psychosocial risk factors, including depressive symptoms,[30] fear of falling (ie, a lasting concern about falling that leads an individual to avoid activities that he/she remains capable of performing)[31] and low falls self-efficacy (ie, perceived self-efficacy or confidence to avoid falls during essential, nonhazardous activities of daily living)[32] also may place community dwelling older adults at increased risk for falls. Growing evidence suggests that fear of falling and low falls-self efficacy are experienced by both fallers and nonfallers.[33,34]

With respect to extrinsic fall risk factors for community-dwelling older adults, polypharmacy (ie, four or more medications) and certain classes of drugs, especially psychotropic medications, increase the risk of fall.[35–37] Although home hazards have received wide attention as an extrinsic fall risk factor, no consistent association has been found between common household hazards and falls in several prospective studies.[8,24,38–40] Current thinking suggests that most falls in the home result from an interaction between environmental stressors and physical abilities or risk-taking behaviors.[23] Furthermore, hazards in the home may not present equal risk to all older adults. Findings from secondary analyses of data from two prospective studies suggest that environmental hazards contribute to falls to a greater extent in older vigorous people than in older frail people.[41,42]

Fall Risk Factors Among People Aging with Physical Disability

Multiple sclerosis

Three studies were identified that examined risk factors for falls among people with MS, two cross-sectional ones[14,16] and one longitudinal.[7] With the exception of the large study by Finlayson and colleagues,[16] which used self-report through telephone interviews, the other studies used a combination of self-report instruments and performance-based evaluations. The variability in sample size, age range, study designs, data collection methods, and time periods examined may explain the variability in fall risk factors identified across these studies (**Table 1**). Despite the variability in findings, several consistencies are noteworthy.

All studies found that mobility devices were in some way associated with falling. Cattaneo and colleagues[14] found that more fallers used a cane than nonfallers, and Nilsågard and colleagues[7] found that individuals who used walking aids either indoors or out had double the risk of a fall compared with those who used no walking aid. Compared with people who always used a wheelchair for mobility, Finlayson and colleagues[16] found that never users and sometimes users had approximately two times greater risk of a fall. Together with other findings regarding balance and ambulation across these studies, it is clear that further investigation of role of mobility device use in fall risk is warranted. Although the findings simply may reflect that mobility

Table 1
Summary of findings regarding fall risk factors among people with MS

Factors Increasing the Likelihood of Reporting the Dependent Variable	Fall in the Past 2 Months[a,14]	Fall in the Past 6 Months[b,16]	Fall Over 9 Months[c,7]
Age	No	No	No
Gender	No	Being male	Being male
MS status/disability	Not examined	Yes	Yes
Balance	Yes	Yes	No
Cognition	No	Yes	No
Incontinence of bladder	Not examined	Yes	No
Mobility device	Yes	Yes	Yes
Fear of falling	Not examined	Yes	No
Fatigue	Not examined	No	No
Spasticity	No	No	Yes
Disturbed proprioception	Not examined	Not examined	Yes
Ambulation	Yes	Not examined	Yes
ADL abilities	No	Not examined	Not examined

[a] Retrospective recall, cross-sectional design, n = 50.
[b] Retrospective recall, cross-sectional design, n = 1089.
[c] Prospective monitoring, longitudinal design, n = 76.

device users are more disabled, and therefore at greater risk, Finlayson and colleagues[16] also suggest that mobility device decision-making (eg, to use any device, to use a more supportive device under specific circumstances) also may be playing a role.

Other factors that were found to increase risk of a fall in at least two of the studies include being male and MS status/disability. Findings about the role of specific symptoms are variable, and will require further investigation in the future.

Late effects of polio
Only one study was identified that examined risk factors for falls among people previously affected by polio,[17] and it focused primarily on the role of lower extremity strength. The study included 40 people with prior polio and 38 age- and sex-matched controls. To examine predictors of falls within the polio group, researchers divided the group into people experiencing zero falls or one fall in the past year (n = 13), those who fell twice (n = 8), and those who fell multiple times (n = 19). Compared with people who fell twice, the multiple fallers had reduced strength in ankle dorsiflexors, greater lower extremity weakness, slower hand and foot reaction times, slower foot-tapping speed, and increased body sway on a compliant surface under both eyes-open and eyes-closed conditions. Of these differences, the ones with the greatest discriminating power were body sway and composite strength. The authors concluded that weakness has a direct association with falls among people with prior polio, as well as an indirect effect mediated through increased body sway.

Muscular dystrophies
Only one study was identified that examined fall risk factors among people with myotonic dystrophy type 1.[19] The study included 13 people with myotonic dystrophy and 12 healthy volunteers matched for sex, weight, and body mass index. In bivariate analyses, fallers (n = 6) and nonfallers (n = 7) within the myotonic dystrophy group were compared. Findings showed that fallers were more likely to have a lower Rivermead Mobility Index score, more likely to use mobility devices or a person to aid mobility indoors or outdoors, have a slower self-selected gait speed, and higher depression.[19] Although the authors also report regression analysis, the small sample size and large number of variables raise questions about the validity of the findings.

Spinal cord injuries
Only one study was identified that examined fall risk factors among people with spinal cord injury, specifically those with incomplete injury. Using a mail-out survey, researchers gathered information on falls and fall risk factors among 119 people. Three multivariable logistic regression models evaluated differences between fallers and nonfallers.

The first model examined differences in demographic and injury characteristics, and no statistically significant differences were found. The second model examined differences in health-related data, and found that fallers were more likely to

Have had more days of poor physical health in the past year
Have greater numbers of medical conditions
Have arthritis
Experience dizziness
Report lower self-rated health
Report worse health compared with the previous year.

The third model examined differences in physical activity and found that fallers exercised less frequently, were fearful of falling, limited activities because of fear of falling, used a cane (vs not), and used a walker (vs not). When the significant variables from all three models were combined into a final model, the most significant factors associated with a fall among people with incomplete spinal cord injuries were exercising less than 8 times per month and not using a walker.

Summary and Comparison

A surge in fall-related research over the past 10 to 15 years has dramatically enhanced understanding of fall risk factors, particularly among community-dwelling older adults. It is clear that knowledge related to fall risks among people aging with physical disability is lagging far behind. To date, the literature on fall risk factors among people aging with multiple sclerosis, late effects of polio, muscular dystrophies, or spinal cord injuries has not addressed extrinsic risk factors, including the potential role of multiple medication use and home hazards in increasing fall risk. Among intrinsic factors across these four groups, vision has not been investigated, and the evaluation of the role of cognition, fear of falling, falls self-efficacy, depression, and functional status has been inconsistent at best. Future work needs to address these gaps in knowledge, and consider the application of consistent frameworks for organizing thinking about risk factors (eg, intrinsic vs extrinsic, modifiable vs not) and how they interact and build on each other to influence an individual's fall-related risk.

CONSEQUENCES OF FALLS

Overall, the incidence and severity of fall-related consequences increases with age, level of disability, and extent of functional impairment.[43,44] Consequences range from physical, psychological, and broader social impacts.

Consequences of Falls Among Community-Dwelling Older Adults

Consequences of falls among older adults range from loss of confidence and fear of falling[33,34,45] to overt physical injuries, activity curtailment, and deconditioning,[46,47] to the loss of functional ability and, in some cases, the need for supervision or institutionalization,[48,49] to death.[50] For many older adults, a fall can represent the introduction to old age and a decline in quality of life.[51,52]

Physical consequences

Many of the physical consequences of falls among older adults occur as a result of the combination of high incidence and high susceptibility to trauma.[53] Although only about 10% of falls among the elderly result in major injuries,[8,40,54] the effects of injurious falls can be devastating.

Fall-related mortality is high in older adults. Sampalis and colleagues[55] compared mortality between two groups of older adults who were treated at regional Level 1 (tertiary) trauma centers—those who sustained trauma from a fall and those who experienced motor vehicle collision-related injuries. Researchers found that being injured in a fall was a strong predictor for mortality, with an odds ratio (OR) of 5.11 (95% confidence interval [CI] = 1.84 to 14.17, $P = .002$). Furthermore, among individuals at least 65 years of age, falls are the leading cause of head injuries,[56] and a factor in over 90% of fractures of the distal forearm, proximal humerus, and hip.[57]

In 2006, nearly 1.8 million (nearly 5% of all older adults) sustained some type of fall-related injury.[12] Schiller and colleagues[48] found that 32% of older adults who sustained a fall-related injury required help with activities of daily living afterwards. Of these individuals, 58.5% were expected to require help for at least 6 months. Other researchers have observed that fall-induced injuries are one of the most common causes of restricted activity and disability in older adult populations.[47,58]

Psychological consequences

Many older people experience psychological difficulties related to falls. These difficulties often are operationalized as fear of falling and reductions in falls self-efficacy. The concept of falls self-efficacy originally was defined by Tinetti and colleagues,[32] who developed the Falls Efficacy Scale. When introduced, the Falls Efficacy Scale was intended as a measure of fear of falling; however, evidence now suggests that falls self-efficacy and fear of falling are separate constructs[59] and that falls self-efficacy may act as a mediator to reduce fear of falling.[60]

Overall, the etiology of fear of falling and falls self-efficacy is not understood well. Two qualitative studies among community-dwelling older adults have explored the nature of fear of falling and provide some insights regarding the development of this fear. Tischler and Hobson[61] and Lee and colleauges[62] found that fear of falling is expressed as fear of losing independence or becoming dependent upon others. It also was experienced as fear of physical injury, fear of being unable to get up or get help after a fall, fear of being institutionalized, and fear of bring confined to a wheelchair or unable to walk.[61]

Prospective research involving community-dwelling older adults suggests that people who are afraid of falling or who have low falls-self-efficacy enter a debilitating spiral characterized by restriction of physical activities and social participation, physical frailty, falls, and loss of independence.[33,34,45] For these reasons, fear of falling and low falls self-efficacy are critical to understanding falls among older adults and considering the potential consequences of a fall experience.

Consequences of Falls Among People Aging with Physical Disability

Rates of fatal falls in the United States are rising for white men and women aged greater than or equal to 45 years and in black and Asian women aged greater than or equal to 65 years.[50] The increase has been attributed partially to a greater proportion of older adults living with chronic diseases, which leave them at greater risk for falling and less likely to survive the injuries resulting from a fall.[63] Despite this knowledge, there is a remarkable lack of documentation about the consequences of falls among people aging with multiple sclerosis, late effects of polio, muscular dystrophy, or spinal cord injury. Across all four conditions, four papers were found that explicitly addressed the physical consequences of falls.[15,64–66] Three others discuss the issues of fear of falling and activity curtailment.[18,65,67] Both of these issues have been identified as psychological consequences of falls in the literature on community-dwelling older adults.

Physical consequences

The studies of fall-related injuries have examined middle-aged and older adults with MS (age 55 to 94 years),[15] people with incomplete spinal cord injury (average age of 51.6 years),[65] and veterans with spinal cord injuries (average age at time of fall 57 years).[64] In the first two studies, injury data as a consequence of a fall were self-reported. The study of veterans was based on retrospective chart review over a 10-year period. Another study of fatal accidents among people with MS in Denmark included analysis of fall-related deaths.[66]

In an interview study, a total of 177 of 354 (50%) of people with MS reported fall-related injuries that required medical attention, with 41 of these individuals doing so in the 6 months before the interview.[15] Injuries sustained included fractures, soft tissue injuries (eg, bruises, sprains), lacerations requiring stitches, and head injuries. Across the 177 individuals, 12 hip fractures, 40 lower extremity fractures (not including hip), and 28 other fractures were reported. In multivariable analysis, only two factors increased the risk of a recent injurious fall: fear of falling (OR = 1.94, 95% CI = 1.27 to 2.96) and osteoporosis (OR = 1.65, 95% CI = 1.03 to 2.62).[15]

Among people with spinal cord injuries, two studies address fall-related injuries. In the first study, 89 of 119 (75%) individuals with incomplete spinal cord injuries reported experiencing at least one fall in the previous year, and 18% (n = 16) of fallers sustained a fracture as a result. Other reported injuries included soft tissue injuries (eg, bruises, cuts, scrapes), strains or sprains, dislocations, and loss of consciousness. Overall, 32 people required medical attention for their injuries.[65] In another study of people with spinal cord injuries, fall-related fractures were identified through a retrospective chart review of records from a Veteran's Health Administration orthopedic department.[64] Over a 10-year period, 45 people sustained a fracture, and 24 of these were the consequence of a fall (53%). These 24 individuals represented 2.7% of the population of spinal cord patients from the center (n = 889). Thirty-one fractures were reported, with four people experiencing two fractures each. In all four cases, both fractures occurred in the lower extremities. All but one of the fractures occurred in the lower extremity; the remaining one was of the seventh rib. Tibia and/or fibula fractures accounted for 55% of the lower extremity fractures.[64]

The most extreme consequence of a fall is death. This physical consequence was examined in one study that linked data from the Danish Multiple Sclerosis Registry to the Cause of Death Registry (1953 to 1996). Information was obtained about 10,174 people with MS. Standardized mortality ratios were calculated for several types of fatal accidents, including falls. Across the time period, 76 people with MS died from an accident; 17 of these accidents were falls. Although the researchers found that the overall risk of death from an accident was higher for people with MS compared with the general population, the risk for falls was elevated but not statistically significant (standardized mortality ratios = 1.29).[66]

Psychological consequences

In addition to injuries, the 89 people with partial spinal cord injury in the study by Brotherton and colleagues[65] also reported high levels of restricted activity as a consequence of their fall experience. For example, 45% of fallers restricted getting out into the community; 46% restricted productive activities, and 35% restricted social interactions.[65] In study of 1064 people aging with MS (aged 45 to 90 years), cross-sectional data indicated that fear of falling and activity curtailment associated with fear of falling were very prevalent. Overall, 64% reported fear of falling,[67] and among those with fear of falling, 83% curtailed activities because of their fear.[67] Individuals who reported fear of falling were more likely to have had a fall in the 6 months before their interview (OR = 1.38, 95% CI = 1.03 to 1.86).

One study has examined fear of falling among people with postpolio syndrome,[18] although no analyses were reported about the association between fear of falling and actual falls experiences. Nevertheless, 95% of 172 people reported fear of falling. Fear of falling negatively affected quality of life and contributed to activity restriction among 80% and 82% of respondents, respectively. Fear of falling affected participants the most when they were tired, when they were outside, and when they felt weak.[18]

Summary and Comparison

Research on the consequences of falls among community-dwelling older adults has examined a broad range of physical and psychological consequences. To date, very little has been documented about the consequences of falls among people aging with physical disability. In fact, no articles were found about the consequences of falls among people aging with muscular dystrophy, and the paper on fear of falling among people with late effects of polio did not directly examine whether this fear was associated with actual fall experiences. Risk of mortality from falls only has been documented in one study of people with MS.[66] Other consequences that may occur as a result of an accidental fall such as activity curtailment, deconditioning, need for supervision, or institutionalization have not been documented for people aging with MS, late effects of polio, muscular dystrophy, and spinal cord injury. Given the prevalence of these consequences among community-dwelling older adults, examination of these consequences among people aging with physical disability is warranted, especially because their disease processes and related secondary conditions are likely to compromise their bone strength or ability to recover from injury.

FALL PREVENTION INTERVENTIONS
Fall Prevention Interventions Among Community-Dwelling Older Adults

Prevention of falls and injuries has been a major focus of research over the past 10–15 years, and there are now more than 100 high-quality randomized trials that offer strong evidence that falls can be prevented among community-dwelling older adults. The recent Cochrane review[68] provides a useful framework for organizing these interventions. A single intervention consists of only one major type of intervention that is delivered to all participants (eg, exercise programs, withdrawal of some types of drugs for improving sleep, reducing anxiety and treating depression, cataract surgery, and pacemaker insertion). Multiple interventions consist of a fixed combination of two or more major types of intervention delivered to all participants (eg, exercise plus home safety education). Multifactorial interventions include several types of interventions, but participants receive different combinations of interventions based on an individual assessment of fall risk.

Meta-analyses of clinical trials have concluded that both single interventions and multiple interventions are effective in preventing falls among community-dwelling older adults.[68,69] The meta-analysis conducted by Gillespie and colleagues[68] concluded that multifactorial interventions do reduce rate (as opposed to risk) of falls in older people living in the community. Across the existing body of knowledge, it appears that many effective fall prevention programs share common features, including:

Completing a comprehensive home assessment,[70–72]
Using an environment–person approach that considers the interactions among personal capacities, behaviors, and environment[72,73]
Providing assistance in mitigating identified hazards[70–72]
Providing follow-up visits or contacts as part of the intervention. Intensity seems to have a direct influence on the effectiveness of interventions. The more effective interventions also include a maintenance or follow-up phase.[71,72,74,75]
Raising awareness of fall safety principles and generalization of that knowledge to other situations.[72,75]

There are several notable examples of multiple interventions focused on fall prevention, which provide excellent illustrations of how the previously mentioned recommendations can be incorporated into a program. Both the Stepping On program[75] and the Matter of Balance program[76] are multiple interventions that incorporate a self-management approach in their delivery.

Both programs are structured group interventions that use the group process as a mechanism to provide emotional support to participants as they explore their concerns about falls and build fall prevention skills. Both programs also use experiential activities to encourage participants to explore and practice safer ways to accomplish valued activities that expose them to some fall risk. The programs emphasize the importance of building relationships with health care providers and using assertive communication skills to get medical (and other) needs met, as needed.

For multifactorial fall prevention interventions, members of the American Geriatrics Society/British Geriatrics Society Expert Panel on Fall Prevention[77] recommended (based on literature review) that the following components be included, as indicated by individual risk factor assessment:

Environmental assessment and adaptation conducted by a health care professional
Balance training, resistive (strengthening) exercises, and gait training
Reductions in psychoactive medications and other medications
Management of vision problems
Management of postural hypotension and other cardiovascular and medical problems.

The *ABLE* program provides an illustration of some of these recommendations and also incorporates a self-management perspective. This multifactorial, home-based intervention targeting community-dwelling older adults (aged 70 years and older) with chronic conditions had two primary objectives: (1) reduce functional difficulties, fear of falling, and home hazards, and (2) enhance self-efficacy and adaptive coping.[78] Two of the outcomes of interest were fear of falling and home hazards. The 6-month intervention consisted of five occupational therapy contacts (four 90-minute visits, one 20-minute telephone contact) and one physical therapy visit (90 minutes).[78] Using a randomized trial, several positive findings were observed, including reduced fear of falling, reduced home hazards, and enhanced adaptive coping (eg, home modifications).[78,79] The program also positively influenced mortality. People who received the intervention gained an average of 3.5 years of lifespan.[80]

Fall Prevention Interventions for People Aging with Physical Disability

The evidence to support fall prevention interventions for people who are aging with multiple sclerosis, late effects of polio, muscular dystrophies, or spinal cord injuries is only beginning to be developed. A search of MEDLINE was unable to identify any interventions for people with late effects of polio, muscular dystrophy, or spinal cord injuries that explicitly targeted reduction in accidental falls. Although several single interventions were located that could be hypothesized to reduce fall risk (eg, exercise interventions, balance retraining), falls were not an evaluated outcome. One notable exception is a balance exercise program for people with MS that recently was published by an Italian research team.[81] In this study, 44 people with MS, with an average age of 46 years (SD = 10.2), were allocated randomly to one of three groups—a balance retaining program to improve motor and sensory strategies, a task-oriented balance retraining program to improve motor strategies, or a conventional therapy program not specifically aimed at improving balance. Falls were one of the primary study outcomes and were experienced frequently by the participants (all groups) before intervention. Upon conclusion of the intervention (frequency and duration not specified), all three groups experienced a significant decline in fall rates. Both groups 1 and 2 experienced significant improvement in balance, and group 1 improved in dynamic gait.

One example of a multiple intervention was identified for middle aged and older adults with MS.[82] The Safe at Home BAASE program was developed using knowledge of fall risk in MS,[15,16,67] evidence supporting fall prevention with other populations,[83] and the input of an international work group. The BAASE acronym reflects areas that are addressed during the program, and their influence on falls and fall risk: behavior (B), attitudes (A), activity (A), symptoms (S), and the environment (E). The overarching goals of the program are to increase knowledge of fall risk factors, increase knowledge and skills to manage falls and fall risk, and modify current behaviors to reduce personal fall risk. This group-based program is delivered through six 2-hour sessions. The first five sessions are conducted over five consecutive weeks. The final booster session is held 1 month after the fifth session.

A pilot feasibility study included 30 people with MS (mean age 56.7 plus or minus 7.4 years). Twenty-three people completed at least five out of six sessions. A pre-/post-intervention design was used, without a control or comparison condition. Participants increased their knowledge and skills to manage falls and fall risk, and reported modification of behaviors to reduce personal fall risk. The most notable behavioral changes reported by participants as a consequence of the intervention included developing an emergency plan in case of a fall, planning the order of daily activities to manage MS symptoms and reduce fall risk, choosing not to do an activity because it may lead to a fall, and selecting and checking mobility devices to reduce fall risk.[82]

Summary and Comparison

Although current practice in fall prevention for community-dwelling older adults now is informed by findings from over 100 randomized trials and meta-analyses of the most scientifically rigorous studies,[68] very little is known about fall prevention interventions for people aging with MS, late effects of polio, muscular dystrophies, or spinal cord injuries. Limited fall prevention research involving people who have experienced a stroke and people living with Parkinson's disease has been conducted[84–87]; however, the interventions tested in those studies (ie, vitamin D analog and exercise-based approaches to fall prevention) have failed to yield to the desired outcomes. Thus, the state of current literature suggests that fall rates need to be added as outcome measures (either primary or secondary) to studies evaluating balance and strengthening programs, general exercise interventions, and other potential single intervention approaches to fall prevention that involve people aging with physical disabilities. In addition, there would be value in attempting to replicate multiple interventions for community-dwelling older adults (eg, Stepping On, Matter of Balance) to determine if they are effective and efficacious for people aging with physical disability. The Safe at Home BAASE program also warrants additional evaluation. Finally, programs that target the specific fall risk factors experienced by a given group must be developed and tested.[1] To move in this direction, additional knowledge will be required about fall risk factors and the context under which falls among people aging with physical disability occur.

IMPLICATIONS AND CONCLUSION

The US Department of Health and Human Services specifically targeted fall-related deaths, hip fractures, and nonfatal head injuries for reduction in the Healthy People 2010 Objectives for Improving Health.[88] In 2005, the National Council on Aging (NCOA), in collaboration with other top US health and safety organizations, launched the Falls Free Initiative. The initiative led to the development of a national action plan that outlines key strategies and action steps to help reduce fall dangers for older adults.[89] Although these efforts primarily target community-dwelling older adults, they do not specifically exclude people aging with physical disability, and attention to these individuals needs to occur.

With improvements in health care and life expectancy, the number of people aging with physical disability and chronic conditions is expected to increase. These individuals are experiencing many challenges associated with the interaction of aging and disability, and these challenges may increase their risk of falls, and the severity of the falls that they experience. Yet, this article demonstrates that knowledge of falls and their consequences among people aging with physical disability falls far behind the knowledge for community-dwelling older adults.

To develop and evaluate theoretically sound and evidence-based fall prevention programs for people aging with physical disability, there is a desperate need for more epidemiologic research on falls in these groups. More knowledge is needed about who is falling, when and where they are falling, and what factors are contributing to their falls. Without this information, it will be difficult to prioritize intervention development and choose or develop appropriate outcome measures, regardless of whether interventions are single, multiple, or multifactorial.

In addition to these efforts, there is also a need to increase awareness of both people aging with physical disability and their health care providers about the problem of falls and the potential to manage these events (ie, reduce number and severity). As Wagner and colleagues[90,91] have noted, improved health outcomes for people with chronic illness depends upon the interactions between informed, activated patients and prepared, proactive health care teams. Barr and colleagues[92] have argued further that it is not simply the patients and the health care teams that must be interacting, but entire communities. When applied to the problem of falls among people aging with physical disability, the expanded chronic care model[92] points to the need for multilevel and multifactorial fall prevention interventions that can develop personal skills, reorient health services, build healthy public policy, and create supportive communities that can reduce fall rates and the severity of falls that are experienced. Such complex health interventions must be theoretically driven so that mechanisms of action and expected outcomes can be clearly explicated and appropriately tested.[93]

Falls are a serious problem for people aging with physical disability. Understanding the problem must occur to inform effective prevention and management interventions.

REFERENCES

1. Sleet DA, Moffett DB, Stevens J. CDC's research portfolio in older adult fall prevention: a review of progress, 1985–2005, and future research directions. J Safety Res 2008;39(3):259–67.
2. Sterling DA, O'Connor JA, Bonadies J. Geriatric falls: injury severity is high and disproportionate to mechanism. J Trauma 2001;50(1):116–9.
3. Hendrie D, Hall SE, Arena G, et al. Health system costs of falls of older adults in Western Australia. Aust Health Rev 2004;28(3):363–73.
4. Englander F, Hodson TJ, Terregrossa RA. Economic dimensions of slip and fall injuries. J Forensic Sci 1996;41(5):733–46.
5. Lamb SE, Jorstad-Stein EC, Hauer K, et al. Prevention of Falls Network Europe and Outcomes Consensus Group. Development of a common outcome data set for fall injury prevention trials: the Prevention of Falls Network Europe consensus. J Am Geriatr Soc 2005;53(9):1618–22.

6. Nachreiner NM, Findorff MJ, Wyman JF, et al. Circumstances and consequences of falls in community-dwelling older women. J Women's Health (Larchmt) 2007; 16(10):1437–46.

7. Nilsagård Y, Lundholm C, Denison E, et al. Predicting accidental falls in people with multiple sclerosis—a longitudinal study. Clin Rehabil 2009;23(3):259–69.

8. Tinetti ME, Speechley M, Ginter SF. Risk factors for falls among elderly people living in the community. N Engl J Med 1988;319:1701–7.

9. Hausdorff JM, Rios DA, Edelberg HK. Gait variability and fall risk in community-living older adults: a 1-year prospective study. Arch Phys Med Rehabil 2001;82: 1050–6.

10. Hornbrook MC, Stevens VJ, Wingfield DJ, et al. Preventing falls among community-dwelling older persons: results from a randomized trial. Gerontologist 1994; 34(1):16–23.

11. Bergland A, Wyller TB. Risk factors for serious fall-related injuries in elderly women living at home. Inj Prev 2004;10(308):313.

12. Stevens JA, Mack KA, Paulozzi LJ, et al. Self-reported falls and fall-related injuries among persons aged >or=65 years—United States, 2006. J Safety Res 2008;39(3):345–9.

13. O'Loughlin JL, Robitaille Y, Boivin JF, et al. Incidence of risk factors for falls and injurious falls among community-dwelling elderly. Am J Epidemiol 1993;137: 342–54.

14. Cattaneo D, De Nuzzo C, Fascia T, et al. Risks of falls in subjects with multiple sclerosis. Arch Phys Med Rehabil 2002;83(6):864–7.

15. Peterson EW, Cho C, von Koch L, et al. Injurious falls among middle aged and older adults with multiple sclerosis. Arch Phys Med Rehabil 2008;89:1031–7.

16. Finlayson M, Peterson E, Cho C. Risk factors for falling among people with multiple sclerosis aged 45 to 90. Arch Phys Med Rehabil 2006;87:1274–9.

17. Lord SR, Allen GM, Williams P, et al. Risk of falling: predictors based on reduced strength in persons previously affected by polio. Arch Phys Med Rehabil 2002; 83(6):757–63.

18. Legters K, Verbus NB, Kitchen S, et al. Fear of falling, balance confidence, and health-related quality of life in individuals with postpolio syndrome. Physiother Theory Pract 2006;22(3):127–35.

19. Wiles CM, Busse ME, Sampson CM, et al. Falls and stumbles in myotonic dystrophy. J Neurol Neurosurg Psychiatry 2006;77(3):393–6.

20. Brotherton SS, Krause JS, Nietert PJ. A pilot study of factors associated with falls in individuals with incomplete spinal cord injury. J Spinal Cord Med 2007;30(3): 243–50.

21. Campbell AJ, Robertson MC. Implementation of multifactorial interventions for fall and fracture prevention. Age Ageing 2006;35(Suppl 2):ii60–4.

22. American Geriatrics Society, British Geriatrics Society, American Academy of Orthopedic Surgeons. Guidelines for the prevention of falls in older persons. J Am Geriatr Soc 2001;49(5):664–72.

23. Lord SR, Menz HB, Sherrington C. Home environment risk factors for falls in older people and the efficacy of home modifications. Age Ageing 2006;35(Suppl 2): ii55–9.

24. Nevitt MC, Cummings SR, Kidd S, et al. Risk factors for recurrent nonsyncopal falls. A prospective study. JAMA 1989;261(18):2663–8.

25. Campbell AJ, Spears GF, Borrie MJ. Examination by logistic regression modeling of the variables which increase the relative risk of elderly women falling compared to elderly men. J Clin Epidemiol 1990;43(12):1415–20.

26. Yasamura S, Haga H, Nagai H, et al. Rate of falls and correlates among elderly people living in urban community Japan. Age Ageing 1994;23:323–7.
27. Tromp AM, Pluijm SM, Smit JH, et al. Fall risk screening test: a prospective study on predictors for falls in community-dwelling elderly. J Clin Epidemiol 2001;54(8): 837–44.
28. Campbell AJ, Borrie MJ, Spears GF. Risk factors for falls in a community-based prospective study of people 70 years and older. J Gerontol 1989;44(4):M112–7.
29. Chu LW, Chi I, Chiu AY. Incidence and predictors of falls in the Chinese elderly. Ann Acad Med Singapore 2005;34(1):60–72.
30. Anstey KJ, Burns R, von SC, et al. Psychological well-being is an independent predictor of falling in an 8-year follow-up of older adults. J Gerontol B Psychol Sci Soc Sci 2008;63(4):249–57.
31. Tinetti ME, Powell L. Fear of falling and low self-efficacy: a case of dependence in elderly persons. J Gerontol 1993;48:35–8.
32. Tinetti ME, Richman D, Powell L. Falls efficacy as a measure of fear of falling. J Gerontol 1990;45(6):239–43.
33. Friedman SM, Munoz B, West SK, et al. Falls and fear of falling: which comes first? A longitudinal prediction model suggests strategies for primary and secondary prevention. J Am Geriatr Soc 2002;50(8):1329–35.
34. Cumming RG, Salkeld G, Thomas M, et al. Prospective study of the impact of fear of falling on activities of daily living, SF-36 scores, and nursing home admission. J Gerontol A Biol Sci Med Sci 2000;55(5):M299–305.
35. Ray WA, Griffin MR, Schaffner W, et al. Psychotropic drug use and the risk of hip fracture. N Engl J Med 1987;316(7):363–9.
36. Robbins AS, Rubenstein LZ, Josephson KR, et al. Predictors of falls among elderly people. Results of two population-based studies. Arch Intern Med 1989; 149(7):1628–33.
37. Leipzig RM, Cumming RG, Tinetti ME. Drugs and falls in older people: a systematic review and meta-analysis: I. Psychotropic drugs. J Am Geriatr Soc 1999; 47(1):30–9.
38. Gill TM, Williams CS, Tinetti ME. Environmental hazards and the risk of nonsyncopal falls in the homes of community-living older persons. Med Care 2000;38(12): 1174–83.
39. Teno J, Kiel DP, Mor V. Multiple stumbles: a risk factor for falls in community-dwelling elderly. A prospective study. J Am Geriatr Soc 1990;38(12): 1321–5.
40. Campbell AJ, Borrie MJ, Spears GF, et al. Circumstances and consequences of falls experienced by a community population 70 years and over during a prospective study. Age Ageing 1990;19(2):136–41.
41. Northridge ME, Nevitt MC, Kelsey JL, et al. Home hazards and falls in the elderly: the role of health and functional status. Am J Public Health 1995; 85(4):509–15.
42. Speechley M, Tinetti M. Falls and injuries in frail and vigorous community elderly persons. J Am Geriatr Soc 1991;39(1):46–52.
43. Oakley A, France-Dawson M, Fullerton D, et al. Preventing falls and subsequent injury in older people. Eff Health Care 1996;2:1–16.
44. van Weel C, Vermeulen H, van den Bosch W. Falls: a community care perspective. Lancet 1995;345:1549–51.
45. Delbaere K, Crombez G, Vanderstraeten G, et al. Fear-related avoidance of activities, falls, and physical frailty. A prospective community-based cohort study. Age Ageing 2004;33:368–73.

46. Scuffham P, Chaplin S, Legood R. Incidence and costs of unintentional falls in older people in the United Kingdom. J Epidemiol Community Health 2003; 57(9):740–4.
47. Gill TM, Allore HG, Holford TR, et al. Hospitalization, restricted activity, and the development of disability among older persons. JAMA 2004;292(17): 2115–24.
48. Schiller JS, Kramarow EA, Dey AN. Fall injury episodes among noninstitutionalized older adults: United States, 2001–2003. Adv Data 2007;392:1–16.
49. Sattin RW, Lambert Huber DA, DeVito CA, et al. The incidence of fall injury events among the elderly in a defined population. Am J Epidemiol 1990;131(6):1028–37.
50. Hu G, Baker SP. Trends in unintentional injury deaths, US, 1999–2005. Age, gender, and racial/ethnic differences. Am J Prev Med 2009;37(3):188–94.
51. Boyd R, Stevens JA. Falls and fear of falling: burden, beliefs, and behaviours. Age Ageing 2009;38(4):423–8.
52. Roe B, Howell F, Riniotis K, et al. Older people and falls: health status, quality of life, lifestyle, care networks, prevention, and views on service use following a recent fall. J Clin Nurs 2009;18(16):2261–72.
53. Rubenstein LZ. Falls in older people: epidemiology, risk factors and strategies for prevention. Age Ageing 2006;35(S2):37–41.
54. von Heideken Wagert P, Gustafson Y, Kallin K, et al. Falls in very old people: the population-based Umeå 85+ study in Sweden. Arch Gerontol Geriatr 2009;49(3): 390–6.
55. Sampalis JS, Nathanson R, Vaillancourt J, et al. Assessment of mortality in older trauma patients sustaining injuries from falls or motor vehicle collisions treated in regional level I trauma centers. Ann Surg 2009;249(3):488–95.
56. Coronado VG, Thomas KE, Sattin R, et al. The CDC traumatic brain injury surveillance system: characteristics of persons aged 65 years and older hospitalized with TBI. J Head Trauma Rehabil 2005;20(3):215–28.
57. Nevitt MC. Falls in the elderly: risk factors and prevention. In: Masdeu JC, Sudarsky L, Wolfson L, editors. Gait disorders of aging. Philadelphia: Lippincott-Raven; 1997. p. 13–36.
58. Kannus P, Sievanen H, Palvanen M, et al. Prevention of falls and consequent injuries in elderly people. Lancet 2005;366:1885–93.
59. McKee KJ, Orbell S, Austin CA, et al. Fear of falling, falls efficacy, and health outcomes in older people following hip fracture. Disabil Rehabil 2002;24(6): 327–33.
60. Li F, Fisher KJ, Harmer P, et al. Falls self-efficacy as a mediator of fear of falling in an exercise intervention for older adults. J Gerontol B Psychol Sci Soc Sci 2005; 60:34–40.
61. Tischler L, Hobson S. Fear of falling: a qualitative study among community-dwelling older adults. Phys Occup Ther Geriatr 2005;23:37–53.
62. Lee F, Mackenzie L, James C. Perceptions of older people living in the community about their fear of falling. Disabil Rehabil 2008;30(23):1803–11.
63. Centers for Disease Control and Prevention. Fatal occupational injuries—United States, 2005. MMWR Morb Mortal Wkly Rep 2007;56(13):297–310.
64. Nelson A, Ahmed S, Harrow J, et al. Fall-related fractures in persons with spinal cord impairment: a descriptive analysis. SCI Nurs 2003;20(1):30–7.
65. Brotherton SS, Krause JS, Nietert PJ. Falls in individuals with incomplete spinal cord injury. Spinal Cord 2007;45(1):37–40.
66. Bronnum-Hansen H, Hansen T, Koch-Henriksen N, et al. Fatal accidents among Danes with multiple sclerosis. Mult Scler 2006;12(3):329–32.

67. Peterson EW, Cho C, Finlayson M. Fear of falling and associated activity curtailment among middle aged and older adults with multiple sclerosis. Mult Scler 2007;13:1168–75.

68. Gillespie LD, Robertson MC, Gillespie WJ, et al. Interventions for preventing falls in older people living in the community. Cochrane Database Syst Rev 2009;(2):CD007146.

69. Chang JT, Morton SC, Rubenstein LZ, et al. Interventions for the prevention of falls in older adults: systematic review and meta-analysis of randomised clinical trials. BMJ 2004;328(7441):680.

70. Close J, Ellis M, Hooper R, et al. Prevention of falls in the elderly trial (PROFET): a randomised controlled trial. Lancet 1999;353(9147):93–7.

71. Tinetti ME, Baker DI, McAvay G, et al. A multifactorial intervention to reduce the risk of falling among elderly people living in the community. N Engl J Med 1994; 331(13):821–7.

72. Cumming RG, Thomas M, Szonyi G, et al. Home visits by an occupational therapist for assessment and modification of environmental hazards: a randomized trial of falls prevention. J Am Geriatr Soc 1999;47(12):1397–402.

73. Campbell AJ, Robertson MC, La Grow SJ, et al. Randomised controlled trial of prevention of falls in people aged > or = 75 with severe visual impairment: the VIP trial. BMJ 2005;331(7520):817.

74. Nikolaus T, Bach M. Preventing falls in community-dwelling frail older people using a home intervention team (HIT): results from the randomized Falls-HIT trial. J Am Geriatr Soc 2003;51(3):300–5.

75. Clemson L, Cumming RG, Kendig H, et al. The effectiveness of a community-based program for reducing the incidence of falls among the elderly: a randomized trial. J Am Geriatr Soc 2004;52:1487–92.

76. Tennstedt S, Howland J, Lachman M, et al. A randomized, controlled trial of a group intervention to reduce fear of falling and associated activity restriction in older adults. J Gerontol B Psychol Sci Soc Sci 1998;53(6):384–92.

77. Tinetti ME, Gordon C, Sogolow E, et al. Fall-risk evaluation and management: challenges in adopting geriatric care practices. Gerontologist 2006;46(6):717–25.

78. Gitlin LN, Winter L, Dennis MP, et al. A randomized trial of a multicomponent home intervention to reduce functional difficulties in older adults. J Am Geriatr Soc 2006;54(5):809–16.

79. Gitlin LN, Winter L, Dennis MP, et al. Variation in response to a home intervention to support daily function by age, race, sex, and education. J Gerontol A Biol Sci Med Sci 2008;63(7):745–50.

80. Gitlin LN, Hauck WW, Dennis MP, et al. Long-term effect on mortality of a home intervention that reduces functional difficulties in older adults: results from a randomized trial. J Am Geriatr Soc 2009;57(3):476–81.

81. Cattaneo D, Jonsdottir J, Zocchi M, et al. Effects of balance exercises on people with multiple sclerosis: a pilot study. Clin Rehabil 2007;21(9):771–81.

82. Finlayson M, Peterson EW, Cho C. Pilot study of a fall risk management program for middle aged and older adults with MS. Neurorehabilitation 2009;25(2):107–15.

83. Gillespie LD, Gillespie WJ, Robertson MC, et al. Interventions for preventing falls in elderly people. Cochrane Database Syst Rev 2006;(2).

84. Sato Y, Manabe S, Kuno H, et al. Amelioration of osteopenia and hypovitaminosis D by 1alpha-hydroxyvitamin D3 in elderly patients with Parkinson's disease. J Neurol Neurosurg Psychiatry 1999;66(1):64–8.

85. Protas EJ, Mitchell K, Williams A, et al. Gait and step training to reduce falls in Parkinson's disease. NeuroRehabilitation 2005;20(3):183–90.

86. Ashburn A, Fazakarley L, Ballinger C, et al. A randomised controlled trial of a home based exercise programme to reduce the risk of falling among people with Parkinson's disease. J Neurol Neurosurg Psychiatry 2007;78(7):678–84.

87. Green J, Forster A, Bogle S, et al. Physiotherapy for patients with mobility problems more than 1 year after stroke: a randomised controlled trial. Lancet 2002; 359(9302):199–203.

88. US Department of Health and Human Services. Healthy people 2010. 2nd edition. Washington, DC: US Government Printing Office; 2000.

89. National Council on Aging. Health and safety leadership launch national action plan to reduce the risk of fall-related injuries for older adults 2005. Available at: http://www.healthyagingprograms.org. Accessed July 8, 2009.

90. Wagner EH, Austin BT, Davis C, et al. Improving chronic illness care: translating evidence into action. Health Aff (Millwood) 2001;20(6):64–78.

91. Wagner EH. Chronic disease management: what will it take to improve care for chronic illness? Eff Clin Pract 1998;1(1):2–4.

92. Barr VH, Robinson S, Marin-Link B, et al. The expanded chronic care model: an integration of concepts and strategies from population health promotion and the chronic care model. Hosp Q 2003;7(1):73–82.

93. Campbell M, Fitzpatrick R, Haines A, et al. Framework for design and evaluation of complex interventions to improve health. BMJ 2000;321(7262):694–6.

Cognition, Aging, and Disabilities: Conceptual Issues

Soo Borson, MD

KEYWORDS

• Normal aging • Cognitive decline • Executive dysfunction

Cognitive impairment is the primary determinant of disability in late life[1] and, at all ages, cognitive function is the foundation of an individual's capacity to meet the challenges of disabling conditions. This article reviews normative changes in cognition that are observed across the adult life span and considers how specific disabilities may interact with aging processes to increase functional decline in later life. Disabling conditions that directly affect the brain are contrasted with those that do not; specific exemplars are used to illustrate these points. The author considers that, whereas some cognitive aging processes may impair the capacity of disabled persons to cope with their lives, others may enhance it. The goal of the approach taken here is twofold: to create a framework for thinking about how cognitive changes, aging, and disability may interact to help explain individual differences in coping, and to promote the inclusion of cognition in a comprehensive approach to assessment and care.

WHAT IS COGNITION?

"Cognition" refers to a broad range of largely invisible activities performed by the human brain. Perceiving, thinking, knowing, reasoning, remembering, analyzing, planning, paying attention, generating and synthesizing ideas, creating, judging, being aware, having insight—all these and more—are aspects of cognition. The following is a working definition: cognition includes any and all process by which a person becomes aware of his or her situation, needs, goals, and required actions, and uses this information to implement problem-solving strategies for optimal living. Motivation, usually considered a quality of affect rather than of thought, would, by this definition, be an aspect of cognition and is included as such here.

This research was supported, in part, by a grant from the Department of Education, National Institute on Disability and Rehabilitation Research (H133B080024). The contents of this article do not necessarily represent the policy of the Department of Education and the reader should not assume endorsement by the Federal Government.
Memory Disorders Program, University of Washington School of Medicine, 1959 NE Pacific Street, Box 356560, Seattle, WA 98195, USA
E-mail address: soob@uw.edu

Phys Med Rehabil Clin N Am 21 (2010) 375–382
doi:10.1016/j.pmr.2010.01.001
1047-9651/10/$ – see front matter © 2010 Elsevier Inc. All rights reserved.

HOW DOES COGNITION CHANGE WITH AGE?

Recent critical reviews of cognitive aging distinguish between processes showing gradual declines across the life span and those that remain stable until advanced age.[2] Basic mechanisms common to many cognitive processes, including perceptual and thinking speed, numerical ability, working memory, and encoding and retrieval of new information, appear to show small but continuous, more or less linear declines across the entire adult life span from the early 20s through the 80s, though the magnitude and precise trajectory of these normal changes is debated. Most functions that depend on stable knowledge stores and well-practiced tasks remain stable into old age, and some improve with age, including wisdom—the superior judgment and insight born of life experience and resulting strategic efficiencies. When cognitive decline departs from its relatively linear path to follow an accelerated pattern of loss, the influence of disease processes must be suspected and makes distinctions between pathology and normal aging very difficult to disentangle. The pathologies that account for much of the accelerated cognitive decline that may be observed in elderly people include both systemic diseases with cerebral effects, such as cardiovascular disease and diabetes, and diseases manifested primarily by their cognitive signs and symptoms, such as Alzheimer's disease. Though studies of brain integrity (eg, those based on neuroimaging technologies, such as structural and functional MRI, positron emission tomography and single-photon emission computed tomography, and MR spectroscopy) provide additional insight into normal versus pathologic aging, it is likely that these distinctions will remain somewhat blurred.[3]

BRAIN AGING: THE SUBSTRATE OF COGNITIVE CHANGE

A concise review of the evidence regarding neural changes associated with brain aging[2] provides a useful working model emphasizing two critical systems subserving cognitive processes. The first component involves changes in the frontostriatal system, broadly associated with executive abilities and adaptation to new environmental inputs and changes in one's physical and mental self, and the second, changes in the medial temporal lobes and the bidirectional relays that link the hippocampus and association cortices. By and large, neurobiological data are generated and interpreted through the one-way glass of a "deficit" model of aging: progressive decay of neural tissues, based on "toxic hits" to vulnerable macromolecules, cumulative oxidative stress, diminished bioreparative mechanisms, subtle disease processes, and disuse, produces impairment in cognitive abilities. The deficit model is the basis for investment in brain aging research aimed at identifying preventive and therapeutic interventions that can delay the onset of a particular disease (eg, Alzheimer's dementia) or mitigate the decline that results. Findings from basic and clinical neurobiology can be most broadly informative if separated, to the extent possible, from specific disease categories, as progress in research has found overlapping molecular mechanisms across a broad spectrum of clinical diagnostic entities. Such findings support a reorientation of research toward locating factors that retard or accelerate brain aging and account for wide variations among individuals in the rate at which brain systems age. The reader is referred to the excellent review cited earlier[2] for a detailed discussion and citation of extensive data supporting a two-component model of brain aging, sketched below. Note that any disease process or injury that affects these age-vulnerable systems is likely to intensify, and be made more disabling as a result of, the age-related changes described here.

Frontostriatal Systems

The prefrontal cortex is particularly expressive of age-related changes, which, like a number of cognitive abilities, shows a linear decline in volume detectable by the 20s (possibly at first the result of extensive synaptic pruning that occurs during the transition from adolescence to early adulthood). Similar volume changes occur in the striatum, to which the prefrontal cortex is linked by a series of parallel pathways that have been associated with cognitive, affective, and motor functions. Not surprisingly, since these pathways use signature neurotransmitters (most prominently, but not limited to, dopamine) as part of their communication systems, neurochemical changes also occur (eg, reductions in dopamine transmission, affecting frontal activation, movement, and motivation). Volumetric changes in frontostriatal systems have been associated with reduced cognitive flexibility, working memory, suppression of unwanted or irrelevant responses, and strategic encoding of time-linked episodic memories. All of these are elements of cognition that underpin everyday multitasking, behavioral regulation, and adaptive functioning.

Medial Temporal Lobes, Hippocampus, and Associated Neocortical Systems

To a far lesser extent than the frontostriatal systems, the volume of medial temporal lobe structures tends to decline a little across the lifespan, but there are few cognitive correlates of such changes until later midlife (eg, age 60) and beyond, when explicit (declarative) memory performance tends to correlate with hippocampal volumes. However, in the healthy aging hippocampus and elsewhere, dendritic branching still occurs and new neural connections form in response to experience (neural plasticity). Functional imaging techniques have shown reductions in hippocampal and corresponding changes in the pattern of prefrontal activation during specific kinds of cognitive tasks in healthy older persons, suggesting altered pathways for at least some information management tasks. The significance of many of the observed changes for everyday function have not been specifically queried, but likely they relate to the gradual declines and shifts in motivation, overall cognitive and motor activity, and efficiency of learning that have been recognized as part of late life throughout history.

What Accounts for the Decreased Volume of Some Aging Brain Structures?

The clearest answer to this question from existing neurobiological research is that brain cells decrease in size (rather than die out) and that the communication highways between regions, the long, myelinated, white matter tracts, undergo gradual thinning and reduced efficiency. Damage to white matter has been extensively attributed to vascular ischemia associated with reduced small-caliber vessel perfusion and the size of the cerebrovascular bed during aging, and to pathologic changes caused by vascular occlusive disease, hypertension, and other cerebrovascular risk factors, and even a form of vascular disease most often recognized as part of Alzheimer's disease, known as amyloid angiopathy. Amyloid angiopathy is receiving renewed research interest because of the development of neuroimaging techniques capable of identifying its presence and consequences in living patients. Other mechanisms for both white matter and neuronal cell body and axonal damage are also under investigation.

Individual Differences, Choices, and Training Matter

Despite good evidence for some decline in many cognitive functions, reductions in brain tissue volumes, and changes in tissue composition that occur with apparently normal aging, there are large individual differences that increase after late midlife, with the mechanisms responsible for these differences remaining largely unaccounted for.[4] Among the factors that may account for some individual differences are two that can be potentially modified by choice and are prompting revisions in the deficit model of brain and cognitive aging. The two are aerobic fitness and specific cognitive training. Six months of sustained aerobic fitness training increases the volume of both gray and white matter in older persons, reducing or reversing tissue losses previously thought to be inevitable.[5] Is sustaining the level of activity required to bring fitness to the effective level practical for most older adults? Can its brain effects be realized for average older people, and its benefits be maintained over prolonged periods of time? These questions have yet to be explored.

Specialized cognitive training has also been shown, first in uncontrolled studies and more recently in randomized controlled trials, to improve a variety of cognitive processes, including memory, speed, and reasoning and problem solving, among others. "Strategy training," based on identification of weaker abilities to be targeted for training and teaching of explicit strategies for improving performance, describes a variety of training models and successful approaches. Most improvements resulting from training paradigms are modality-specific, showing little or no transfer or generalization to other cognitive abilities. Reasoning training, however, has been found to cross modalities more effectively than memory and speed-of-processing training and to be associated with less decline in instrumental activities of daily living over a prolonged (5 year) period of follow-up.[6] The reader is referred to a recent comprehensive review of both mental and physical training approaches to sustaining cognitive abilities in normally aging individuals.[7]

APPLICATION OF BRAIN AGING PRINCIPLES TO SPECIFIC DISABILITIES

Recent discoveries that age-related structural and functional brain changes can be mitigated or reversed by aerobic and cognitive training point to a crucial dilemma for persons aging with a disability. Conditions that directly impair the function of the brain, or of the large muscle groups needed to enhance fitness and forestall age-related losses, may prevent successful participation in aerobic conditioning or cognitive training, or both. Many disabling conditions affect both brain and neuromuscular control mechanisms, including multiple sclerosis (MS), cerebral palsy, and many traumatic brain injuries, whereas others have no recognized cognitive (eg, post-polio syndrome) or neuromotor (eg, permanent amnesia in survivors of herpes encephalitis) component. While a full review of the emerging evidence about cognitive and physical training for individuals aging with disabilities is beyond the scope of this article, the high prevalence of MS, and the extensive literature on the heterogeneity of cognitive and motor aspects of the disease, make it a useful exemplar of how aging principles may be applied to a specific condition.

MS

Impairment in complex attention, processing speed and efficiency, executive functioning, and memory are increasingly appreciated as features of MS that may occur with the first recognized neurologic episode, independent of the more familiar motor and neuropsychiatric signs, and in a wide variety of clinical types and symptom arrays that differ from person to person and over time.[8] While overt dementia has been considered a rare outcome in MS, deficits consistent with an MS form of mild cognitive impairment are not. Evolution in the concept of what constitutes dementia—and a concomitant shift away from using the features of Alzheimer's disease as the paradigm for all dementias—may prompt increased attention to cognitive impairment as a source of disability in MS in the future. Such a shift has already occurred in thinking about Parkinson's disease (PD), another neurologic condition that, like MS, was initially defined solely by its hallmark motor features. Somewhat later, depression and anxiety disorders came to be recognized as much more common in PD than could be accounted for by psychological factors alone, and depression, anxiety, and neuro-behavioral disturbances have now been incorporated into the standardized approach to staging PD and rating the disability it causes. Later, cognitive impairment of some degree was discovered to occur in most patients with PD who live 2 decades or more with disease and it too has become part of the standard way of assessing PD as a motor-neuropsychiatric-cognitive syndrome. In MS, impaired processing speed, learning and memory, impulse sorting and suppression, self-appraisal, and executive function (occurring variably in 10%–70% of patients depending on clinical form and duration of disease) are common enough to indicate that cognitive dysfunction should be considered a core feature of the MS syndrome. Cognitive impairments are more frequent and chronic among persons classified as having primary or secondary progressive MS than those with relapsing-remitting forms of disease. Secondary progressive MS increases in prevalence with age, as remissions become shorter and less complete. The reasons for this change in course are not fully understood, but likely result from accumulation of permanent central nervous system damage over time, age-related diminution in brain repair mechanisms, and overall loss of brain and body fitness.

Cognitive deficits are associated with functional impairment in everyday life, inde-pendent of the effects of depression, fatigue, and motor disability.[8] These deficits can impair day-to-day decision making, motivation, and new learning sufficient to affect self-care in both higher order and basic activities of daily living and to impact capacity for gainful employment and promote the transition to permanent disability status. As data accrue and thinking continues to evolve about cognition and its relationship to functionality, and as the clinical course of MS is modified by newer treatments and those still to be developed, cognitive function will likely come to be incorporated into standard methods for assessing and staging MS disability, as it has in PD.

WHAT COGNITIVE ABILITIES ARE CENTRAL TO AGING WELL WITH A DISABILITY?

Many cognitive abilities, such as remembering important conversations (auditory and verbal memory) and balancing a checkbook (arithmetic skills), are convenient, time-saving skills that make everyday life more efficient. However, many such skills have acceptable substitutes (voice recorders, written notes, calculators), and most cogni-tive measures are poor predictors of everyday functioning. In a comprehensive review published by a working group of the American Neuropsychiatric Association,[9] very few specific cognitive abilities were associated with everyday functional capacity. Measures that accounted for the largest amount of variance were tests of general cognitive ability and executive control. Broadly, executive control functions encom-pass many "general purpose mechanisms for goal-oriented organization and manip-ulation of information stored in working memory."[2] Executive function encompasses those cognitive activities that relate to making plans, thinking ahead, suppressing irrelevant sensory, cognitive, and emotional intrusions, imagining, evaluating, and comparing possible consequences of alternative actions, managing time and space, changing or correcting behavior in light of its results, organizing and sequencing tasks in service to specific goals, and sustaining the necessary motivation to follow through to their accomplishment. In health care, impaired executive function is most easily appreciated "in the breach"—when a patient unintentionally omits a necessary medication several days a week, resulting in a relapse of a treatable chronic condition, or a young adult in rehabilitation for a traumatic brain injury neglects to practice his or her problem-solving and impulse-management exercises. Patients with impaired executive control functions cope poorly with many other disabilities, and when impairment is not recognized, such patients may considered bad, intentionally noncompliant, passive-aggressive, or just plain frustrating to their families, partners, providers, and even themselves.

Executive function, representing an integrated composite of many related elemental cognitive activities, is most often linked in common clinical parlance and neuroscience research to the frontal lobes, which, as we have seen earlier, are particularly vulnerable to age-related changes: across the human lifespan, the frontal lobes are last to finish their development and first to decay. However, the extensive synaptic connections that link various subregions of the frontal lobes to other cortical and subcortical structures imply that brain lesions occurring outside the frontal lobes may have exaggerated impact on frontal functioning as individuals age. This mechanism is recognized in certain stroke syndromes, where damage to one area of the brain causes functional deficits in otherwise normal tissue that is synaptically linked to the region of the stroke (referred to as diaschisis), but is also commonly seen in subcortical vascular ischemic disease of the brain, which affects executive function and cognitive speed to a greater extent than it does formal memory processing. The same can occur in MS and other brain diseases with distributed lesion foci.

FUTURE PERSPECTIVES: FINDING OPPORTUNITIES TO PRESERVE OR IMPROVE COGNITION IN AGING PEOPLE WITH DISABILITIES
Uniform Assessments

A key step toward improving the recognition of the cognitive components of disability in aging individuals is a core set of assessment tools that can be applied across a broad range of ages, disorders, and conditions, and supplemented with disease-specific measures when needed. Progress toward that goal is represented by the National Institutes of Health Toolbox Initiative, to be completed by 2011, which aims to offer "efficient, flexible, and responsive assessment of cognitive functions such as learning, memory, executive function, language/lexical retrieval, visuospatial abilities, attention, and speed of processing"[10] in addition to similarly uniform assessments of emotion and motor and sensory function.

Testing and Adapting Emerging Antiaging Strategies for Persons with Disabilities

The most promising avenues currently identified for preserving cognitive health in aging are physical and cognitive fitness training. The goals are to maximize and support the function of healthy brain and, despite some research, there is currently no convincing evidence that they can delay or prevent any specific disease that causes cognitive decline. In persons with chronic disabilities, studies showing the potential of cognitive and physical training to improve important dimensions of functionality yield inconsistent results, at least partly because of the variability inherent between persons and conditions. Whereas one study reported better "cortical and cognitive plasticity" in relapsing-remitting MS patients with higher baseline cardiorespiratory fitness,[11] other work finds cognitive impairment a limiting factor in the success of exercise-based approaches to rehabilitation.[12] A new pilot trial of intensive, computer-assisted cognitive training for relapsing-remitting patients with MS, relatively low levels of disability, and deficits in attention, information processing, and executive function, found significant improvements in all domains, and in depressive symptoms, after 3 months of training, compared with a usual-care, nonmatched control group.[13] As the value, limitations, and necessary adaptations of both physical and neuropsychological training approaches are better defined by research in specific disabled populations, the case for incorporating them into standard care will become more compelling.

Pharmacologic Approaches to Enhancing Cognition

Alzheimer's disease has led the way in drug development for cognitive impairments of late life and remains the principal condition for which cognitive enhancing medications have received Food and Drug Administration indication. The recognized antidementia medications, which are known by their pharmacologic actions as inhibitors of acetylcholinesterase or glutamate in the brain, do not affect basic causal processes and do not have significant disease-modifying effects in Alzheimer's disease or other disorders. Donepezil, an acetylcholinesterase inhibitor approved for treating all stages of Alzheimer's disease, has shown some promise for improving memory processing and subjective cognition in MS, in a small randomized placebo-controlled trial of moderate quality.[14] Other pharmacologic agents, generally classed as stimulants and alerting, rather than cognitive-enhancing, drugs, can have cognitive benefits in persons with suitable conditions. Such conditions span a broad range of diagnoses, including attention deficit disorder in children and adults, attention deficits in MS, and disorders of wakefulness such as narcolepsy and sleep apnea. Drugs in the stimulant-alerting class generally act on dopaminergic and noradrenergic brain systems, which provide strong neurochemical inputs to the frontal lobes. No fundamentally new molecular entities having cognitive impairment as their principal target have been approved for use in over 6 years, despite large worldwide investment in drug discovery and development and a willing and eager aging population. Such facts encourage (and demand) enduring respect for the many secrets still held by the aging brain and the dysfunctions that come with living long.

REFERENCES

1. Agüero-Torres H, Thomas VS, Winblad B, et al. The impact of somatic and cognitive disorders on the functional status of the elderly. J Clin Epidemiol 2002;55: 1007–12.
2. Hedden T, Gabrieli JDE. Insights into the aging mind: a view from cognitive neuroscience. Nat Rev Neurosci 2004;5:87–96.
3. Whitehouse P, George D. The myth of Alzheimer's: what you aren't being told about today's most dreaded diagnosis. New York: St Martin's Press; 2008.
4. Wilson RS, Beckett LA, Barnes LL, et al. Individual differences in rates of change in cognitive abilities of older persons. Psychol Aging 2002;17(2):179–93.
5. Colcombe SJ, Erickson KI, Scalf PE, et al. Aerobic exercise training increases brain volume in aging humans. J Gerontol A Biol Sci Med Sci 2006;61(11): 1166–70.
6. Willis SL, Tennstedt SL, Marsiske M, et al. Long-term effects of cognitive training on everyday functional outcomes in older adults. J Am Med Assoc 2006;296(23): 2805–14.
7. Lustig C, Shah P, Seidler R, et al. Aging, training, and the brain: a review and future directions. Neuropsychol Rev 2009;19:504–22.
8. Chiaravalloti ND, DeLuca J. Cognitive impairment in multiple sclerosis. Lancet Neurol 2008;7:1139–51.

9. Royall DR, Lauterbach EC, Kaufer D, et al. The cognitive correlates of functional status: a review from the Committee on Research of the American Neuropsychiatric Association. J Neuropsychiatry Clin Neurosci 2007;19(3):249–65.

10. NIH Toolbox Initiative. Available at: http://www.nihtoolbox.org. Accessed December 13, 2009.

11. Prakash RS, Snook EM, Erickson KI, et al. Cardiorespiratory fitness: a predictor of cortical plasticity in multiple sclerosis. Neuroimage 2007;34(3):1238–44.

12. Brown TR, Kraft GH. Exercise and rehabilitation for individuals with multiple sclerosis. Phys Med Rehabil Clin N Am 2005;16(2):513–55.

13. Flavia M, Stampatori C, Zanotti D, et al. Efficacy and specificity of intensive cognitive rehabilitation on attention and executive functions in multiple sclerosis. J Neurol Sci 2010;288(1–2):101–5.

14. Krupp LB, Christodoulou C, Melville RN, et al. Donepezil improved memory in multiple sclerosis in a randomized clinical trial. Neurology 2004;63(1):1579–85.

Aging with Spinal Cord Injury

Susan Charlifue, PhD[a],*, Amitabh Jha, MD, MPH[a,b],
Daniel Lammertse, MD[a]

KEYWORDS

• Aging • Consequences of aging • Spinal cord injury
• Quality of life

Traumatic spinal cord injury (SCI) was long ago thought of as "an ailment not to be treated."[1] Since World War II, this once always fatal condition has reaped the benefits from advances in emergency and acute management, to the extent that people with SCI are surviving the early years posttrauma. Further advances in rehabilitative interventions, assistive technology to enhance independence, and early identification of secondary conditions enables those with SCI to live many years, often into their seventh and eighth decades. Several studies suggest that survival is influenced by the level and severity of injury,[2–4] age at injury,[5–8] and decade of injury.[9–12] Individuals with higher level, more neurologically complete lesions (ie, no or limited motor or sensory preservation below the level of lesion), and those injured at older ages have higher mortality rates in general. Those that live into their middle and older years with relatively stable health and functional abilities, however, experience the physical deterioration that naturally occurs with aging. Of note, the recent pattern of individuals incurring SCI is shifting with the mean age at onset increasing.[13–15] With this trend, the effects of aging may appear more quickly post-SCI.

In addition, there may be numerous psychosocial changes associated with functional decline, alterations in family and social support structures, and potential depletion of economic resources. It is useful for individuals with SCI and their health care team to know what changes may be expected as the individual ages, to identify possible preventive strategies to minimize the effects of aging.

PHYSICAL AGING

SCI can have a major affect on organ system functioning, both in the acute phase and long-term. Autonomic and somatic nervous system dysfunction may result in lasting impairment of many organ systems. Cumulatively, this is likely to result in the

[a] Research Department, Craig Hospital, 3425 South Clarkson Street, Englewood, CO 80113, USA
[b] Department of Physical Medicine and Rehabilitation, University of Colorado at Denver, Denver, CO, USA
* Corresponding author.
E-mail address: susie@craighospital.org

Phys Med Rehabil Clin N Am 21 (2010) 383–402
doi:10.1016/j.pmr.2009.12.002
1047-9651/10/$ – see front matter © 2010 Elsevier Inc. All rights reserved.

development of secondary complications that become increasingly prevalent with longer duration of impairment. This phenomenon has been confirmed in several studies describing health complications associated with aging and SCI.[16–18]

Gastrointestinal System

The most obvious alteration in gastrointestinal physiology after SCI is loss of volitional control over bowel emptying. Surveys of people with SCI have documented numerous gastrointestinal complications that accompany the aging process and have been associated with an increased need for assistance with activities of daily living.[19,20] Colorectal function is significantly altered by SCI, typically requiring a "bowel program" that induces (using a combination of various intestinal reflexes, diet, and pharmaceuticals) bowel movements and scheduled, predictable intervals. The altered colorectal function is expected to be a source of problems in the aging SCI population. Specifically, constipation is a problem in individuals with SCI, regardless of age; but when accompanied by the aging process, constipation is likely to be more prevalent in older or longer-injured individuals.[21] For example, one longitudinal study that involved people more than 20 years post-SCI in the United Kingdom indicated that 42% had difficulties with constipation, 27% reported fecal incontinence, and 35% had general gastrointestinal pain.[16,19] An even greater prevalence of constipation and fecal incontinence in up to 86% of individuals with SCI has been reported by others.[22]

Newer modalities, such as transanal irrigation techniques, show some promise in treating bowel evacuation difficulties.[23–26] If other methods become ineffective or difficult to manage for the person with SCI, elective colostomy may be an option, and numerous studies suggest that this approach, although less desirable for some, is not generally detrimental to perceived quality of life.[27,28] Rosito and colleagues,[29] in a study of 27 individuals who had undergone emergency or elective colostomy following injury, reported that colostomy significantly improved perceived quality of life.

Hemorrhoids and periodic rectal bleeding are common complications for those with chronic SCI,[30] which may worsen as the years progress and as the rectal tissue thins. Topical therapy is the least invasive intervention, but surgical options, including banding or hemorrhoidectomy, have shown reasonably good results with few complications.[31]

There is no evidence suggesting that people with SCI are at increased risk of colon cancer, but it is reasonable to assume they are at no less risk than the general population. Periodic screening for colon and rectal cancer, consistent with general population guidelines, is appropriate.[32] This screening can be problematic for the person with SCI, because the typical preparation for colonoscopy is very difficult for those with neurogenic bowel. In addition, insurance may not cover the costs of the colonoscopy preparation and related care. Because of the frequent presence of hemorrhoids, rectal prolapse, and other distal rectal pathology, fecal occult blood may not be a reliable screening tool, and endoscopy may provide more accurate information.

Genitourinary System

Diminished bladder capacity and urethral compliance, an increase in uninhibited detrusor contractions and residual bladder volumes, and a gradual decline in kidney function are associated with normal human aging in the general population.[33–35] In addition, elderly individuals seem to be at increased risk for urinary tract infections, presumably related to the decline in immune function, postmenopausal changes, and the effects of prostatism.[36–38]

Genitourinary function following SCI is characterized by the loss of volitional control over micturition and the loss of coordination of detrusor and sphincter reflexes. These reflexes recover, but over time there is a tendency to develop detrusor sphincter dyssynergia and elevated lower urinary tract pressure that can lead to hypertrophy of the detrusor muscle and decreased bladder compliance. Cumulatively, these changes can also result in the development of hydronephrosis and upper urinary tract deterioration.[39] SCI-related changes in urinary tract physiology can be significant risks to health. Urinary tract complications, formerly the leading cause of death in those with SCI, now account for only 3.8% to 5.4% of deaths,[15,40] probably because of advances in urologic management and a wide range of antibiotic treatment options. Nonetheless, urologic complications continue to be common,[41,42] with urinary tract infections among the most frequent reasons for rehospitalization in the years following SCI.[43,44]

Bladder management methods seem to be associated with certain urinary complications. Individuals using indwelling catheters are shown to have higher rates of bladder stones, urinary tract infections, and bladder cancer.[45,46] The use of anticholinergic medications may improve some health outcomes for these individuals.[47,48] For many years, studies have suggested that the incidence of bladder cancer is increased by the presence of SCI,[49–52] although this finding has not been supported by others.[53,54] Bladder management technique is implicated in one study, which showed that indwelling catheter management resulted in a fourfold higher risk for the development of bladder cancer than nonindwelling catheter methods of management.[45] Additional risk factors for the development of bladder cancer likely related to the SCI and consequent neurogenic bladder include irritation to the bladder from recurrent urinary tract infections and bladder stones.[45,55,56] It does seem that malignant degeneration requires the cumulative effects of various risk factor exposure (eg, recurrent infections, indwelling catheter management, urinary tract stones, and cigarette smoking) over a long period of time. SCI survivors who develop bladder carcinoma typically present with hematuria; however, this sign alone is not a reliable indicator of bladder cancer. Bladder tumors are commonly metastatic and invasive at the time of diagnosis in people with SCI; the importance of identifying and using the most effective screening methods available cannot be underestimated. Urine cytology and biochemical markers of urinary tract malignancy are problematic in that they have high false-positive rates, possibly because of concomitant urinary tract infections and related hematuria. Most clinicians agree that screening cystoscopy to detect these tumors in chronically catheterized individuals is an option for early detection of bladder cancer in SCI,[55,57] although there is a lack of evidence that screening by cystoscopy or other methods has had an impact on mortality from bladder cancer in this population.

Other forms of bladder management also may pose difficulties, and it has been shown that those who have used intermittent catheterization for many years may increase their risk for developing urethral strictures and epididymo-orchitis.[58]

Because of the relationship of chronic prostatitis to recurrent urinary tract infection, there may be some added risk of prostate cancer in men with chronic SCI. To date, however, there is no compelling evidence that such an association exists. One study found that there was a lower incidence of carcinoma of the prostate in individuals with SCI.[59] Nonetheless, when prostate cancer is diagnosed in men with SCI, it is usually at a more advanced grade and stage[60]; men aging with SCI should be considered at risk and be provided with the same age-specific prostate cancer screening that is recommended for the general population.

Skin and Subcutaneous Tissues

SCI predisposes many individuals to an increased risk for skin trauma, which can result in pressure ulcers. Immobility, lack of sensory protection, and spasticity all contribute to the common occurrence of pressure ulcers in this population. Analysis of US Model Spinal Cord Injury Systems data showed a statistically significant increase in the average number of pressure ulcers from 5 to 20 years of follow-up.[61] Other investigators using these data found the incidence of pressure ulcers to increase from 15% at 1 year postinjury to nearly 30% at 20 years postinjury.[41] A Canadian study showed similar findings, with the odds ratio for developing pressure ulcers increasing for every year postinjury.[18]

The clinical approach to prevention and management of pressure ulcers in SCI is paramount, given the high economic and personal costs associated with this complication. Primary prevention of pressure ulcers through education focuses on skin protection, pressure relief, hygiene, and routine surveillance. Most studies of preventive interventions are limited by small sample sizes and inconsistent findings, but there is a suggestion that seating assessments and focused educational interventions may be most beneficial.[62,63] Once pressure ulcers occur, the basic principles of pressure relief, debridement, and asepsis are still the foundation of successful conservative management.[64,65] Depending on severity, clinicians may opt to use these conservative approaches, which include dressings, debridement, or electrical stimulation.[65] Anecdotal clinical experience and published data suggest that vacuum-assisted wound closure may help clear drainage from these sites and promote wound healing.[66] Conservative management, however, may not be sufficient for large and deep skin sores, which may require myocutaneous flap closure. Even with successful surgical management, the recurrence rate of pressure ulcers is high, and one of the strongest predictors of having a pressure ulcer is having had a previous ulcer.[67–69] Because of the high frequency of pressure ulcer occurrence in the chronic SCI population, prevention is paramount and periodic assessment should include a thorough evaluation of the skin and reinforcement of prevention education.

Musculoskeletal System

In the general population, musculoskeletal system aging is characterized by deterioration of articular cartilage function. This ultimately leads to degenerative arthritic changes, both in the spine and in joints of the appendicular skeleton.[70] People with SCI experience unique physical stresses during mobility activities, and it is not surprising that overuse syndromes and pain in the upper extremities are common in this population. Surveys document that upper extremity pain is reported by more than 50% of SCI survivors.[71] Not only is there is a positive association between shoulder pain and age, but pain occurs at a younger age in those with SCI compared with the general population.[72] Maneuvers, such as transfers, wheelchair propulsion, and pressure relief, may contribute to upper extremity discomfort.

When individuals with SCI identify shoulder pain, conservative management includes a review of mobility mechanics and how the individual engages in daily activities, which may result in suggestions for modifying those aspects of functioning and mobility to avoid pain-causing maneuvers.[73] Specific diagnosis of upper extremity joint pain can be difficult. Acromioclavicular degenerative changes may be seen on radiograph but plain radiographs are commonly of little value in the assessment of shoulder pain in these individuals. For more optimal diagnostic capabilities, arthrography, MRI, and ultrasound can commonly show impingement syndromes, tendinopathies, and rotator cuff tears in both symptomatic and asymptomatic individuals with SCI reporting shoulder pain.[74–76]

Overuse syndrome at the shoulders may present as a muscular imbalance across the glenohumeral joint with anterior musculature development significantly greater than posterior to the shoulder. Muscular balance across the joint to restore an optimal glenohumeral geometric relationship can be facilitated with exercises designed to address the posterior shoulder girdle.[71] Surgery for impingement or rotator cuff tears may be an option when a conservative approach cannot resolve the problem; however, studies reporting on postsurgical outcomes for shoulder surgery in SCI are few and limited by small sample sizes.[77–79] The postoperative rehabilitation period can be prolonged and potentially difficult for the person with SCI, and temporary limitations in independence because of the postoperative shoulder activity restrictions may necessitate the use of personal assistance services.[77,78] A balance between the potential benefits of surgical intervention and the temporary postoperative functional limitations is a realistic consideration, and the long-term benefits of such intervention require more study.

Osteoporosis is common to the aging process, most typically associated with postmenopausal women but also occurring in aging men.[80,81] Osteoporosis related to paralysis and disuse is commonly believed to be the underlying risk factor for pathologic fractures following SCI. Lower extremity osteoporosis develops rapidly in the first year postinjury, with approximately one third of original bone mass being lost by 16 months postinjury before relative stability is achieved.[82] A lower extremity fracture rate and extremity fracture rate of over 30% for individuals followed for several decades has been reported.[83] Various interventions have been proposed to limit further bone loss and potentially enhance bone growth, including standing, functional electrical stimulation, and treatment with bisphosphonates. There is some evidence that high-volume functional electrical stimulation cycling induces bone formation at the distal femur, although other areas of the lower extremities do not show the same benefit.[84] Frotzler and colleagues[85] studied five individuals with motor and sensory complete SCI who had participated in high-volume functional electrical stimulation cycling and after detraining or reduced cycling, found that the bone mass gained was maintained longer term with reduced cycling. Furthermore, preliminary trials of pamidronate showed some promise in reducing bone loss in the acute-phase post-SCI,[86] but more recent evidence suggested limited efficacy in preventing long-term bone loss.[87]

Because of both the frequency of musculoskeletal complaints in this population and increased fracture risk, a reasonable monitoring approach is to incorporate a thorough symptom review and examination as a part of periodic reassessment. Equipment modifications, assessment of and changes to posture, and techniques used in performing functional activities may be necessary for individuals with SCI as they age. In addition, periodic bone density evaluations may be warranted, particularly for menopausal women with SCI.

Nervous System

Histologic changes in the normal spinal cord demonstrate continual neuronal loss with aging.[88] Physiologic changes related to the nervous system in the aging general population have been reported to include loss of vibratory sensation, muscle mass, and strength; slower reaction time; decreased fine coordination and agility; decreased deep tendon reflexes; and deteriorating stability in station and gait.[89–92]

With the combination of age and SCI, it is reasonable to expect a progressive deterioration of neurologic function above and beyond that imposed by the original injury. A study of individuals aging with SCI of more than 20 years duration showed that 12% reported some sensory loss, and more than 20% reported increasing motor deficits over the years.[93] Similarly, a Canadian study found self-reported prevalence of neurologic deterioration in 11% of 633 individuals with traumatic SCI.[18] Although these data are compelling, it is not possible to state with certainty that an age-related loss of myelinated tracts and dropout of anterior horn cells may contribute to these reported symptoms, and further research regarding age-related neurologic decline in SCI is needed.

A high incidence of upper extremity entrapment neuropathies has been reported in studies of people with long-term SCI, with up to 63% of those with paraplegia showing evidence of neuropathies, both on electrodiagnostic testing and on symptom surveys.[94,95] The most frequent site of involvement is the median nerve at the wrist, but ulnar nerve entrapments at the elbow and wrist are also common. Repeated hand contact with wheelchair rims, and positioning of the wrist during transfer activities and pressure relief, may predispose individuals with SCI to increased risk for nerve entrapments in the upper extremities. It is suspected that the incidence of significant entrapment increases with duration of injury, although this has not been conclusively proved. The functional implications for this type of upper extremity injury are profound and may pose significant limitations to mobility and independence.

Treatment includes assessing the mechanics of mobility and daily living activities to determine any underlying sources of repetitive trauma. Some individuals may need to modify activities to minimize further trauma to conserve and protect wrist function. Wrist splinting may be beneficial in reducing repetitive trauma at the extremes of wrist flexion and extension, which are known to contribute to carpal tunnel symptomatology. Individuals with SCI usually are successfully treated with activity and equipment modification and rarely require surgical intervention. When conservative measures fail to provide a relief of symptoms in people with significant entrapments, however, surgical release of the entrapped nerve may be necessary. Similar to those who undergo procedures for musculoskeletal problems, such as rotator cuff tears, individuals undergoing carpal tunnel surgery should anticipate a postoperative period of restricted activity, which may temporarily require increased assistance from others.

Individuals with chronic SCI may experience a new onset of more marked neurologic deterioration, most commonly the result of progressive posttraumatic cystic myelopathy.[96–98] This condition is also referred to as "posttraumatic syrinx," and is characterized by the progressive enlargement of a cystic cavity originating at the site of injury and extending in either a cephalad or caudal direction in the spinal cord. The concept of progressive cystic myelopathy recently has been broadened to include progressive noncystic or myelomalacic myelopathies. These conditions are thought to be a part of a pathophysiologic continuum. The onset of this neurologic complication may vary from several months to several decades after injury, but most commonly occurs within the first 5 to 10 years postinjury. Signs and symptoms of late progressive neurologic deterioration include losses of sensory or motor function; increasing spasticity; neuropathic pain; increasing autonomic dysreflexia; increasing sweating; and the development of a variable, positional Horner syndrome. Confirmation of this diagnosis includes a combination of the typical history and physical findings and MRI. Arachnoid scarring, which interferes with spinal fluid flow and spinal cord mobility, seems to be the underlying mechanism of progressive spinal cord pathology. When neurologic deterioration is progressive, surgical treatment, including untethering of the arachnoid scar and, in some cases, shunting of the cyst cavity fluid, is warranted.[98,99] All individuals with SCI have the potential for late neurologic change; the assessment of motor and sensory function, and a neurologic review of systems, should be included in periodic follow-up. Appropriate electrodiagnostic and imaging studies are indicated in the presence of signs or symptoms of neurologic deterioration.[98,100]

Unlike nociceptive mechanical or musculoskeletal pain, neuropathic pain can be initiated or caused by a primary lesion or dysfunction in the spinal cord, such as that which occurs with SCI.[101] The clinical manifestation of this is an abnormal pain perception, characterized by burning, stabbing, and electric shock–like pain.[102] Neuropathic pain can occur above, at, or below the level of injury. That which occurs below the level of injury occurs in a diffuse distribution, compared with at-level, which typically occurs in a dermatomal or segmental distribution at the level of injury.[103] Neuropathic pain is typically constant; unrelated to position or movement; and may be exacerbated by other conditions, such as urinary tract infections or bowel function disturbances.[104] The prevalence of neuropathic pain following SCI has not been well-described, because most surveys combine all types of pain (including musculoskeletal) in their estimates.

There is no specific evidence to suggest that neuropathic pain in the person with SCI worsens with age; however, there may be age-related differences in the response to pharmacologic interventions for this type of pain, which commonly include gabapentin; pregabalin; tricyclic antidepressants; or weak opioids, such as tramadol. A study of 66 individuals without SCI, aged 5 to 84 years with a variety of conditions including neuropathic pain, found a significantly higher gabapentin blood pharmcodynamics in those aged 65 and older.[105] The authors posited that the higher concentrations of gabapentin in the elderly may be the result of slower bowel transit time leading to better absorption and a decline in renal function leading to decreased clearance. It is reasonable to suspect that as individuals with SCI using drugs, such as gabapentin, age, smaller doses may be indicated to provide the desired therapeutic response.

Cardiovascular System

Cardiovascular diseases (CVDs) are the most common causes of death in the United States among both men and women of all racial and ethnic groups.[106] Although age is the most important risk factor for manifest ischemic heart disease, the contribution of other risk factors is significant.[107] Notably, physical inactivity, common in older individuals, is associated with cardiovascular deconditioning.[108]

Heart disease is known to be one of the leading causes of mortality in long-term SCI, accounting for more than 20% of deaths.[40,109,110] A longitudinal study of long-term SCI survivors showed the risk of developing CVD was associated with both level and completeness of injury.[111] A number of studies have documented abnormalities of glucose and lipid metabolism and other risk factors for the development of CVD in people with SCI.[112–115] Individuals with SCI tend to have a lipid profile characterized by low high-density lipoprotein, compared with matched nondisabled controls.[116] Nonetheless, a report from the Agency for Healthcare Research and Quality concluded that there was insufficient evidence to suggest that adults with SCI are at greater risk of carbohydrate and lipid disorders, nor did it support the use of different thresholds to define or treat lipid abnormalities in this population.

It has been suggested that diabetes is an independent risk factor for mortality in people with SCI.[40] In a study of male veterans with SCI, 22% were found to be diabetic on oral glucose tolerance testing, compared with 6% in nondisabled control subjects, and 82% of the control subjects had normal glucose tolerance, compared with 50% of those with paraplegia and 38% of those with tetraplegia.[114] It has been suggested that changes in body composition, which are common in SCI, may contribute to impaired glucose metabolism.[113] Spinal-injured individuals typically have a reduction of lean muscle mass and a corresponding increase of fat mass. In addition, the diminished activity level of people with SCI may also contribute to insulin resistance.

These alterations in lipid and glucose metabolism indicate that people with SCI may have an elevated risk of coronary heart disease and other manifestations of CVD. Routine follow-up should include periodic assessment of blood lipids, glucose, weight, blood pressure, dietary habits, smoking, activity level, and alcohol consumption to identify potentially modifiable risk factors. Recommendations to reduce cardiac risk do not differ from those for the general population and include diets that limit the intake of saturated fats and cholesterol, weight management, smoking cessation, and medications to manage lipid abnormalities. There has been some evidence to suggest that functional electrical stimulation may improve arterial function and metabolic profiles in people with SCI,[117,118] and promotion of exercise and a general increase in physical activity may prove beneficial.

Respiratory System

In the general population, studies have shown a number of changes that result in a gradual loss of respiratory system function with advancing age.[119,120] Elderly men, in particular, are likely to experience sleep-disordered breathing associated with age-related increases in body weight, loss of upper airway muscle tone, and other factors.[121–123]

Individuals with SCI may experience respiratory complications both in the immediate postinjury period and during long-term follow-up.[18,41] The highest risk of respiratory complications is in those with neurologically complete tetraplegia, because of respiratory muscle paralysis and dysfunction. Older age at the time of injury is also associated with a higher risk of respiratory complications.[18] The combined effects of SCI and older age are likely to pose a significant risk for respiratory tract complications, such as pneumonia and atelectasis, and sleep-disordered breathing. This is particularly concerning because the leading causes of rehospitalization and death in people with both acute and chronic SCI are respiratory disorders.[124] Stolzmann and colleagues,[125] in a longitudinal study of 174 men with SCI, found no relationship between neurologic level and completeness in predicting a negative change in forced expiratory volume or forced vital capacity. They did, however, identify an age-related acceleration of decline in these two respiratory parameters. Other studies have investigated the incidence of respiratory tract morbidity in persons aging with SCI. A longitudinal study of 834 British individuals with SCI of at least 20 years' duration found the incidence of pneumonia and atelectasis to increase with age (going from 1.6% in those <30 years of age to 5.4% in those >60 years), but not with duration of injury.[16] US Model System data reveal similar findings, with pneumonia incidence increasing from 1.5% per year in the 16- to 30-year age group to 8.2% in the over 76–year-old group.[126] It seems from these studies that the risk of respiratory complications is associated with age rather than duration of injury.

Several investigators have identified a higher rate of sleep-disordered breathing in individuals with SCI, noted within weeks of injury and continuing in the follow-up years, with prevalence ranging from 25% to 53%.[127–130] Further study is needed to identify the factors contributing to this potentially life-threatening condition in SCI, because level of impairment, increased abdominal girth, neck circumference, and duration of injury have not consistently predicted those at greater risk of sleep apnea.

Based on data showing an increased risk of respiratory complications, clinical follow-up of individuals aging with SCI should include periodic assessment of vital capacity, especially in those with cervical levels of injury who are at the highest risk.[131] Annual immunizations against influenza and pneumococcus as appropriate are also recommended. Diagnosis and treatment of sleep-disordered breathing may also be indicated in symptomatic individuals.[132] In terms of personal behavioral modifications, maintenance of an appropriate weight to reduce the risk of further respiratory compromise is optimal, and smoking cessation programs should be encouraged. Aggressive management of community-acquired pneumonia, including hospitalization, mobilizing pulmonary secretions by manually assisted coughing, and mechanical cough assistance, and prompt administration of antibiotics are recommended.[124]

Immune System

The constellation of health conditions associated with aging in each of the body systems includes many factors related to immune system function. In the general population, function of the immune system declines with age and the risk of infection increases.[133,134] Aging of the immune system is likely influenced by multiple factors including the pathogen load that individuals are exposed to throughout their lives.[135] This relationship may be circular, in that although aging is a major risk factor for infection, it has been suggested that infection may also contribute to the aging process.[136]

There is evidence of diminished immune function in people with SCI above the T-10 neurologic level, which is demonstrated by impaired bacterial phagocytosis.[137] The previously cited British longitudinal study of aging with SCI showed a dramatic increase in urinary tract infections among those aged 60 and over and a slight increase in frequency of infection between the tenth and thirtieth postinjury year.[16] Other factors, such as the use of indwelling urinary catheters and pressure ulcers, may be associated with an ongoing systemic inflammatory response.[138]

The high incidence of urinary infection in SCI, and the likely increase of respiratory and other infectious processes with aging, calls for aggressive management and preventive strategies. Education regarding optimal health maintenance, appropriate immunizations, and early identification of infectious processes is critical. It is possible that advances in immunologic assessment and treatment will identify therapies that can improve immune defenses in individuals aging with SCI.

FUNCTIONAL AND PSYCHOSOCIAL AGING

People aging with SCI clearly face the possibility of numerous physical issues. The physical decline, often anticipated because of the consideration that time does take its toll on the body, regardless of disability, however, does not negatively affect the person with SCI if the functional consequences of such declines are negligible. In addition, when physical problems do arise, much can be done to intervene and either delay, minimize, or eliminate potential negative consequences. Of great importance is how the individual perceives the changes and is able to adapt his or her lifestyle in response to such changes. Also experienced by the person growing older with SCI are economic factors, the impact of environmental barriers and facilitators, cultural issues, and changes in intimate and more remote social relationships. Consideration of these multiple factors in the evaluation of individuals aging with SCI is critical to understand the multiple issues that underlie this complex phenomenon.

Independence

In the general population, advancing age is often accompanied by a loss of physical independence resulting from diminished muscle strength, decreased sensory acuity, slowed reflexes, decreased coordination, inadequate aerobic capacity, and lower energy levels.[139–144] Data from the National Center for Health Statistics showed that nearly 20% of the civilian community-dwelling population of the United States aged 55 to 64 and more than 34% of those aged 65 and older reported some degree of activity limitation.[145]

Aging may magnify issues of physical dependency for the person with SCI, because abilities change over time. The issues of concern to people aging with SCI include their overall health, their ability to remain independent, and their ability to sustain a satisfying lifestyle,[146] and research suggests that some of these concerns are well-founded. In the study of British individuals aging with SCI, increasing age was a significant predictor of functional decline. The average age when additional functional assistance was first needed was 49 years for those with tetraplegia and 54 years for those with paraplegia.[147] This study also found that 22% of the participants reported a functional decline or decreasing physical independence over a 3-year time span.[148] Other studies identified similar significant cross-sectional and longitudinal increases in the need for assistance among older individuals with SCI.[149]

Preserving or maintaining functional ability and independence can be facilitated through modifications in how activities are performed or the use of adaptive equipment and other technology. When assistance from others is necessary, the individual with SCI can still make decisions and direct his or her own care, optimizing independence.

Quality of Life

Quality of life may be related to how well a person copes with changes that occur as a result of aging. Stress and poor health have been linked with depression in older individuals.[150] For example, prospective cohort studies have demonstrated evidence that psychosocial factors, such as depression, are independent, etiologic, and prognostic factors for coronary heart disease.[151,152]

The relationship between increasing age and depression is often inconsistent, reflecting the complexities of affect management in older age. Older adults living in nursing homes, and those with dementia and other deteriorating health conditions, typically have higher rates of depression than do their younger or healthier counterparts.[153,154] Community-dwelling older adults in good health seem to be at no greater risk of depression than are younger adults, however, and apparent age-effects on depression in this population are often linked to health-related impairments in functioning[155,156] and to birth-cohort effects in terms of exposure to social risk factors (eg, economic deprivation).[157] Although findings on prevalence of geriatric depression are equivocal, there is evidence that perceived overall quality of life may not be negatively affected for older individuals.[158] For some individuals, quality of life may be determined by financial security; for others, maintaining health or having good relationships with others are determinants of life satisfaction. Rather than aging itself, maintaining good health, social support, and participation in activities have been found to more predictive of higher quality of life[158] and a person's sense of contentment has been suggested as an underlying factor of life satisfaction.[159]

Studies have shown that depression is common among individuals with SCI[160–162] and is greater for those who are older and who have been injured longer.[163] This suggests that life satisfaction may also be diminished for older individuals, a finding consistent with research by the authors and others, showing significant differences in self-perceived quality of life with younger individuals and those injured shorter periods of time rating their quality of life higher than older individuals.[16,164,165] Longitudinal and cross-sectional studies indicate that life satisfaction is not necessarily negatively impacted by aging, finding mixed patterns of change over time.[149,166,167] The variation in these findings may be a consequence of the differences in how older and younger individuals assess quality of life. The general message, nonetheless, is that individuals with SCI maintain relatively good and reportedly stable life satisfaction over time, even after many years of living with SCI.[168] Identifying the multitude of underlying factors that might contribute to declines in perceived quality of life or increased depressive symptoms is difficult; health care providers should assess both the physical health of the individual aging with SCI, and the psychologic status, social situation, and environment, because all have an impact on successful aging.

Family Issues

SCI can have a far-reaching impact on family members, friends, and others in the community close to the individual, particularly when that person requires physical assistance. Evidence suggests that SCI survivors' need for help increases as they age.[147] Complicating this issue, however, is the fact that many SCI caregivers are also aging, and facing their own age-related health issues. Potentially, poor health of the caregiver can negatively affect the care recipient, and with the advancing age of both, these consequences are likely to be magnified. On-going assessment of not only the person with SCI, but the physical and emotional health of family members, particularly if they provide personal assistance services to their loved one with SCI, is important. Detecting potential difficulties early and offering appropriate interventions, such as seeking occasional respite care or employing home health agency assistance, can help families maintain a positive focus on issues other than caregiving. Even with these efforts, all may not progress smoothly. There is evidence that assistance provided by a caregiving spouse is not always perceived positively by the recipient, and increasing age is a significant predictor of negative reactions to receiving assistance.[169] This may be of particular concern for those individuals with SCI who, having been independent when younger, need assistance as they age. Beneficial strategies to incorporating the need for more help include encouraging people with SCI to prioritize those activities that are most time consuming, difficult, or tedious as those that can be delegated to others, such as dressing, bathtub transfers, or bowel programs. Small steps can help individuals with SCI preserve their energy to use in more desirable personal and social activities. Ultimately, it is the shared responsibility of health care providers, people with SCI, and their families to work cooperatively in identifying the underlying issues that may negatively affect quality of life and community participation. This involves evaluating many issues, including the living situation, resources, and environment, because all play an important role in successful aging for the person with SCI.

SUMMARY

New challenges facilitating success for people aging with SCI aging are being encountered by health care providers. There remain substantial gaps in the literature regarding the numerous issues related to organ system aging in this unique population. Although this article has identified some key findings through various longitudinal and cross-sectional observational studies and limited clinical trials, research with larger, diverse samples allowing greater generalizability of findings is needed. In addition, knowledge of aging in SCI is enhanced through contacts with and liaisons to gerontologists and other professionals with an expertise in general population aging.

Strategies to minimize conditions and complications that occur with aging should be identified and implemented as early as possible to more effectively manage and assist people aging with SCI. The first critical component involves systematic surveillance by an experienced SCI team to identify potential problems at their earliest onset. Second and no less important is ongoing education for health care providers, involving learning about the physical, psychologic, social, and environmental consequences of aging and their potential impact on people with SCI. Education for the person with SCI is widely enhanced by electronic access to information. Unfortunately, much of this information is inaccurate and potentially damaging. Encouraging an open atmosphere of mutual dialog can help guide people with SCI through the maze of information is critical to ensure that the best practices are adopted. There may be indications for "re-rehabilitation" or equipment modifications as physical needs and independence change over time.

Aging is another step along the continuum of life with SCI, equal in importance to initial rehabilitation, returning to work, developing relationships, and engaging in other life activities. Through research, clinical experience, and self-reported outcomes from those living with SCI, a much greater insight has been gained into this phenomenon. When both clinicians and people with SCI are apprised of the natural likely trajectory of health and psychosocial issues and the research that supports best practices, successful aging can be greatly enhanced.

REFERENCES

1. Breasted JH. The Edwin Smith surgical papyrus: hieroglyphic transliteration, translation and commentary. Chicago: University of Chicago Press; 1930.
2. Vaidyanathan S, Soni BM, Gopalan L, et al. A review of the readmissions of patients with tetraplegia to the Regional Spinal Injuries Centre, Southport, United Kingdom, between January 1994 and December 1995. Spinal Cord 1998;36:838.
3. Yeo JD, Walsh J, Rutkowski S, et al. Mortality following spinal cord injury. Spinal Cord 1998;36:329.
4. Strauss D, DeVivo M, Shavelle R, et al. Economic factors and longevity in spinal cord injury: a reappraisal. Arch Phys Med Rehabil 2008;89:572.
5. Alander DH, Parker J, Stauffer ES. Intermediate-term outcome of cervical spinal cord-injured patients older than 50 years of age. Spine 1997;22:1189.
6. Shavelle RM, DeVivo MJ, Paculdo DR, et al. Long-term survival after childhood spinal cord injury. J Spinal Cord Med 2007;30:S48.
7. Fassett DR, Harrop JS, Maltenfort M, et al. Mortality rates in geriatric patients with spinal cord injuries. J Neurosurg Spine 2007;7:277.
8. Furlan JC, Bracken MB, Fehlings MG. Is age a key determinant of mortality and neurological outcome after acute traumatic spinal cord injury? Neurobiol Aging 2008. [Epub ahead of print].
9. DeVivo MJ, Ivie CS. Life expectancy of ventilator-dependent persons with spinal cord injuries. Chest 1995;108:226.
10. Frankel HL, Coll JR, Charlifue SW, et al. Long-term survival in spinal cord injury: a fifty year investigation. Spinal Cord 1998;36:266.
11. Shavelle RM, DeVivo MJ, Strauss DJ, et al. Long-term survival of persons ventilator dependent after spinal cord injury. J Spinal Cord Med 2006;29:511.
12. Strauss DJ, Devivo MJ, Paculdo DR, et al. Trends in life expectancy after spinal cord injury. Arch Phys Med Rehabil 2006;87:1079.
13. Jackson AB, Dijkers M, Devivo MJ, et al. A demographic profile of new traumatic spinal cord injuries: change and stability over 30 years. Arch Phys Med Rehabil 2004;85:1740.
14. Ahoniemi E, Alaranta H, Hokkinen EM, et al. Incidence of traumatic spinal cord injuries in Finland over a 30-year period. Spinal Cord 2008;46:781.
15. National Spinal Cord Injury Statistical Center. The 2008 annual statistical report for the spinal cord injury model systems. Birmingham (AL): University of Alabama at Birmingham; 2009.
16. Whiteneck GG, Charlifue SW, Frankel HL, et al. Mortality, morbidity, and psychosocial outcomes of persons spinal cord injured more than 20 years ago. Paraplegia 1992;30:617.

17. Whiteneck GG, Charlifue SW, Gerhart KA, et al, editors. Aging with spinal cord injury. New York: Demos Medical Publishers; 1993.
18. Hitzig SL, Tonack M, Campbell KA, et al. Secondary health complications in an aging Canadian spinal cord injury sample. Am J Phys Med Rehabil 2008;87: 545.
19. Menter R, Weitzenkamp D, Cooper D, et al. Bowel management outcomes in individuals with long-term spinal cord injuries. Spinal Cord 1997;35:608.
20. Liem NR, McColl MA, King W, et al. Aging with a spinal cord injury: factors associated with the need for more help with activities of daily living. Arch Phys Med Rehabil 2004;85:1567.
21. Faaborg PM, Christensen P, Finnerup N, et al. The pattern of colorectal dysfunction changes with time since spinal cord injury. Spinal Cord 2008;46:234.
22. Valles M, Vidal J, Clave P, et al. Bowel dysfunction in patients with motor complete spinal cord injury: clinical, neurological, and pathophysiological associations. Am J Gastroenterol 2006;101:2290.
23. Christensen P, Bazzocchi G, Coggrave M, et al. A randomized, controlled trial of transanal irrigation versus conservative bowel management in spinal cord-injured patients. Gastroenterology 2006;131:738.
24. Del Popolo G, Mosiello G, Pilati C, et al. Treatment of neurogenic bowel dysfunction using transanal irrigation: a multicenter Italian study. Spinal Cord 2008;46:517.
25. Christensen P, Andreasen J, Ehlers L. Cost-effectiveness of transanal irrigation versus conservative bowel management for spinal cord injury patients. Spinal Cord 2009;47:138.
26. Faaborg PM, Christensen P, Kvitsau B, et al. Long-term outcome and safety of transanal colonic irrigation for neurogenic bowel dysfunction. Spinal Cord 2009; 47:545.
27. Branagan G, Tromans A, Finnis D. Effect of stoma formation on bowel care and quality of life in patients with spinal cord injury. Spinal Cord 2003;41:680.
28. Munck J, Simoens C, Thill V, et al. Intestinal stoma in patients with spinal cord injury: a retrospective study of 23 patients. Hepatogastroenterology 2008;55: 2125.
29. Rosito O, Nino-Murcia M, Wolfe VA, et al. The effects of colostomy on the quality of life in patients with spinal cord injury: a retrospective analysis. J Spinal Cord Med 2002;25:174.
30. Stone JM, Nino-Murcia M, Wolfe VA, et al. Chronic gastrointestinal problems in spinal cord injury patients: a prospective analysis. Am J Gastroenterol 1990;85: 1114.
31. Scott D, Papa MZ, Sareli M, et al. Management of hemorrhoidal disease in patients with chronic spinal cord injury. Tech Coloproctol 2002;6:19.
32. Johnston MV, Diab ME, Chu BC, et al. Preventive services and health behaviors among people with spinal cord injury. J Spinal Cord Med 2005;28:43.
33. Resnick NM, Yalla SV. Aging and its effect on the bladder. Semin Urol 1987;5:82.
34. Madersbacher S, Pycha A, Klingler CH, et al. Interrelationships of bladder compliance with age, detrusor instability, and obstruction in elderly men with lower urinary tract symptoms. Neurourol Urodyn 1999;18:3.
35. Pfisterer MH, Griffiths DJ, Schaefer W, et al. The effect of age on lower urinary tract function: a study in women. J Am Geriatr Soc 2006;54:405.
36. Liang SY, Mackowiak PA. Infections in the elderly. Clin Geriatr Med 2007;23:441.
37. Htwe TH, Mushtaq A, Robinson SB, et al. Infection in the elderly. Infect Dis Clin North Am 2007;21:711.

38. Truzzi JC, Almeida FM, Nunes EC, et al. Residual urinary volume and urinary tract infection–when are they linked? J Urol 2008;180:182.
39. Madersbacher G, Oberwalder M. The elderly para- and tetraplegic: special aspects of the urological care. Paraplegia 1987;25:318.
40. Garshick E, Kelley A, Cohen SA, et al. A prospective assessment of mortality in chronic spinal cord injury. Spinal Cord 2005;43:408.
41. McKinley WO, Jackson AB, Cardenas DD, et al. Long-term medical complications after traumatic spinal cord injury: a regional model systems analysis. Arch Phys Med Rehabil 1999;80:1402.
42. Cardenas DD, Hoffman JM, Kirshblum S, et al. Etiology and incidence of rehospitalization after traumatic spinal cord injury: a multicenter analysis. Arch Phys Med Rehabil 2004;85:1757.
43. Savic G, Short DJ, Weitzenkamp D, et al. Hospital readmissions in people with chronic spinal cord injury. Spinal Cord 2000;38:371.
44. Haisma JA, van der Woude LH, Stam HJ, et al. Complications following spinal cord injury: occurrence and risk factors in a longitudinal study during and after inpatient rehabilitation. J Rehabil Med 2007;39:393.
45. Groah SL, Weitzenkamp DA, Lammertse DP, et al. Excess risk of bladder cancer in spinal cord injury: evidence for an association between indwelling catheter use and bladder cancer. Arch Phys Med Rehabil 2002;83:346.
46. Drake MJ, Cortina-Borja M, Savic G, et al. Prospective evaluation of urological effects of aging in chronic spinal cord injury by method of bladder management. Neurourol Urodyn 2005;24:111.
47. O'Leary M, Erickson JR, Smith CP, et al. Effect of controlled-release oxybutynin on neurogenic bladder function in spinal cord injury. J Spinal Cord Med 2003;26:159.
48. Bennett N, O'Leary M, Patel AS, et al. Can higher doses of oxybutynin improve efficacy in neurogenic bladder? J Urol 2004;171:749.
49. Melzak J. The incidence of bladder cancer in paraplegia. Paraplegia 1966;4:85.
50. Kaufman JM, Fam B, Jacobs SC, et al. Bladder cancer and squamous metaplasia in spinal cord injury patients. J Urol 1977;118:967.
51. El-Masri WS, Fellows G. Bladder cancer after spinal cord injury. Paraplegia 1981;19:265.
52. Stonehill WH, Dmochowski RR, Patterson AL, et al. Risk factors for bladder tumors in spinal cord injury patients. J Urol 1996;155:1248.
53. Pannek J. Transitional cell carcinoma in patients with spinal cord injury: a high risk malignancy? Urology 2002;59:240.
54. Subramonian K, Cartwright RA, Harnden P, et al. Bladder cancer in patients with spinal cord injuries. BJU Int 2004;93:739.
55. Yang CC, Clowers DE. Screening cystoscopy in chronically catheterized spinal cord injury patients. Spinal Cord 1999;37:204.
56. Castillo CM, Ha CY, Gater DR, et al. Prophylactic radical cystectomy for the management of keratinizing squamous metaplasia of the bladder in a man with tetraplegia. J Spinal Cord Med 2007;30:389.
57. Navon JD, Soliman H, Khonsari F, et al. Screening cystoscopy and survival of spinal cord injured patients with squamous cell cancer of the bladder. J Urol 1997;157:2109.
58. Ku JH, Jung TY, Lee JK, et al. Influence of bladder management on epididymoorchitis in patients with spinal cord injury: clean intermittent catheterization is a risk factor for epididymo-orchitis. Spinal Cord 2006;44:165.
59. Frisbie JH, Binard J. Low prevalence of prostatic cancer among myelopathy patients. J Am Paraplegia Soc 1994;17:148.

60. Scott PAS, Perkash I, Mode D, et al. Prostate cancer diagnosed in spinal cord-injured patients is more commonly advanced stage than in able-bodied patients. Urology 2004;63:509.

61. Charlifue S, Lammertse DP, Adkins RH. Aging with spinal cord injury: changes in selected health indices and life satisfaction. Arch Phys Med Rehabil 2004;85:1848.

62. Rintala DH, Garber SL, Friedman JD, et al. Preventing recurrent pressure ulcers in veterans with spinal cord injury: impact of a structured education and follow-up intervention. Arch Phys Med Rehabil 2008;89:1429.

63. Regan MA, Teasell RW, Wolfe DL, et al. A systematic review of therapeutic interventions for pressure ulcers after spinal cord injury. Arch Phys Med Rehabil 2009;90:213.

64. Yarkony GM. Aging skin, pressure ulcerations, and spinal cord injury. In: Whiteneck GG, Charlifue SW, Gerhart KA, et al, editors. Aging with spinal cord injury. New York: Demos Publications; 1993.

65. Consortium for Spinal Cord Medicine Clinical Practice Guidelines. Pressure ulcer prevention and treatment following spinal cord injury: a clinical practice guideline for health-care professionals. J Spinal Cord Med 2001;(24 Suppl 1):S40.

66. Vicario C, de Juan J, Esclarin A, et al. Treatment of deep wound infections after spinal fusion with a vacuum-assisted device in patients with spinal cord injury. Acta Orthop Belg 2007;73:102.

67. Schryvers OI, Stranc MF, Nance PW. Surgical treatment of pressure ulcers: 20-year experience. Arch Phys Med Rehabil 2000;81:1556.

68. Krause JS, Broderick L. Patterns of recurrent pressure ulcers after spinal cord injury: identification of risk and protective factors 5 or more years after onset. Arch Phys Med Rehabil 2004;85(8):1257–64.

69. Dorsett P, Geraghty T. Health-related outcomes of people with spinal cord injury: –a 10 year longitudinal study. Spinal Cord 2008;46:386.

70. Waters RL, Sie IH, Adkins RH. The musculoskeletal system. In: Whiteneck GG, Charlifue SW, Gerhart KA, et al, editors. Aging with spinal cord injury. New York: Demos Publications; 1993.

71. Consortium for Spinal Cord Medicine. Preservation of upper limb function following spinal cord injury: a clinical practice guideline for health-care professionals. J Spinal Cord Med 2005;28:434.

72. Alm M, Saraste H, Norrbrink C. Shoulder pain in persons with thoracic spinal cord injury: prevalence and characteristics. J Rehabil Med 2008;40:277.

73. Boninger ML, Koontz AM, Sisto SA, et al. Pushrim biomechanics and injury prevention in spinal cord injury: recommendations based on CULP-SCI investigations. J Rehabil R D 2005;42:9.

74. Bayley JC, Cochran TP, Sledge CB. The weight-bearing shoulder: the impingement syndrome in paraplegics. J Bone Joint Surg Am 1987;69:676.

75. Escobedo EM, Hunter JC, Hollister MC, et al. MR imaging of rotator cuff tears in individuals with paraplegia. AJR Am J Roentgenol 1997;168:919.

76. Brose SW, Boninger ML, Fullerton B, et al. Shoulder ultrasound abnormalities, physical examination findings, and pain in manual wheelchair users with spinal cord injury. Arch Phys Med Rehabil 2008;89:2086.

77. Robinson MD, Hussey RW, Ha CY. Surgical decompression of impingement in the weightbearing shoulder. Arch Phys Med Rehabil 1993;74:324.

78. Goldstein B, Young J, Escobedo EM. Rotator cuff repairs in individuals with paraplegia. Am J Phys Med Rehabil 1997;76:316.

79. Popowitz RL, Zvijac JE, Uribe JW, et al. Rotator cuff repair in spinal cord injury patients. J Shoulder Elbow Surg 2003;12:327.
80. Wright VJ. Osteoporosis in men. J Am Acad Orthop Surg 2006;14:347.
81. Gennari L, Bilezikian JP. Osteoporosis in men. Endocrinol Metab Clin North Am 2007;36:399.
82. Garland DE, Stewart CA, Adkins RH, et al. Osteoporosis after spinal cord injury. J Orthop Res 1992;10:371.
83. Frisbie JH. Fractures after myelopathy: the risk quantified. J Spinal Cord Med 1997;20:66.
84. Frotzler A, Coupaud S, Perret C, et al. High-volume FES-cycling partially reverses bone loss in people with chronic spinal cord injury. Bone 2008;43:169.
85. Frotzler A, Coupaud S, Perret C, et al. Effect of detraining on bone and muscle tissue in subjects with chronic spinal cord injury after a period of electrically-stimulated cycling: a small cohort study. J Rehabil Med 2009;41:282.
86. Nance PW, Schryvers O, Leslie W, et al. Intravenous pamidronate attenuates bone density loss after acute spinal cord injury. Arch Phys Med Rehabil 1999; 80:243.
87. Bauman WA, Wecht JM, Kirshblum S, et al. Effect of pamidronate administration on bone in patients with acute spinal cord injury. J Rehabil Res Dev 2005;42:305.
88. Cruz-Sanchez FF, Moral A, Tolosa E, et al. Evaluation of neuronal loss, astrocytosis and abnormalities of cytoskeletal components of large motor neurons in the human anterior horn in aging. J Neural Transm 1998;105:689.
89. Hatzitaki V, Amiridis IG, Arabatzi F. Aging effects on postural responses to self-imposed balance perturbations. Gait Posture 2005;22:250.
90. Lauretani F, Bandinelli S, Bartali B, et al. Axonal degeneration affects muscle density in older men and women. Neurobiol Aging 2006;27:1145.
91. Olafsdottir H, Yoshida N, Zatsiorsky VM, et al. Elderly show decreased adjustments of motor synergies in preparation to action. Clin Biomech (Bristol, Avon) 2007;22:44.
92. Shaffer SW, Harrison AL. Aging of the somatosensory system: a translational perspective. Phys Ther 2007;87:193.
93. Lammertse DP. The nervous system. In: Whiteneck GG, Charlifue SW, Gerhart KA, et al, editors. Aging with spinal cord injury. New York: Demos Publications; 1993.
94. Gellman H, Sie I, Waters RL. Late complications of the weight-bearing upper extremity in the paraplegic patient. Clin Orthop Relat Res 1988;(233):132–5.
95. Davidoff G, Werner R, Waring W. Compressive mononeuropathies of the upper extremity in chronic paraplegia. Paraplegia 1991;29:17.
96. Edgar R, Quail P. Progressive post-traumatic cystic and non-cystic myelopathy. Br J Neurosurg 1994;8:7.
97. Falci S, Holtz A, Akesson E, et al. Obliteration of a posttraumatic spinal cord cyst with solid human embryonic spinal cord grafts: first clinical attempt. J Neurotrauma 1997;14:875.
98. Falci SP, Lammertse DP, Best L, et al. Surgical treatment of posttraumatic cystic and tethered spinal cords. J Spinal Cord Med 1999;22:173.
99. Lee TT, Arias JM, Andrus HL, et al. Progressive posttraumatic myelomalacic myelopathy: treatment with untethering and expansive duraplasty. J Neurosurg 1997;86:624.
100. Bursell JP, Little JW, Stiens SA. Electrodiagnosis in spinal cord injured persons with new weakness or sensory loss: central and peripheral etiologies. Arch Phys Med Rehabil 1999;80:904.

101. Mellegers MA, Furlan AD, Mailis A. Gabapentin for neuropathic pain: systematic review of controlled and uncontrolled literature. Clin J Pain 2001;17:284.

102. Jensen TS, Gottrup H, Sindrup SH, et al. The clinical picture of neuropathic pain. Eur J Pharmacol 2001;429:1.

103. Siddall PJ. Management of neuropathic pain following spinal cord injury: now and in the future. Spinal Cord 2009;47:352.

104. Widerstrom-Noga EG, Finnerup NB, Siddall PJ. Biopsychosocial perspective on a mechanisms-based approach to assessment and treatment of pain following spinal cord injury. J Rehabil Res Dev 2009;46:1.

105. Armijo JA, Pena MA, Adin J, et al. Association between patient age and gabapentin serum concentration-to-dose ratio: a preliminary multivariate analysis. Ther Drug Monit 2004;26:633.

106. Lloyd-Jones D, Adams R, Carnethon M, et al. Heart disease and stroke statistics–2009 update: a report from the American Heart Association Statistics Committee and Stroke Statistics Subcommittee. Circulation 2009;119:e21.

107. Ferdinandy P, Schulz R, Baxter GF. Interaction of cardiovascular risk factors with myocardial ischemia/reperfusion injury, preconditioning, and postconditioning. Pharmacol Rev 2007;59:418.

108. Ragnarsson KT. The cardiovascular system. In: Whiteneck GG, Charlifue SW, Gerhart KA, et al, editors. Aging with spinal cord injury. New York: Demos Publications; 1993. p. 73.

109. DeVivo MJ, Stover SL. Long-term survival and causes of death. In: Stover SL, DeLisa JA, Whiteneck GG, editors. Spinal cord injury: clinical outcomes from the model systems. Gaithersburg (MD): Aspen Publishers, Inc; 1995.

110. National Spinal Cord Injury Statistical Center. The 2007 annual statistical report for the spinal cord injury model systems. Birmingham (AL): University of Alabama, 2007.

111. Groah SL, Weitzenkamp D, Sett P, et al. The relationship between neurological level of injury and symptomatic cardiovascular disease risk in the aging spinal injured. Spinal Cord 2001;39:310.

112. Brenes G, Dearwater S, Shapera R, et al. High density lipoprotein cholesterol concentrations in physically active and sedentary spinal cord injured patients. Arch Phys Med Rehabil 1986;67:445.

113. Bauman WA, Kahn NN, Grimm DR, et al. Risk factors for atherogenesis and cardiovascular autonomic function in persons with spinal cord injury. Spinal Cord 1999;37:601.

114. Bauman WA, Spungen AM. Disorders of carbohydrate and lipid metabolism in veterans with paraplegia or quadriplegia: a model of premature aging. Metabolism 1994;43:749.

115. Banerjea R, Sambamoorthi U, Weaver F, et al. Risk of stroke, heart attack, and diabetes complications among veterans with spinal cord injury. Arch Phys Med Rehabil 2008;89:1448.

116. Liang H, Chen D, Wang Y, et al. Different risk factor patterns for metabolic syndrome in men with spinal cord injury compared with able-bodied men despite similar prevalence rates. Arch Phys Med Rehabil 2007;88:1198.

117. Davis GM, Hamzaid NA, Fornusek C. Cardiorespiratory, metabolic, and biomechanical responses during functional electrical stimulation leg exercise: health and fitness benefits. Artif Organs 2008;32:625.

118. Zbogar D, Eng JJ, Krassioukov AV, et al. The effects of functional electrical stimulation leg cycle ergometry training on arterial compliance in individuals with spinal cord injury. Spinal Cord 2008;46:722.

119. Wilmot CB, Hall KM. The respiratory system. In: Whiteneck GG, Charlifue SW, Gerhart KA, et al, editors. Aging with spinal cord injury. New York: Demos Publications; 1993.

120. Katial R, Zheng W. Allergy and immunology of the aging lung. Clin Chest Med 2007;28:663.

121. Wolkove N, Elkholy O, Baltzan M, et al. Sleep and aging: 1. Sleep disorders commonly found in older people. CMAJ 2007;176:1299.

122. Martinez D. Effects of aging on peripheral chemoreceptor CO2 response during sleep and wakefulness in healthy men. Respir Physiolo Neurobiol 2008;162:138.

123. Eckert DJ, Malhotra A. Pathophysiology of adult obstructive sleep apnea. Proc Am Thorac Soc 2008;5:144.

124. Burns SP. Acute respiratory infections in persons with spinal cord injury. Phys Med Rehabil Clin N Am 2007;18:203.

125. Stolzmann KL, Gagnon DR, Brown R, et al. Longitudinal change in FEV1 and FVC in chronic spinal cord injury. Am J Respir Crit Care Med 2008; 177:781.

126. Menter RR, Hudson LM. Effects of age at injury and the aging process. In: Stover SL, DeLisa JA, Whiteneck GG, editors. Spinal cord injury: clinical outcomes from the model systems. Gaithersburg (MD): Aspen Publishers, Inc; 1995. p. 272.

127. Short DJ, Stradling JR, Williams SJ. Prevalence of sleep apnoea in patients over 40 years of age with spinal cord lesions. J Neurol Neurosurg Psychiatr 1992;55: 1032.

128. Burns SP, Little JW, Hussey JD, et al. Sleep apnea syndrome in chronic spinal cord injury: associated factors and treatment. Arch Phys Med Rehabil 2000; 81:1334.

129. Consortium for Spinal Cord Medicine. Respiratory management following spinal cord injury: a clinical practice guideline for health-care professionals. J Spinal Cord Med 2005;28:259.

130. Leduc BE, Dagher JH, Mayer P, et al. Estimated prevalence of obstructive sleep apnea-hypopnea syndrome after cervical cord injury. Arch Phys Med Rehabil 2007;88:333.

131. Lanig IS, Peterson WP. The respiratory system in spinal cord injury. Phys Med Rehabil Clin N Am 2000;11:29.

132. Burns SP, Rad MY, Bryant S, et al. Long-term treatment of sleep apnea in persons with spinal cord injury. Am J Phys Med Rehabil 2005;84:620.

133. Ershler WB. Biomarkers of aging: immunological events. Exp Gerontol 1988;23: 387.

134. Weksler ME. Immune senescence. Ann Neurol 1994;(Suppl 35):S35–7.

135. Pawelec G, Derhovanessian E, Larbi A, et al. Cytomegalovirus and human immunosenescence. Rev Med Virol 2009;19:47.

136. Gavazzi G, Krause KH. Ageing and infection. Lancet Infect Dis 2002;2:659.

137. Campagnolo DI, Bartlett JA, Chatterton RJ, et al. Adrenal and pituitary hormone patterns after spinal cord injury. Am J Phys Med Rehabil 1999;78:361.

138. Frost F, Roach MJ, Kushner I, et al. Inflammatory c-reactive protein and cytokine levels in asymptomatic people with chronic spinal cord injury. Arch Phys Med Rehabil 2005;86:312.

139. Couture M, Lariviere N, Lefrancois R. Psychological distress in older adults with low functional independence: a multidimensional perspective. Arch Gerontol Geriatr 2005;41:101.

140. Rejeski WJ, Fielding RA, Blair SN, et al. The lifestyle interventions and independence for elders (life) pilot study: design and methods. Contemp Clin Trials 2005;26:141.

141. Bear-Lehman J, Albert SM, Burkhardt A. Cutaneous sensitivity and functional limitation. Topics in Geriatric Rehabilitation 2006;22:61.

142. Song J, Chang RW, Dunlop DD. Population impact of arthritis on disability in older adults. Arthritis Rheum 2006;55:248.

143. Arnett SW, Laity JH, Agrawal SK, et al. Aerobic reserve and physical functional performance in older adults. Age Ageing 2008;37:384.

144. Tanaka H. Habitual exercise for the elderly. Fam Community Health 2009;32:S57.

145. National Center for Health Statistics. Health, United States, 2006 with chartbook on trends in the health of Americans. Hyattsville (MD): US Department of Health and Human Services; 2006.

146. McColl MA, Rosenthal C. A model of resource needs of aging spinal cord injured men. Paraplegia 1994;32:261.

147. Gerhart KA, Bergstrom E, Charlifue SW, et al. Long-term spinal cord injury: functional changes over time. Arch Phys Med Rehabil 1993;74:1030.

148. Gerhart KA, Charlifue SW, Weitzenkamp DA, et al. Aging with spinal cord injury. Am Rehabil 1997;23:19.

149. Charlifue SW, Weitzenkamp DA, Whiteneck GG. Longitudinal outcomes in spinal cord injury: aging, secondary conditions, and well-being. Arch Phys Med Rehabil 1999;80:1429.

150. Jorm AF, Windsor TD, Dear KB, et al. Age group differences in psychological distress: the role of psychosocial risk factors that vary with age. Psychol Med 2005;35:1253.

151. Rafanelli C, Roncuzzi R, Milaneschi Y, et al. Stressful life events, depression and demoralization as risk factors for acute coronary heart disease. Psychother Psychosom 2005;74:179.

152. Frasure-Smith N, Lesperance F. Recent evidence linking coronary heart disease and depression. Can J Psychiatry 2006;51:730.

153. Ames D. Depressive disorders among elderly people in long-term institutional care. Aust N Z J Psychiatry 1993;27:379.

154. Djernes JK. Prevalence and predictors of depression in populations of elderly: a review. Acta Psychiatr Scand 2006;113:372.

155. Prince MJ, Harwood RH, Blizard RA, et al. Social support deficits, loneliness and life events as risk factors for depression in old age. The Gospel Oak Project VI. Psychol Med 1997;27:323.

156. Roberts RE, Kaplan GA, Shema SJ, et al. Does growing old increase the risk for depression? Am J Psychiatry 1997;154:1384.

157. Yang Y. Is old age depressing? Growth trajectories and cohort variations in late-life depression. J Health Soc Behav 2007;48:16.

158. Lachman ME, Rocke C, Rosnick C, et al. Realism and illusion in Americans' temporal views of their life satisfaction: age differences in reconstructing the past and anticipating the future. Psychol Sci 2008;19:889.

159. Fisher BJ. Successful aging, life satisfaction, and generativity in later life. Int J Aging Hum Dev 1995;41:239.

160. Kemp BJ, Kahan JS, Krause JS, et al. Treatment of major depression in individuals with spinal cord injury. J Spinal Cord Med 2004;27:22.

161. Dryden DM, Saunders LD, Rowe BH, et al. Depression following traumatic spinal cord injury. Neuroepidemiology 2005;25(25):55.

162. Osteraker AL, Levi R. Indicators of psychological distress in postacute spinal cord injured individuals. Spinal Cord 2005;43:223.

163. Krause JS, Kemp B, Coker J. Depression after spinal cord injury: relation to gender, ethnicity, aging, and socioeconomic indicators. Arch Phys Med Rehabil 2000;81:1099.

164. Charlifue SW, Gerhart KA, Whiteneck GG. Conceptualizing and quantifying functional change: an examination of aging with spinal cord injury. Topics in Geriatric Rehabilitation 1998;13:35.

165. Post MW, de Witte LP, van Asbeck FW, et al. Predictors of health status and life satisfaction in spinal cord injury. Arch Phys Med Rehabil 1998;79:395.

166. Krause JS, Broderick L. A 25-year longitudinal study of the natural course of aging after spinal cord injury. Spinal Cord 2005;43:349.

167. Krause JS, Coker JL. Aging after spinal cord injury: a 30-year longitudinal study. J Spinal Cord Med 2006;29:371.

168. Charlifue S, Gerhart K. Changing psychosocial morbidity in people aging with spinal cord injury. NeuroRehabilitation 2004;19:15.

169. Newsom JT, Schulz R. Caregiving from the recipient's perspective: negative reactions to being helped. Health Psychol 1998;17:172.

Aging with Multiple Sclerosis

Michelle Stern, MD[a],*, Lyssa Sorkin, MD[b], Kelly Milton, MS[c],
Kevin Sperber, MD[c]

KEYWORDS

• MS • Aging • Disability • Pain • Progressive condition

Multiple sclerosis (MS) is the most common cause of acquired neurologic disability in young adults. In 70% of cases, symptoms first emerge between the ages of 20 and 40 years. The exact cause is not known, but current theories suggest that MS is an inflammatory autoimmune disorder. The hallmarks of MS are central nervous system (CNS) inflammation, demyelination, axonal degeneration, and gliosis, which can cause a wide array of brain and spinal cord syndromes. Although MS is generally considered a chronic progressive illness, the timing and the severity of progression is highly variable and unpredictable. As the patient with MS ages, the morbidities and physiologic changes associated with the normal aging process have an effect on the severity of impairment and disability. Older patients with MS have been observed to have a faster rate of disease progression leading to irreversible disability. This finding is suspected to be related to progressive axonal loss. The synergistic effects of age and neurologic illness bring a unique challenge to the clinician and patient.[1–4]

Major clinical manifestations of MS include sensory deficits, weakness, visual disturbances, cognitive impairment, depression, spasticity, ataxia, heat intolerance, fatigue, pain, and bowel and genitourinary dysfunction. The normal aging process can have similar effects. Weakness and fatigue from MS may also be compounded by age-related changes including muscle atrophy, reduced cardiopulmonary reserve, and impaired temperature regulation. In addition, older individuals are more sensitive to side effects of medication because of their decreased ability to distribute and eliminate metabolites. The risk/benefit ratio of medication use in elderly MS patients needs to be considered thoroughly. Thus, there are many issues the clinician must address in the management of the older patient with MS to help minimize the disability caused by aging with this chronic and progressive disease.[5–7]

[a] Department of Physical Medicine and Rehabilitation, Columbia University College of Physicians and Surgeons, New York Presbyterian Hospital, 180 Fort Washington Avenue, Harkness Pavilion, Suite 199, NY 10032, USA
[b] New York Presbyterian Columbia Cornell Residency Program, NY, USA
[c] Columbia University College of Physicians and Surgeons, New York Presbyterian Hospital, NY, USA
* Corresponding author.
E-mail address: ms1127@columbia.edu

Phys Med Rehabil Clin N Am 21 (2010) 403–417
doi:10.1016/j.pmr.2009.12.008
1047-9651/10/$ – see front matter © 2010 Elsevier Inc. All rights reserved.

pmr.theclinics.com

A diagnosis of MS does not confer mortality, however, there is significant morbidity associated with MS. There are limited studies looking at the effect of MS on life expectancy. One recent study suggested that patients with MS were 3 times more likely to die prematurely relative to the general population, and the most common cause of death was respiratory distress.[8]

Although the course of MS is variable, many prognostic indicators have been identified. Indicators of a poor prognosis include male gender, late onset, initial motor, cerebellar, and sphincter involvement, a progressive course at onset, shorter inter-attack intervals, and a large number of early attacks with residual disability.[9] Indicators of a favorable prognosis include minimal disability 5 years after onset, complete and rapid remission of initial symptoms, relapsing remitting type, age 35 years or less at onset, only 1 symptom in the first year, and onset with sensory symptoms or mild optic neuritis.[2,10,11]

CLASSIFICATION OF MS

The diagnosis of MS is usually clinical and is defined by discrete neurologic events separated in time. The McDonald Criteria, which were revised in 2005, combine clinical presentation with findings on magnetic resonance imaging (MRI) that are characteristic of the disease. Improved imaging techniques help to evaluate the brain, and the spinal cord can show lesions disseminated in time and in space. This can assist in making the diagnosis.

There are 4 major subtypes of MS that can be characterized by their disease course: relapsing remitting multiple sclerosis (RRMS), secondary progressive multiple sclerosis (SPMS), progressive relapsing multiple sclerosis (PRMS), and primary progressive multiple sclerosis (PPMS).[12-14]

RRMS is diagnosed in 85% of patients on initial diagnoses and overall 55% have this subtype. The relapses occur with or without complete recovery and the patient is clinically stable between these episodes. Most patients will recover from relapses within 4 weeks. The longer a patient has MS, the greater the chance that the relapses will be associated with residual deficits and increasing disability. There is a subtype of RRMS called benign MS. Benign MS occurs in 10% to 20% of patients. This group has few attacks and excellent recovery between attacks. There is usually minimal disability 20 years after onset, but several patients develop significant disability after 25 years. RRMS patients usually transit to secondary progressive disease.[3,13,14]

SPMS occurs in 30% of patients and is characterized by gradual progression of disability with or without superimposed relapses. If RRMS is left untreated, 50% of patients will develop SPMS in 10 years and 90% in 25 years. It is speculated that disease progression is secondary to ongoing axonal loss despite a lower rate of inflammatory lesions compared with RRMS.[3,13,14]

PPMS is defined by the gradual progression of disability from onset without superimposed relapses. This form occurs in 10% of patients and onset is most likely at an older age (40–60 years) and fewer cognitive changes due to primary involvement of the spinal cord.[3,13,14] PRMS affects 5% of patients and is characterized by the gradual accumulation of neurologic deficits from initial disease onset with additional intermittent exacerbations.[3,13,14]

STUDIES USED IN THE DIAGNOSIS OF MS

MRI with gadolinium is commonly used to aid in the diagnosis of MS by showing disseminated white matter lesions in the CNS with a characteristic demyelination pattern. Gadolinium enhancement can show the breakdown in the blood-brain barrier that occurs during active MS. T1 gadolinium enhancing lesions indicate acute disease activity (<6 weeks). T2 hyperintense lesions indicate the extent of MS lesions. Demyelination on MRI is not a unique finding for MS. MRI studies have revealed that aging is associated with increased prevalence of subcortical hyperintense foci in T2-weighted images. These hyperintense lesions develop mainly in periventricular deep white matter. Subcortical white matter hyperintensities in the brain increase by 5% to 9% per year in older adults. Lesions in MS are commonly found extending outward from the ventricular surface, within the brainstem, corpus callosum, cerebellum, and spinal cord. Lesions of the anterior corpus callosum are particularly useful diagnostically because this site is usually spared in cerebrovascular disease. Older patients may present a challenge in differentiating between a new MS lesion and a stroke, but changes in MRI due to an ischemic stroke typically follow a vascular territory.[3,15]

Examination of the cerebrospinal fluid (CSF) and evoked potentials (visual evoked potential , brainstem auditory evoked potential and somatosensory evoked potential) are also used in diagnosing MS. The presence of oligoclonal bands in the CSF is not exclusive to MS. Evoked potentials will reveal an increase in latency that is indicative of a demyelinating process. With late onset MS, there will be a higher frequency of oligoclonal banding in the CSF and asymptomatic evoked potential abnormalities compared with a younger age-matched MS population.[16,17]

SYMPTOMS OF MS
Sensory Disturbance and Pain

Sensory disturbances are common at presentation and affect several patients with MS at some point during the course of their disease. Patients may experience numbness, tingling, the sensation of pins-and-needles, coldness, and feelings of tightness or swelling in the limbs and trunk.

More than half of all patients experience chronic or acute pain syndromes as either a direct consequence of MS, or indirectly as a consequence of the disability created by the disease process. Pain can be characterized into 4 categories: neuropathic pain, acute pain due to the inflammatory process, pain caused by increased muscle tone, and musculoskeletal pain from poor body posture, improper positioning, or paraplegic shoulder. Patients with MS may experience trigeminal neuralgia, the sensation of electric shock radiating down the spine or into limbs on neck flexion (Lhermitte sign), dysesthetic pain, back pain, visceral pain, and pain secondary to muscle spasms.[18]

Pain is associated with longer disease duration and spinal cord involvement. The older population often reports pain as the most distressing symptom. Aging is associated with musculoskeletal degeneration, which can further aggravate painful conditions. Studies have shown that patients with MS are often under-treated for pain, which can result in increased morbidity.[19–21]

Medication useful for treating pain in this population includes opioid analgesics, nonsteroidal antiinflammatory drugs (NSAIDS), antiseizure medication, antidepressants, antispasticity agents, and cannibiods. An intrathecal pump may also be beneficial for intractable pain and spasms.

It is important to consider side effects when prescribing medication to the elderly, and dose adjustments may be necessary. Side effects of opioids include constipation, respiratory depression, confusion, and lethargy. Carbamazepine and other anticonvulsants may increase confusion and ataxia in the elderly. Tricyclic antidepressants (TCAS) or other medications with anticholinergic effects may lead to urinary retention, confusion, cardiac symptoms, and autonomic instability. The NSAIDS should be used with caution in the elderly because of the increase risk of hypertension, myocardial infarction, stroke, gastrointestinal bleeding, and renal insufficiency.[22]

The antidepressant duloxetine, which is a selective serotonin and a norepinephrine reuptake inhibitor, is approved for treatment of pain from secondary diabetic neuropathy and fibromyalgia. It has been used off label for other types of neuropathic pain. Studies have shown duloxetine to be safe and effective in the geriatric population although most of these studies involved the use of duloxetine for conditions other than pain. Nausea and headache are the most common side effects, but the drug can also cause orthostatic hypotension and hyponatremia, both of which may affect the aging population more prominently. (Duloxetine for Multiple Sclerosis Pain. http://www.ClinicalTrials.gov).[23]

Although many pain syndromes are solely caused by MS, pain complaints in an aging population should be evaluated for other possible causes. Cervical and lumbar spondylosis may occur in conjunction with MS. Clues to help identify cases of spondylosis include neck or back pain, radicular pain in the extremities, muscle atrophy in a segmental distribution, and the loss of deep tendon reflexes. MRI of the cervical or lumbar spine should be part of the diagnostic work-up. Surgery may be beneficial for select patients.[12]

Fatigue

Fatigue is present in two-thirds of patients with one half describing fatigue as the most disabling symptom. Common features of MS fatigue include malaise, motor weakness during sustained activity, and difficulty maintaining concentration. An aging patient with MS who complains of fatigue should be evaluated to rule out other potential causes including infection, cancer, anemia, hypothyroidism, rheumatologic disorders, sleep apnea, and diseases of the cardiovascular, pulmonary, renal, or hepatic system. Medications that can contribute to fatigue include TCAS, selective serotonin reuptake inhibitors, benzodiazepines, opioids, anticonvulsants, β-blockers, interferons, and antispasticity medications. Other factors that can lead to fatigue include depression, pain, physical deconditioning, disrupted sleep secondary to neurogenic bladder, and exposure to a heated environment. Once other causes have been ruled out, treatment of fatigue includes energy conservation, exercise program, and medication. Aerobic exercises in particular have been shown to be beneficial in reducing fatigue.[24] Medications include amantadine, modafinil, and methylphenidate. The use of stimulants in the aging population should be used with caution because of the increased risk of cardiac side effects. Methylphenidate has been associated with increased heart rate, but has been shown to be safe and effective in adult populations with traumatic brain injuries.[25] Amantadine has been associated with an increase in risk of confusion and edema in the elderly.[26,27]

Depression

Depression is the most common mood disorder affecting more than half of patients. The incidence of depression in MS is 3 times higher than in the general population and more common even compared with other chronic disease states. Depression may be overlooked as there are symptoms common to both, such as fatigue, reduced activity, decreased appetite, and poor concentration. MS is associated with a 7.5 times higher suicide rate than in the general population, which cannot be explained fully by a reactive depression. In general, suicide rates increase with age. Risk factors for suicide include major depression, living alone, and alcohol abuse. Duration of MS, severity of physical disability, and cognitive impairment do not affect the risk of suicide. Drugs that can cause depressive symptoms include anxiolytics, β-blockers, methyldopa, clonidine, reserpine, interferon, and steroids. Depression rating scales that are currently used may have limited use in the MS population. The widely used

Beck Depression Inventory evaluates depression based on responses to 21 questions, but the questions may overlap with the symptoms of MS itself, such as fatigue. The same is also true for the Geriatric Depression Scale. How common depression scales should be modified to better evaluate the MS patient is still unclear at this time.[19,28–30]

Cognitive Dysfunction

Fifty percent of patients with MS suffer from some form of cognitive dysfunction. Changes in cognitive ability can significantly impair the ability to work and live independently. Even though mild cognitive dysfunction occurs frequently, only 5% to 10% of patients will develop a severe cognitive dysfunction.[19] Cognitive deficits involve loss of short-term memory, reasoning, verbal fluency, visuospatial functions, abstract reasoning, and speed of processing information whereas intellectual functions and language skills are generally unaffected. Decreased short-term memory is the most common finding. Patients show slowed retrieval of formed memories and often require cueing. Aging itself causes a slowing in the frontal lobe, which can lead to a slower learning rate and difficulty with memory. Thus, the aging patient with MS may be at an even greater risk for significant cognitive disturbance. Patients should be encouraged to use lists, daily journals, and appointment books for activities. The Mini-mental Examination may be useful in tracking changes in cognition but it may be insensitive to detect subtle cognitive changes occurring in most patients with MS. The patient's medications should be assessed for possible effects on cognitive function. Medications that can contribute to cognitive slowing, especially in the aging population, include anticholinergics, antispasmodics, opioids, benzodiazepines, and TCAS. Consideration should be given to a change to long-acting anticholinergic preparations for bladder dysfunction. The use of intrathecal medications or botulinum toxin injections may be used to reduce high doses of oral antispasticity agents. As always, it is important to monitor for signs of depression, anxiety, or fatigue, which may exacerbate cognitive difficulties.[31–37]

Opthomalogical Dysfunction

Disturbances of the visual system are among the most common manifestations of MS, affecting up to 80% of patients at some time during the disease course. These abnormalities can result in significant disability, culminating in an inability to work and compromising the patient's activities of daily living. The most common visual manifestations of MS are optic neuritis, internuclear ophthalmoplegia, and nystagmus. Symptoms may include blurred vision, scotoma, impaired color vision, and diminished contrast sensitivity. Visual changes are also common in the aging population with the development of cataracts, presbyopia, macular degeneration, and glaucoma, which can lead to further social isolation and difficulty in self-care. Useful recommendations may include the outlining of doorways, steps, and wall switches with tape or markers, the use of magnifiers, and glare reduction. Using eyeglasses with prisms, or having the patient patch one eye, may minimize diplopia.[19,38]

Cerebellar Symptoms

Cerebellar lesions are seen in one-third of patients with MS. Tremor in MS can be one of the more disabling symptoms of the disease and can affect any muscle group. Tremors can increase fatigue by causing an increase in energy consumption. Although there is no effective treatment, medications used include propranolol (Inderal), clonazepam (Klonopin), primidone (Mysoline), and isoniazid (risk of hepatitis increases with age >35 years). Stereotactic surgery is not recommended.[19]

Motor Loss and Spasticity

Corticospinal tract involvement is present in 62% of patients with progressive disease. Spasticity and weakness usually have a greater effect on the lower extremities. The weakness associated with aging is a result of lower motor neuron denervation and muscle atrophy.

The energy requirement for an activity is increased with the presence of spasticity. The aging patient with increased spasticity needs to be evaluated to rule out secondary causes such as infections, skin breakdown, spinal stenosis with myelopathy, or other disease processes. Oral antispasticity medication may be poorly tolerated by the older population and should be monitored closely. Baclofen use in an elderly patient will require an initial lower dose and a slower titration to decrease the risk of sedation and confusion. Tizanidine should also be used with caution in the elderly because clearance of the drug is decreased fourfold. Monitoring for hypotension and sedation is essential. The benzodiazepines are traditionally poorly tolerated in the older population and are associated with an increased half-life and a higher association of paradoxic reactions, agitation, and disequilibrium.[6,19]

Bladder Disturbance

Ninety-six percent of patients for have had MS for more than 10 years will develop urological symptoms, with detrusor hyperreflexia being the most common. Using oxybutynin or tolterodine for the treatment of detrusor hyperreflexia in clinical studies was found to be safe in older and younger patients. Anatomic and physiologic changes because of aging can cause urinary frequency, incontinence, hesitancy, retention, and nocturia. Incontinence may also be due to delirium, atrophic vaginitis, enlarged prostrate, constipation, and endocrine disorders. Women should be evaluated for estrogen replacement and men should have routine prostate evaluation. The elderly are especially sensitive to the urological side effects of medications. Alpha blocking agents used to treat sphincter dysnergia may cause a higher incidence of orthostasis in the elderly. Urinary tract dysfunction can lead to the formation of bladder and renal stones and frequent urinary tract infections. Urinary retention or frequent catheterization can lead to frequent urinary tract infections, commonly with antibiotic-resistant organisms. Treatment of urological symptoms should take into account the patient's level of disability, degree of reversibility of symptom, ability to function independently, other medical problems, and social support networks. For instance, before initiating a program of clean intermittent catheterization, a careful assessment of coordination, vision, cognitive function, and manual dexterity needs to be completed. If intermittent catheterization is impractical, a suprapubic or urethral indwelling catheter can be used. Chronic indwelling catheters can lead to colonization of the urinary tract, which may lead to chronically positive urine cultures, even in the absence of infections. Other disadvantages include increased risk of bladder calculi and bladder cancer. In patients with poor mobility, dexterity, or significant lower extremity spasticity, an augmentation cystoplasty with a catheterizable abdominal stoma may facilitate catheterization.[19,39]

Bowel Disturbance

Constipation as a result of pelvic floor spasticity, decreased gastro-colic reflex, inadequate hydration, medication, immobility, and weak abdominal muscles, is the most common bowel dysfunction. The elderly are also at risk for constipation because of slowed motility of the gastrointestinal tract. Many medications can exacerbate constipation, especially in the elderly. The TCAS or other medications with anticholinergic side effects, antihypertensives (especially the calcium channel blockers), iron, calcium, and opioid agents are common offenders. Fecal incontinence can result from sphincter dysfunction, constipation with rectal overflow, and diminished rectal sensation. A regular bowel program including stool softeners, promotility agents, and timed evacuation may be necessary. Changes in bowel habit need to be investigated to exclude colon cancer, diverticular disease, thyroid disease, or other medical causes.[19,40]

Sexual Disturbance

Most patients with MS and their partners suffer from some form of sexual dysfunction. Primary sexual dysfunction is due to lesions in the CNS that cause loss of libido, decreased genital sensation, decreased orgasmic response, difficulty in achieving an erection, or decreased vaginal lubrication. Secondary sexual dysfunction occurs due to other symptoms of MS such as bowel and bladder problems, spasticity, and so forth. Tertiary sexual dysfunction is related to psychosocial and cultural issues. Sexual changes that occur commonly in the elderly include impotence, orgasmic dysfunction, and dyspareunia. A sexual history should be taken routinely and treatment options should be discussed with the patient and their partner. Phosphodiesterase 5 inhibitors should be used with caution in the elderly due to possible cardiac side effects.[39,41]

Heat Intolerance

MS is associated with an increase in severity of symptoms with heat caused by environmental factors, over exertion, or pyrexia. The elderly are vulnerable to hyperthermia due to loss of homeostatic temperature regulation, declining function of the autonomic nervous system, decrease in sweat gland function, and loss of subcutaneous fat. To help manage heat intolerance, outside activities should be timed for early morning, energy conservation techniques should be used, and air conditioning should be used in homes and cars. Cooling vests and light-colored clothes may be useful, saunas and hot tubs should be avoided, and pool temperatures should be less than 30°C (86°F).[7,19]

Swallowing Difficulties

Swallowing disorders have been estimated to affect 3% to 20% of patients with MS. Oral intake and nutritional status should be closely monitored in these patients. Swallowing studies may be needed for evaluation and patients with severe dysphagia may require enterostomal feedings. Elderly patients may develop deficits, such as ineffective pharyngeal peristalsis and reduced motility of the esophagus leading to reflux, achalasia, and hiatal hernia, and this can exacerbate the dysphagia associated with MS.[19]

Other Related Conditions

Falls

Older age, leg weakness, and impaired balance lead to an increased fall risk. Recent studies suggested that gait speed might predict fall risk in MS, see the article by Finlayson and colleagues elsewhere in this issue for further exploration of this topic. There are limited data on the effects of exercise on reducing fall risk in the MS population. A home-exercise program may help improve lower extremity strength and thus reduce falls. Fall prevention in the elderly MS patient can include a home safety evaluation, proper footwear, orthotic use, and access to a lifeline. Medications that can contribute to fall risk include benzodiazepines, antihypertensives, TCAS, and tizanidine. Home modifications, such as non-slip floors, low carpet, removing area rugs, and a bedside commode may be beneficial.[42]

Osteoporosis

The effects of aging, limited ambulation ability, and the use of corticosteroids are common causes of bone loss. Patients of both genders with MS usually have decreased bone density in the spine and femoral neck. Patients should be screened regularly for osteoporosis. The aging patient with MS with impaired balance and ambulation is at increased risk for fractures. Studies have shown that hip fractures can be reduced with the use of a hip protector in the elderly, but this study did not include patients with MS.[43,44]

Osteoarthritis and degenerative joint disease

Osteoarthritis (OA) is common among patients over the age of 55 years and several patients over the age of 70 years have some evidence of disease. Joints including the knees, hips, spine, and hands are subject to degenerative changes secondary to wear and tear of the articular cartilage. This can be accompanied by osteophyte formation, narrowing of the joint space, sclerosis of bone, and gross joint deformity. Symptoms include pain, joint stiffness, and limited range of motion all of which might reduce functional mobility. Patients with MS may be at increased risk for osteoarthritis because of additional stress placed on joints secondary to weakness and spasticity. Furthermore, pain is a common symptom in patients with MS and it is important to differentiate between pain secondary to MS and pain in OA.

Most cases of OA may be treated with conservative methods, including physical therapy, NSAIDS, intra-articular steroids and/or viscosupplementation, however, eventually some patients may warrant a surgical intervention. In the MS population, postoperatively, patients have been found to develop hamstring spasticity, which can lead to a flexion deformity, resulting in pain and decreased range of motion. This may require additional therapy, bracing, muscle relaxants, or subsequent surgery to perform hamstring release. General and regional anesthesia have also been implicated in MS relapses and should be considered when deciding whether to pursue surgical options.[45]

Cardiac disease

Cardiac disease risk increases in the aging population. Some patients with MS have lower participation in physical activity and may be at an increased risk for coronary artery disease as they age. Low- and high-intensity exercise programs have been associated with a reduction in coronary artery disease risk in women with MS. Patients with lower physical activity had higher abdominal fat, and an increase in exercise led to lower glucose and triglyceride levels. Although it has been shown that patients with MS benefit from physical activity, the current research has mainly been conducted on patients below 65 years of age, and its effect on the elderly with MS is unknown.[46]

Diabetes mellitus

The prevalence of diabetes increases with age and has been linked to obesity. As patients with MS age and their disease progresses, their level of physical activity tends to decrease placing them at risk for gaining weight and developing diabetes. One complication of diabetes is increased risk of infections, which poses a problem for MS patients as infections can trigger relapses.[47] Other chronic problems associated with diabetes include microvascular complications, such as nephropathy and retinopathy, neuropathic complications, strokes, and coronary artery disease. Many symptoms of diabetes can overlap or mimic symptoms of MS. For example, the neuropathy of diabetes consists of pain and parasthesias beginning distally and spreading proximally in a typical glove and stocking distribution. Retinopathy can also lead to visual disturbances such as blurry vision, which is also seen in optic neuritis. In patients who have MS and diabetes, treating an acute exacerbation may pose a challenge secondary to the negative effects that high-dose steroids have on glycemic control. Therefore close monitoring and medication adjustment is essential.

Cancer
Cancer is currently the second leading cause of mortality in the United States. In 2009, it is estimated that there will be 1.5 million new cases of cancer diagnosed.[48] According-ing to new studies, patients with MS have a decreased overall cancer risk, however they are at a higher risk for developing CNS or urological tumors. The lower rates of digestive, respiratory, prostate, and ovarian cancer in MS patients may be secondary to lifestyle changes associated with their illness, immunologic changes due to disease activity, or treatment effects. There has been some evidence of an increased risk of breast cancer in women with MS treated with immunosuppressive therapy, but this is still under investigation.[49,50]

The increased risk of brain cancer associated with MS may be related to the chronic neurologic inflammation that accompanies the disease. However, patients with MS undergo imaging frequently and the increased risk may reflect an increase in detection. As for bladder cancer, this may be secondary to chronic bladder inflammation secondary to urological dysfunction.[49]

Although patients with MS may have a lower risk of cancer than the general population, they still require the general screening tests such as annual mammograms for women older than 40 years of age with no risk factors, colonoscopy or flexible sigmoidoscopy in men and women after the age of 50 years, and prostate-specific antigen levels in men older than 50 years.

MEDICATIONS USED TO TREAT MS

There is no cure for MS, but disease-modifying agents are available. If left untreated, 30% of patients with MS will develop significant disability within 20 to 25 years from onset. Exacerbations are usually treated with a short course of intravenous corticosteroids with or without a prednisone taper. Side effects of high-dose steroids include mood changes, hypertension, glucose abnormalities, and fluid retention. Use of steroids can predispose to the development of osteoporosis, avascular necrosis, and cataracts.

Once a patient is diagnosed with RRMS, interferons and glatiramer acetate may be used to decrease the frequency and severity of relapses and reduce the degree of disability. The 3 currently available interferons are interferon beta-1b (Betaseron), interferon beta-1a (Avonex and Rebif). Side effects include flulike symptoms, injection site reaction, elevated liver function tests, and an abnormal complete blood count. Tachyphylaxis may result from the development of neutralizing antibodies.[51]

Glatiramer acetate (Copaxane) is made up of 4 amino acids that form a collection of random peptides designed to mimic myelin basic protein. Side effects include injection site reaction and a short-lived postinjection reaction characterized by chest tightness, palpitations, flushing, and anxiety.[51]

Most studies that have evaluated these disease-modifying agents used patients with a mean age of 34 to 47 years. Therefore the effects of these medications on an aging population are not fully understood and more studies are needed to confirm long-term safety, efficacy, and tolerability.

Immunosuppressants are mainly used for progressive MS, but in the older population, the risks may outweigh the benefits.[51] Mitoxantrone is an anthracycline analog that shows promise for the MS population, although optimal use of this drug is not known. This drug is associated with the development of a cardiomyopathy, which limits its use to 2 years. The long-term effect of this drug on an aging MS population is unknown, but patients should be monitored annually for cardiac dysfunction.[52]

A newer therapy currently being used to treat MS is natalizumab (Tysabri). It is a humanized monoclonal antibody, which binds to the alpha4 beta1 integrins on leukocytes, inhibiting them from crossing the blood-brain barrier, thereby reducing inflammation. Natalizumab is used for treating relapsing multiple sclerosis in patients with an inadequate response to, or who cannot tolerate, other therapies. Natalizumab has been shown to reduce the risk of disability progression and decrease the annual relapse rate. However, most studies looking at natalizumab as monotherapy or an addition to interferon beta-1a included patients younger than 55 years old. Some of its side effects also limit its use. Natalizumab was initially approved in 2004, but was withdrawn in February 2005 secondary to 10 reported cases of progressive multifocal leukoencephalopathy (a viral infection of the brain that usually leads to death or severe disability). However, after safety evaluation, the US Food and Drug Administration approved it in 2006. Because of the risk of these dangerous side effects, the medication can only be given through a special distribution program called the TOUCH Prescribing Program (American Society of Health-System Pharmacists, Bethesda, MD, USA). Other adverse reactions include liver damage, allergic reaction, fatigue, headaches, and infections. Currently, nothing is known about the safety of long-term use of natalizumab or whether additional side effects will emerge in time.[53]

Cladribine, another drug that has shown promise in treating relapsing remitting MS, is an immunosuppressive medication that targets lymphocytes, particularly T cells, thereby decreasing the immune response. In the CLARITY trial, cladribine has been shown to reduce the number and volume of MS lesions, decrease the relapse rate, and slow disability progression. Currently the ONWARD trial and ORACLE MS trial are underway to examine the safety and effectiveness of cladribine. The major side effect is myelosuppression resulting in thrombocytopenia. There is a risk of developing opportunistic infections due to impaired immunity, however only cases of herpes zoster have been reported thus far.[54]

The use of azathioprine as a treatment for MS remains controversial as a result of mixed research results. Side effects include nausea, anemia, leukopenia, liver damage, and a long-term increased risk of developing cancers such as leukemia or lymphoma. This medication is less likely to be tolerated in an older population and if used may require long-term monitoring for cancers. Cyclophosphamide has shown only a modest benefit. It appears to be most effective in patients younger than 40 years, especially in those who have been in the progressive phase for less than 1 year. The duration of treatment is limited by the risk of bladder cancer, which seems to increase with time and may depend upon the total accumulated drug dose.[51,55]

ASSISTIVE DEVICES

Reports have shown that gait disturbance is a result of, in the order of importance, muscle weakness, ataxia, sensory loss, and spasticity.[19] There are many devices available to help the patient with MS in mobilization. Aides include canes, crutches, walkers, scooters, and manual or motorized wheelchairs. Lofstrand crutches (Lofstrand Labs Limited, Gaithersburg, MD, USA) although useful in the younger MS population have limited use in older patients. Older patients generally benefit from canes or walkers.

A rolling walker helps to conserve energy, and the addition of hand brakes, a seat, and a basket can be beneficial. Patients with ataxia may require the use of weighted equipment. Orthotics such as an ankle foot orthosis (AFO) may be helpful in improving toe clearance in patients with foot drop. The ground force reaction AFO can add knee stability without much additional weight. Orthotics with high- energy demands, such as the hip-knee-ankle-foot orthosis should be avoided, especially in the elderly MS patient. Wrist hand orthosis are useful in the treatment of upper extremity paresis and spasticity. Other equipment that may be required for safety or for energy conservation include bathtub benches, shower chairs grab bars, hoyer lifts, and stair lifts.

The use of even light-weight self-propelled wheelchairs can be difficult for MS patients especially as they age, and consideration should be given to a motorized wheelchair. Before prescribing a motorized wheelchair, the patient should be evaluated for deficits in cognition, vision, and manual dexterity, which can affect a patient's ability to safely operate the device. The safety of these devices needs to be reassessed periodically as the disease progresses. Patients may prefer a scooter to a motorized wheelchair, as there is less associated perception of disability. However, a scooter is not designed for prolonged seating and a wheelchair will be more useful for those patients who rely solely on motorized devices for mobility. Patients with MS who have risk factors for a progressive course should be advised to consider wheelchair/handicap accessible housing as early as possible.[56]

DRIVING WITH MS

Patients with MS have a higher number of traffic violations and accidents compared with healthy adults. After the diagnosis of MS 77% of persons continue to drive. As disease severity increases, driving frequency decreases. Assessment for driving ability needs to be done periodically especially as patients age to ensure their cognitive and physical status is sufficient for safe automobile operation. A formal driving evaluation may be necessary. Referral for a handicap parking plaque should be done as early as possible. This will help conserve energy in the early phase of the disease and be useful in the future as ambulation becomes impaired. Car adaptation may be needed as the disability progresses. The clinician should prepare the MS patient for the future if it seems likely they will no longer be able to drive. Alternative transportation options should be discussed.[57–59]

FAMILY

Family dynamics may change after a diagnosis of MS. Compromises from family members are necessary to successfully adapt to the deficits brought on by the disease. There should be open communication of how care will be managed at home as the patient progresses and their caregiver ages. Appropriate referrals to home care agencies and social workers should be arranged. Support groups or counseling can help the patient and family deal with difficult decisions and help with coping strategies. Long-term placement may be explored for patients with severe disability.[19]

SUMMARY

The chronic and progressive nature of MS may be overwhelming to the patient and their family. It is vital for the clinician to develop a system of periodic evaluations as the patient ages with MS, and then suggest or provide interventions that will monitor the disease and address its effects on the patient's physical, psychological, social, and vocational functioning. Moreover, MS does not provide any protection from other disease of aging such as stroke, cancer, heart disease, diabetes, and patients also need to be evaluated and treated for these conditions. Obtaining appropriate routine medical care may become difficult for aging patients who may be less mobile, as many clinicians' offices are unable to accommodate handicapped patients. Careful coordination and referral to handicap accessible centers may be required to ensure adequate treatment.

As a result of advancements in diagnostics and treatments many people are living longer with MS. There are many unanswered questions for the older MS population because of the paucity of research, but future studies will hopefully rectify this situation. Although there is no current cure for MS, the clinician can play a key role in helping the patient and family adapt to this illness and improving quality of life. The following resources are available for the clinician, the patient, and family members:

Multiple Sclerosis Association of America (MSAA) 1 800 532 7667 www.msaa.com
National Multiple Sclerosis Society (NMSS) 1 800 FIGHT MS (1 800 344 4867) www.nmss.org
American Nystagmus Network, www.nystagmus.org
The Lighthouse, 800 829 0500, www.lighthouse.org,
Low Vision Information Center, 301 951 4444, www.lowvisioninfo.org.

REFERENCES

1. Williams R, Rigby AS, Airey M, et al. Multiple sclerosis: its epidemiological, genetic, and health care impact. J Epidemiol Community Health 1995;49:563–9.
2. Frohman E. Multiple sclerosis. Med Clin North Am 2003;87:867–97.
3. Hauser S, Goodkin D. Multiple sclerosis and other demyelinating diseases. In: Braunwald E, Fauci A, Kasper D, et al, editors. Harrison's principles of internal medicine. 15th Edition. Minneapolis (MN): McGraw-Hill; 2001. p. 1096–133.
4. Trojano M. Age-related disability in multiple sclerosis. Ann Neurol 2002;51: 475–80.
5. Joy J, Johnston R. Characteristics and management of major symptoms in multiple sclerosis current status and strategies for the future. Washington, DC: National Academy Press; 2001. p.115–76.
6. Paty D. Initial symptoms. In: Burks J, Johnson K, editors. Multiple sclerosis: diagnosis, medical management, and rehabilitation. New York: Demos; 2000. p. 75–9.
7. Hazelwood M, Fielstein E. Physiological aspects of aging. In: Maloney F, Means K, editors. Physical medicine and rehabilation: state of the art review rehabilitation and the aging population. Philadelphia: Hanley and Belfus 4; 1990. p. 19–28.
8. O'Connor P, Canadian Multiple Sclerosis Working Group. Key issues in the diagnosis and treatment of multiple sclerosis. An overview. Neurology 2002;59:S1–33.
9. Weinshenker BG. Natural history of multiple sclerosis. Ann Neurol 1994; 36(Suppl):S6–11.
10. Bergamaschi R. Prognostic factors in MS. Int Rev Neurobiol 2007;79:423–47.
11. Amato MP, Ponziani G, Bartolozzi ML, et al. A prospective study on the natural history of multiple sclerosis: clues to the conduct and interpretation of clinical trials. J Neurol Sci 1999;168:96–106.
12. Bashir K, Hadley MN, Whitaker JN. Surgery for spinal cord compression in multiple sclerosis. Curr Opin Neurol 2001;14(6):765–9.
13. Lublin FD, Reingold SC. Defining the clinical course of multiple sclerosis: results of an international survey. Neurology 1996;46:907–11.

14. Joy J, Johnston R. Clinical and biological features in multiple sclerosis current status and strategies for the future. Washington, DC: National Academy Press; 2001. p. 29–114.
15. Miller D. Magnetic resonance imaging in multiple sclerosis. In: Cohen J, Rudick R, editors. Multiple sclerosis therapeutics. New York: Martin Dunitz; 2003. p. P81–97.
16. Polliak M, Barak Y, Achiron A. Late-onset multiple sclerosis. J Am Geriatr Soc 2001;49:168–71.
17. Noseworthy J, Paty D, Wonnacott T, et al. Multiple sclerosis after age 50. Neurology 1983;33:1537–44.
18. Solero C. The prevalence of pain in multiple sclerosis: a multicenter cross-sectional study. Neurology 2004;63(5):919–21.
19. Cobble N, Miller E, Grigsby J. Aging with multiple sclerosis. In: Felsenthal G, Garrison S, Steinberg F, editors. Rehabilitation of the aging and elderly patient. Philadelphia: Williams and Wilkins; 1994. p. 427–39.
20. Ehde DM, Jensen MP, Engel JM, et al. Chronic pain secondary to disability: a review. Clin J Pain 2003;19(1):3–17.
21. Jeffrey D. Pain and dysthesia. In: Burks J, Johnson K, editors. Multiple sclerosis: diagnosis, medical management, and rehabilitation. New York: Demos; 2000. p. 425–31.
22. Boop W. Pain management in the geriatric patient. In: Maloney F, Means K, editors. Physical medicine and rehabilation: state of the art review rehabilitation and the aging population. Philadelphia: Hanley and Belfus 4; 1990. p. 83–92.
23. Mancini M. Duloxetine in the management of elderly patients with major depressive disorder: an analysis of published data. Expert Opin Pharmacother 2009; 5(10):847–60.
24. Mostert S, Kesselring J. Effects of a short-term exercise training program on aerobic fitness, fatigue, health perception and activity level of subjects with multiple sclerosis. Mult Scler 2002;8:161–8.
25. Willmott C. Safety of methylphenidate following traumatic brain injury: impact on vital signs and side-effects during inpatient rehabilitation. J Rehabil Med 2009; 41(7):585–7.
26. Krupp L. Fatigue in multiple sclerosis. In: Cohen J, Rudick R, editors. Multiple sclerosis therapeutics. New York: Martin Dunitz; 2003. p. 599–608.
27. Van den Noort, Fisk JD, Pontefract A, et al. The impact of fatigue on patients with MS. Can J Neurol Sci 1994;21:9–14.
28. Minden S, Frumin M, Erb J. Treatment of disorders of mood and affect in multiple sclerosis. In: Cohen J, Rudick R, editors. Multiple sclerosis therapeutics. New York: Martin Dunitz; 2003. p. 651–89.
29. Sadovnick AD, Eisen K, Ebers GC, et al. Cause of death in patients attending multiple sclerosis clinics. Neurology 1991;41:1193–6.
30. Feinstein A. An examination of suicidal intent in patients with multiple sclerosis. Neurology 2002;59:674–8.
31. Rao SM. Neuropsychology of MS. Curr Opin Neurol 1995;8(3):216–20.
32. Bolbholz JA, Rao S. Cognitive decline in MS: an eight year longitudinal study. J Int Neuropsychol Soc 1998;16:435–40.
33. Rao SM, Hammeke TA, McQuillen MP, et al. Memory disturbance in chronic progressive MS. Arch Neurol 1984;41:625–31.
34. Rao S, Leo G, Bernardin L, et al. Cognitive dysfunction in MS: I frequency, patterns and prediction. Neurology 1991;41:685–91.
35. Amato MP, Ponzianni G, Pracucci G, et al. Cognitive impairments in early-onset MS: pattern predictors and impact on every day life in a 4-year follow-up. Arch Neurol 1995;52:168–72.

36. Amato MP, Ponzianni G, Siracusa G, et al. Cognitive dysfunction in early-onset MS: a reappraisal after 10 years. Arch Neurol 2001;58:1602–6.

37. Schwid S. Management of cognitive impairments in MS. In: Cohen J, Rudick R, editors. Multiple sclerosis therapeutics. New York: Martin Dunitz; 2003. p. 715–25.

38. Frohman E, Zimmerman C. Neuro-opthalmic signs and symptoms. In: Burks J, Johnson K, editors. Multiple sclerosis: diagnosis, medical management, and rehabilitation. New York: Demos; 2005. p. 341–77.

39. DasGupta R, Fowler CJ. Sexual and urological dysfunction in multiple sclerosis: better understanding and improved therapies. Curr Opin Neurol 2002;15(3): 271–8.

40. Wiesel PH, Norton C, Glickman S, et al. Pathophysiology and management of bowel dysfunction in multiple sclerosis. Eur J Gastroenterol Hepatol 2001;13(4): 441–8.

41. Zorzon M, Zivadinov R, Bragadin LM, et al. Sexual dysfunction in MS: a 2-year follow-up study. J Neurol Sci 2001;187:1–5.

42. DeBolt L, McCubbin J. The effects of home-based resistance exercise on balance, power and mobility in adults with multiple sclerosis. Arch Phys Med Rehabil 2004;85:290–7.

43. Cosman F, Nieves J, Komar L, et al. Fracture history and bone loss in patients with MS. Neurology 1998;51(4):1161–5.

44. Kannus P, Parkkari J, Niemi S, et al. Prevention of hip fracture in elderly people with the use of a hip protector. N Engl J Med 2000;343:1506–13.

45. Shannon FJ. Total knee replacement in patients with multiple sclerosis. Knee 2004;11:485–7.

46. Slawta JN, McCubbin JA, Wilcox AR, et al. Coronary heart disease risk between active and inactive women with multiple sclerosis. Med Sci Sports Exerc 2002; 34(6):905–12.

47. Metz LM, McGuinness SD, Harris C. Urinary tract infections may trigger relapse in multiple sclerosis. Axone 1998;19(4):67–70.

48. American Cancer Society statistics. 2009.

49. Bahmanyar S, Montgomery SM, Hillert J, et al. Cancer risk among patients with multiple sclerosis and their parents. Neurology 2009;72:1170–7.

50. Lebrun C, Debouverie M, Vermersch P, et al. Cancer risk and impact of disease-modifying treatments in patients with multiple sclerosis. Mult Scler 2008;14: 399–405.

51. Noseworthy JH. Management of multiple sclerosis: current trials and future options. Curr Opin Neurol 2003;16(3):289–97.

52. Ghalie RG, Edan G, Laurent M, et al. Cardiac adverse effects associated with mitoxantrone (Novantrone) therapy in patients with MS. Neurology 2002;59: 909–13.

53. O'Connor P. Natalizumab and the role of alpha 4-integrin antagonism in the treatment of multiple sclerosis. Expert Opin Biol Ther 2007;7(1):123.

54. Beutler E, Sipe JC, Romine JS, et al. The treatment of chronic progressive MS with cladribine. Proc Natl Acad Sci U S A 1996;93(4):1716–20.

55. Galetta SL, Markowitz C, Lee AG. Immunomodulatory agents for the treatment of relapsing multiple sclerosis: a systematic review. Arch Intern Med 2002;162: 2161.

56. Strobel W, Rumrill D Jr, Hennessey M. Multiple sclerosis: a guide for rehabilitation and health care professionals. Springfield (IL): Charles C Thomas; 2002. p. 179–208.

57. Bobholz J, Rao S. Cognitive dysfunction in MS a review of recent developments. Curr Opin Neurol 2003;16(3):283–8.
58. Schultheis M, Garay E, DeLuca J. The influence of cognitive impairment on driving performance in MS. Neurology 2001;56(8):1089–94.
59. Schultheis M, Weisser V, Manning K, et al. Driving behaviors among community-dwelling persons with multiple sclerosis. Arch Phys Med Rehabil 2009;90: 975–81.

Aging and Developmental Disability

Thomas E. Strax, MD[a,b,]*, Lisa Luciano, DO[a,b],
Anna Maria Dunn, MD[a,c], Jonathan P. Quevedo, MD[a,b]

KEYWORDS

• Aging • Cerebral palsy • Disability • Management

This article discusses aging in individuals with developmental disabilities and functional impairment. A developmental disability is defined as a life-long disability attributable to mental and/or physical impairments manifested at birth or in early childhood.[1] Persons with cerebral palsy provide a good working model, and are the second largest group of persons with developmental disabilities.[2] However, the definition of developmental disability applies to a spectrum of causes including brain injury, severe malnutrition during development, genetic abnormalities, prematurity, autism, fetal exposure to drugs and alcohol, child abuse and childhood trauma, and pre- or postnatal infection. In this article most of the text applies to all individuals who are aging with a developmental disability. Most persons with a developmental disability who reach the geriatric age group age like everybody else. However, because they have preexisting neurologic, functional, and physical damage, these persons show signs of aging in their late 40s and 50s that are not present in the normal population until their 70s or 80s. An individual with damage present at or shortly after birth has a faster aging process than the general population. Thus, many physicians do not recognize a problem in a 50-year-old patient with cerebral palsy that they would recognize if the patient were 80 years old.[3]

One in every 10 families knows the tragedy of having a child born who is less than perfect.[4] A birth defect does not happen to one person, it happens to an entire family. People aging with a development disability today were born in the 1940s, 1950s, and

This work was supported by JFK Johnson Rehabilitation Institute.
[a] Department of Physical Medicine & Rehabilitation, UMDNJ-Robert Wood Johnson Medical School, 675 Hoes Lane, Piscataway, NJ 08854, USA
[b] JFK Johnson Rehabilitation Institute, 45 James Street, Edison, NJ 08818, USA
[c] Department of Physical Medicine & Rehabilitation, Robert Wood Johnson University Hospital, NJ, USA
* Corresponding author. Department of Physical Medicine & Rehabilitation, UMDNJ-Robert Wood Johnson Medical School, 675 Hoes Lane, Piscataway, NJ 08854.
E-mail address: tstrax@solarishs.org

Phys Med Rehabil Clin N Am 21 (2010) 419–427
doi:10.1016/j.pmr.2009.12.009
1047-9651/10/$ – see front matter © 2010 Published by Elsevier Inc.

1960s. During these years, society did not accept them. Some individuals living in institutions suffered physical injuries, sexual violence, isolation, and emotional abuse. Many who were institutionalized were not given a proper education, and most of these individuals were not employable and, therefore, continued to live in poverty. Individuals living below the poverty line have decreased access to health care, proper nutrition, and fitness, and many need some assistance with activities of daily living and mobility. Many children with a developmental disability were institutionalized on the recommendations of their physicians. Less than 20% of those who were kept with their families and educated achieved some form of employment.[5] However, many continued to live with their parents. As they aged, their parents and caretakers aged and died, forcing them to spend their aging years in an institution or other isolated setting.[3,6–9]

If we use cerebral palsy as a model, only 20% of these individuals who live in society are able to walk independently. Forty percent are independent in ambulation with some assistance, and 40% require a wheelchair for mobility.[3] These individuals, over time, have decreased strength and become prone to disease. As they enter their 40s, 50s, and 60s, they have an increased incidence of developing secondary conditions because they began life less than perfect. Overeynder and Turk[10] described that pain is one of the most common secondary conditions found in 84% of disabled women surveyed. This statistic was significantly higher than the 25% reported in the general American adult population. Most pain syndromes are musculoskeletal in origin as a result of overuse syndromes, dislocations, fractures, osteoporosis, and entrapment neuropathies.[11–15]

Poor nutrition and lack of exercise lead to reduced muscle mass, muscle weakness, reduced ambulation, hip dislocations and arthritis, early hip and knee replacements, patellar fractures, increasing scoliosis, and other skeletal disabilities found frequently in middle age. Osteoporosis is a common problem in middle-aged individuals with developmental disabilities because many become sedentary, are less ambulatory, and are not involved in exercise programs.[16] Vitamin D levels should be evaluated in these individuals along with bone density studies to delineate those who would benefit from medication and exercise. Physicians should also carefully evaluate exercise programs, and be aware that some individuals can fully participate in programs seated at wheelchair level. Wheelchair Tai Chi increases flexibility, strength, endurance, and self-confidence safely at wheelchair level.[11,12,17]

Persons with neuromuscular disorders often find it difficult to balance their activity level and exercise tolerance without overdoing it. The possibility of overuse syndrome must be taken into account with regard to a person's activity level, musculoskeletal deformity, spasticity, and overall heath.[18] However, the apprehension that can sometimes be present not to overfatigue a muscle group can also severely limit the potential activity level of a person. It is the same principle that we sometimes see in the cardiac population, referred to as the "cardiac crippled." The progress that can be expected needs to be explained to the patient such that the rate of progress depends on the underlying condition. Usually the rate of improvement is much slower than in the able-bodied population and in some cases is tailored simply to try and slow disease progression. However, the benefit of the activity and exercise greatly outweighs the negative effect of inactivity and overall deconditioning that can occur as a result.[17] What is necessary is an interdisciplinary team approach. The physician needs to give the clearance and the encouragement for a particular activity or exercise, and the therapist needs to work with the patient to achieve that activity or exercise level without overfatigue. Sometimes it may also be necessary for the patient to work with a rehabilitation psychologist to overcome fears if the overall program is overwhelming. The ultimate goal is to improve function and quality of life.

Murphy and colleagues[13,17] suggested that early degenerative arthritis in 40-year-old individuals explained the large amount of pain that many had on weight-bearing joints.[13] Musculoskeletal abnormalities, such as abnormal movement across joint surfaces and joint compression, can lead to early degenerative joint disease. Many 40- and 50-year-olds have neuropathies, radiculopathies, and myelopathies. Myelopathies, especially in the cervical spine, are frequently found in individuals with movement disorders, especially athetoid cerebral palsy. Many of these patients are in their 50s and have a slowly progressive increase in balance problems and weakness in the lower extremities.[19] This is followed by progressive atrophy and weakness in the upper extremities. If not diagnosed and treated, spinal stenosis and spinal cord compression can progress to pulmonary failure and ultimately, death. Physicians seeing these patients who do not understand the aging process and effect of movement disorders on the spine do not have a high index of suspicion for myelopathies or cervical spinal stenosis in the event of functional decline.[17,20]

The following case study is just one example of misdiagnosis as a result of underlying developmental disability and points toward specific challenges for these individuals in the health care setting. Alvin was a 54-year-old state employee with mixed athetoid spastic cerebral palsy. He had an IQ of 150, and functioned independently in the community despite significant dysarthria. Six months before admission, he began complaining of increasing difficulty ambulating and fatigue, which was discounted as an outpatient, being attributed to his disability and aging alone. In a 6-month period he was seen by physicians 3 times, each time complaining of progressive decline in his ability to ambulate. He also had limited insurance and limited social support. Ultimately, he presented to the emergency room when he had functionally declined to the point of being nonambulatory. After several days, and severe limitations in communication, he was found to have significant cervical myelopathy with cord compression most severely at C4. By the time he underwent decompression surgery he suffered tetraplegia, respiratory depression, and dysphagia requiring placement of a percutaneous endoscopic gastrostomy tube, and was ultimately discharged to a skilled nursing facility. Many physicians feel uncomfortable treating a patient with a developmental disability and do not take the time to understand or to realize that the symptoms described are real. Therefore, they miss diagnosing fractures, spinal stenosis, and other serious illnesses that must be taken care of as soon as possible. Instead they see the patient as a complainer or cognitively impaired or consider that the patient's complaints have nothing to do with the real problem at hand.

Fractures are a well-documented problem in people with developmental disabilities who are aging, especially those with spastic conditions such as spastic cerebral palsy. Fractures are 5 times more likely in patients aging with cerebral palsy.[21] In these patients, severe uncontrollable motion of unbalanced muscle action with superimposed osteoporosis, contractures, and spasticity can cause atraumatic fractures. The most common site is the supracondylar region of the distal femur. Ambulatory persons are at risk for fractures as a result of falls. Individuals with cerebral palsy, ataxia, spasticity, contractures, histories of dislocations, and severe muscle imbalance are unable to protect their joint and soft tissues during activity because they lack precise neurologic control. Basic activities of daily living and ambulation create more wear and tear on their musculoskeletal systems than in the general population without a developmental disability.[10,17]

Persons with developmental disabilities, as they approach middle age, realize they are physiologically 20 years older than their chronologic age. Many who do ambulate notice that small changes in their physiology cause great changes in overall functional ability.[22] Inactivity in a person who used to be active can lead to accelerated cardiac disease, deep vein thrombosis, cellulitis, pressure ulcers, and skin atrophy. A skilled physical exercise program along with proper nutrition can restore people with weakness, osteoporosis, balance, and coordination difficulties to their previous quality of life. Aging patients must be placed on an exercise program that is tailored to their abilities. Immobility decreases strength by 1% to 1.5% per day. Strength decreases 20% to 30% a week for up to 5 weeks. Inactivity can cause as much as 50% loss in overall strength. One muscle contraction a day at 50% of maximum strength is enough to prevent this decline. Muscle loss due to immobility is greatest in the quadriceps and other extensor groups.[23] As previously described, decreased muscle strength and tension on bones leads to loss of bone and osteopenia. Osteoporosis affects 70% of persons with disability and decreased mobility.[21] Persons who are immobile spend a great deal of time indoors and ultimately do not receive enough sunlight. Measuring vitamin D levels and providing supplementation may help prevent ongoing osteopenia. Calcium is excreted in urine specimens on the second or third day of immobilization and peaks at 3 to 7 weeks. Certain medications often prescribed to patients aging with developmental disabilities predisposes them to additional bone loss. Such medications include phenytoin, phenobarbital, heparin, steroids, proton pump inhibitors such as Nexium, Prilosec, Prevacid, and selective serotonin reuptake inhibitors (SSRIs) such as Lexapro, Prozac, and Zoloft. During periods of immobility joints also show decreased periarticular connective tissue and stability. The ligaments undergo biochemical changes that can be noted as early as 2 weeks after immobilization.[24]

The rate of physiologic aging depends on the continued activity of the individual. Along with the musculoskeletal effects of immobility there are cardiopulmonary effects. Volume reduction of body fluids leads to venous retention and venous pooling in the lower extremity. This causes an increased risk of thromboembolism secondary to decreases in blood volume and increases in coagulability. Cardiovascular efficiency decreases, increasing resting heart rate and decreasing stroke volume. The decrease of stroke volume may reach 15% after 2 weeks of complete bed rest. If one does not exercise, there is a progressive decline of maximum heart rate and a decreased strength of contraction and decreased peripheral muscle efficiency. There is an increased incidence of orthostatic hypotension and a gradual decline in maximum oxygen consumption. This decline can be dramatically reduced by ongoing exercise.[24]

With aging, changes in the lung show decreased vital capacity, decreased Po_2, and decreased efficiency of gas exchange. Aspiration is a major problem with many adults with cerebral palsy and developmental disability. It is important to identify people who cough while eating meals and have a high index of suspicion for dysphagia. Dysphasia should be identified and evaluated by modified barium swallow and an appropriate diet given to the patient to reduce the likelihood of aspiration. Referral to speech pathology is appropriate for ongoing oral motor exercise and dysphagia follow-up.[21,24]

Diet is important for those who are nonmobile and spend a great deal of time sedentary. Poor nutrition, especially a diet high in carbohydrates and low in grains and vegetables, can lead to problems with the gastrointestinal system along with obesity. In addition to poor diet, increased reflux and slowing of gastric motility can lead to constipation. To decrease problems with constipation, patients need to increase liquid intake and follow a high-fiber diet. Persons with central neurologic involvement often have difficulty with gastrointestinal motility, which only worsens with age.[22]

Poor dental care because of disability as well as socioeconomic status is commonly seen in patients with developmental disability. Many patients have thickened saliva, abnormal jaw closure, and breathe through the mouth, which causes an increase in poor dental health, gum disease, and early loss of teeth. Few dental offices will accept these patients even if they are accessible. Dentists believe that they have to use general anesthesia even when it is not needed. Some special clinics are able to treat 80% of these patients without general anesthesia.[25]

Patients who are aging with a developmental disability can get any number of neurologic problems found in able-bodied people who are much older. Dementia, myelopathies, Parkinson disease, tumors, and neuropathies can be found as their damaged nervous system ages.[23] Any decline in neurologic function should be evaluated as one would evaluate someone who was able-bodied and 20 years older. An older individual with developmental disability who shows some changes in cognitive or effectual behavior should be reviewed carefully. It should not be assumed that a patient has early dementia or is mentally weaning unless the process has gone on more than 2 years without a complete evaluation. One needs to evaluate if the patient is depressed or has some system failures, such as a heart that has suffered a silent myocardial infarct or pulmonary disease with pneumonia, or whether the patient fell and has a silent subdural hematoma that is now expanding. One must also rule out endocrine problems such as hypothyroidism, or depression because of decline in quality of life, or caused by an undiagnosed neurologic condition. A complete medical work-up is warranted with any decline in cognition or changes in neurologic or behavioral status.[17,23]

Depression is a major problem in this population and needs to be identified and treated promptly. Some individuals aging with disability develop profound depression and require treatment with medication. The efficacy of antidepressants in the aging population was discussed at a National Institute of Mental Health consensus conference.[26] It was concluded that the most studied drug, a tricyclic antidepressant nortriptyline, showed a 78% depression remission rate. SSRIs such as Lexapro showed response rates similar to tricyclic antidepressants. However, morning orthostatic blood pressure and cardiac toxicity have been reported in the elderly on tricyclic antidepressants, which poses limitations on their use in the aging population. Thus serotonin reuptake inhibitors are the most common class prescribed because of their efficacy and favorable side effect profile.[26]

Because this population is often economically depressed, durable medical equipment needed by these individuals may not be available to them as they age.[27] As persons with neuromuscular disorders age, they may experience changes in their functional impairments that make it necessary to make further modifications to their home, work, or leisure environments. Often, people become so accustomed to their way of functioning that they may be less receptive to making changes that would enhance function and safety and minimize possible adverse physical consequences. The health care professional needs to be fully aware of the persons' everyday performance and any changes in their status that would warrant further modifications. Such modifications could include the elimination of steps with a first-floor setup, and/or the use of ramps. To ramp a set of stairs, one requires a foot of ramp space for every inch of stair rise. The use of grab bars in the bathroom, instead of an unsafe towel bar, helps with clothing management and personal hygiene. The need for other equipment such as a tub bench, shower chair, long handled scrub brush, or shoe horn should also be addressed with logic and compassion because such changes are often emotionally perceived as failure or losing ground, as opposed to maintaining a level of independence.

Aging with a developmental disability is just like aging without a developmental disability when we speak of the genitourinary system. Kidney stones, incontinence, decreased bladder and sphincter tone, decreased bladder capacity, and decreased urinary retention require diagnosis through urodynamic evaluation and urinalysis. Strict bladder management decreases the frequency and time of onset of reduction in the glomerular filtration rate. As the kidney ages there is glomerular loss and a decrease in renal tubular cell mass. Incontinence in a previously continent individual is not part of aging and should always prompt the evaluation and ongoing management of the underlying cause.[28]

There are many issues concerning sexuality and the gynecologic care of women aging with developmental disabilities. Because of social prejudice and limited education during the 1940s until the late 1960s, between 50,000 and 100,000 women with disabilities worldwide were sterilized.[29] Major changes that these women with developmental disabilities experience during aging are related to decreased hormonal production, just as found in the general population. Common symptoms include decreased libido, sleep disturbances, emotional lability, and slowing of sexual arousal. Only 88% of women have adequate lubrication, leading to painful sexual intercourse in the remaining.[11] Women with disabilities report that problems with sexual activity are often related to weakness (40%), vaginal dryness (39%), lack of balance (38%), joint pain (32%), and spasticity of the legs (28%).[30] A recent survey showed that 49% of women with a disability over the age of 65 years who have a spouse, report being satisfied with their level of sexual activity. Gynecologic care poses an increased challenge with aging because of difficult pelvic examinations caused by spasticity, limited lower extremity function, contractures, and pain. Many women require sedation for a complete pelvic examination. This factor, combined with inadequate access to health care, places this group of women at a higher risk for undiagnosed cervical, uterine, and ovarian cancers and leads to delayed treatment and early morbidity and mortality.[11,31]

Many men over the age of 65 with a central nervous system–related disability have erectile dysfunction. It is important to recognize that 72% of these men can achieve an erection, whereas only 67% can achieve ejaculation. Men find that it takes longer to have an erection.[19] An aging man, with or without a disability, may require increased physical stimulation to achieve and maintain an erection. He also requires a longer period of rest time before being able to have another erection. Many men may not be able to understand these physiologic changes, which can lead to anxiety and psychogenic erectile dysfunction. Adequate education, pharmacologic management, and counseling with subsequent follow up can alleviate many of these concerns.

During the lifetime of someone living with a developmental disability, the risk of being physically or sexually assaulted is 4 to 10 times higher than it is for the general population.[32] Research, including Centers for Disease Control data, found that 68% to 83% of women with developmental disabilities are sexually assaulted in their lifetime[33]; this rate is 50% higher than women in the rest of the population. Women with developmental disabilities are more likely to be re-victimized by the same person, and 50% never receive assistance. Of the perpetrators of sexual abuse against a person with disabilities, 48.1% gained access to their victims through disability services.[31] Most health care providers are unaware of the prevalence of sexual violence in this population, leading to under-reporting and lack of recognition.[31–34]

With advances in medicine and rehabilitation, long-term survival should be expected for most individuals aging with developmental disability. However, 60% will ultimately die from respiratory complications.[35] Quality of life and personal assistance issues affected by physical and functional changes affect the longevity of a person aging with a disability.[36] Lack of access to routine health care and poverty contributes to early mortality in this population from diseases such as cancer and pulmonary and cardiac diseases, which would otherwise be detected and treated sooner and more routinely. Many patients are closely followed in their pediatric years, but are then never referred to a physiatrist for ongoing management as they age. Physician and health care professional bias toward this population is real and must be overcome by education and self-reflection.[37,38] Health care for this group of patients must not be left entirely to the least experienced practitioner. The proper education and intervention of physicians and health care providers can make the difference between this group of patients living life to their greatest opportunity or suffering early mortality and morbidity.[3,27,35]

REFERENCES

1. Currie DM, Gershkoff AM, Cifu DX. Geriatric rehabilitation. Mid- and late-life effects of early-life disabilities. Arch Phys Med Rehabil 1993;74:s413–6.
2. Roig RL, Worsowicz GM, Cifu DX. Geriatric rehabilitation. Physical medicine and rehabilitation interventions for common disabling disorders. Arch Phys Med Rehabil 2004;85:s12–7.
3. Evans PM, Evans SJW, Alberman E. Cerebral palsy: why we must plan for survival. Arch Dis Child 1990;65:1325–33.
4. McNeil JM. Americans with disabilities: 1994–95. Washington, DC: Department of Commerce, Bureau of the Census; 2001. p. 70–3 Current Population Reports P70–61.
5. Pfeiffer D. Help the disabled work [editorial]. Los Angeles Times. December 13, 1998:M4.
6. Center for Disease Control and Prevention. Healthy people 2010. Washington, DC: US Government Printing Office; 2001. chapter 6 (disability and secondary conditions).
7. Center for Disease Control and Prevention. Prevalence of disabilities and associated health conditions among adults – US. 1999. MMWR Morb Mortal Wkly Rep 2001;50(7):120–5 [Erratum in: MMWR Morb Mortal Wkly Rep 2001;50(8):149].
8. Center for Disease Control and Prevention. Trends in aging – United States and worldwide. MMWR Morb Mortal Wkly Rep 2003;52(6):100–4 106.
9. Basile KC, Saltzman LE. Sexual violence surveillance: uniform definitions and recommended data elements. Version 1.0. Atlanta (GA): National Center for Injury Prevention and Control, Centers for Disease Control and Prevention; 2002.
10. Overeynder JC, Turk MA. Cerebral palsy and aging: a framework for promoting health of older persons with cerebral palsy. Top Geriatric Rehabil 1998;13:19–24.
11. Turk MA, Geremski CA, Rosenbaum PF, et al. The health status of women with cerebral palsy. Arch Phys Med Rehabil 1997;78(Suppl 5):S10–7.
12. Turk MS, Geremski CA, Rosenbaum PF. Secondary conditions of adults with cerebral palsy: final report. Syracuse (NY): State University of New York; 1997.
13. Murphy KP, Molnar GE, Lankasky K. Medical and functional status of adults with cerebral palsy. Dev Med Child Neurol 1995;37:1074–84.
14. Hodgkinson I, Jindrich ML, Duhaut P, et al. Hip pain in 234 non-ambulatory adolescents and young adults with cerebral palsy; a cross-sectional multicentre study. Dev Med Child Neurol 2001;43:806–8.
15. Schwartz L, Engel JM, Jensen MP. Pain in persons with cerebral palsy. Arch Phys Med Rehabil 1999;80:1243–6.

16. Ando N, Ueda S. Functional deterioration in adults with cerebral palsy. Clin Rehabil 2000;14:300–6.
17. Murphy KP. Medical problems in adults with cerebral palsy: case examples. Assist Technol 1999;11:97–104.
18. Gajdosik CG, Cicirello N. Secondary conditions of the musculoskeletal system in adolescents and adults with cerebral palsy. Phys Occup Ther Pediatr 2001;21: 49–68.
19. Klingbeil H, Baer HR, Wilson PE. Aging with a disability. Arch Phys Med Rehabil 2004;7:S68–73.
20. Azuma S, Seichi A, Ohinishi I, et al. Long-term results of operative treatment for cervical spondylotic myelopathy in patients with athetoid cerebral palsy. Spine 2002;27:943–8.
21. King W, Levin R, Scmidt R, et al. Prevalence of reduced bone mass in children and adults with spastic quadriplegia. Dev Med Child Neurol 2003;45: 12–6.
22. Phillips EM, Bodenheimer CF, Roig RL, et al. Physical medicine rehabilitation interventions fro the common age-related disorders and geriatric syndromes. Arch Phys Med Rehabil 2004;85:s18–26.
23. Stewart DG, Phillips EM, Bodenheimer CF, et al. Geriatric rehabilitation. Physiatric approach to the older adult. Arch Phys Med Rehabil 2004;85:S7–11.
24. Cuccurullo SJ. Physical medicine and rehabilitation board review. Physical modalities, Therapeutic exercise, extended bedrest, and aging effects. New York: Demos Medical Publishing; 2004. p. 553–80.
25. Bottos M, Feliciangeli A, Sciuto L, et al. Functional status of adults with cerebral palsy and implications for treatment of children. Dev Med Child Neurol 2001;43: 516–28.
26. Liebowitz BD, Pearson JL, Schneider LS, et al. Diagnosis and treatment of depression in late life. Consensus statement update. JAMA 1997;278(14): 1186–90.
27. McNeil JM. Americans with disabilities: household economic studies, 1997. Washington, DC: Department of Commerce, Bureau of the Census, Current Population Reports; 2001. p. 70–3.
28. Zaffuto-Sforza CD. Aging with cerebral palsy. Phys Med Rehabil Clin N Am 2005; 16(1):235–49.
29. Strax TE. Moral and ethical decision: to be or not to be. The 39th Walter J. Zeiter lecture. Arch Phys Med Rehabil 2008;89:4–9.
30. Nosek MA, Howland CA, Rintala DH, et al. National study of women with physical disabilities. Sex Disabil 2001;19:5–40.
31. Sobsey D. Violence and abuse in the lives of people with disabilities: the end of silent acceptance. Paul H. Brooks Publishing Co; 1994. p. 75–6.
32. California Coalition Against Sexual Assault. Serving survivors of sexual assault with disabilities. Sacramento (CA): CALCASA; 2001.
33. Centers for Disease Control and Prevention. Sexual violence against people with disabilities. Available at: http://www.cdc.gov/ncipc/factsheets. 2002. Accessed November 20, 2002.
34. Klesges L, Pahor M, Shorr R, et al. Financial difficulty in acquiring food among elderly disabled women; results from the Women's Health and Aging Study. Am J Public Health 2001;9:68–75.
35. Crighton J, MacKinney M, Light CP. The life expectancy of persons with cerebral palsy. Dev Med Child Neurol 1995;37:567–76.

36. National Organization on Disability. Methodology for the 2000 N.O.D./Harris Survey of Americans with disabilities. Available at: http://www.nod.org/index.cfm?fuseaction=page.viewPage&pageID=1430&nodeID=1&FeatureID-=152&redirected=1&CFID=27335197&CFTOKEN=51209501. 2001. Accessed April, 2004.
37. Kaiser Permanente National Diversity Council and Kaiser Permanente National Diversity Department. A provider's handbook on culturally competent care: individuals with disabilities. Oakland (CA): Kaiser Permanente; 2004.
38. Examined the conclusions of the 1991 National Institutes of Health consensus panel on diagnosis and treatment of depression in late life in light of current scientific evidence. Available at: www.nimh.nih.gov. Accessed December 14, 2009.

Aging with Muscular Dystrophy: Pathophysiology and Clinical Management

Gregory T. Carter, MD, MS[a,b,*], Michael D. Weiss, MD[c],
Joel R. Chamberlain, PhD[c], Jay J. Han, MD[d],
Richard T. Abresch, MS[d], Jordi Miró, PhD[e], Mark P. Jensen, PhD[a]

KEYWORDS

- Muscular dystrophy • Aging • Pathophysiology • Management

Medical technologic advances can have profound effects on people's lives by extending the life course and creating uncertain futures. This has certainly been the case for persons with various forms of muscular dystrophy (MD), many of which had previously been called "diseases of childhood." Individuals with MD are surviving well into adulthood thanks to advances in the medical management of comorbid problems, such as pneumonia, respiratory failure, and cardiomyopathy. Moreover, advances in rehabilitative technologies have greatly improved the functional capacity and mobility of this group of patients.

Alternatively, due in large part to advances in the care of individuals with MD, clinicians are faced with a new population of aging patients with MD. Adults with Duchenne MD (DMD) have an upward shifting of life expectancy and are experiencing new "personal identities" as they become adults. To a large extent, this is a population at risk of being marginalized in terms of health care and society in

This research was supported by the National Institutes of Health, National Institute of Child Health and Human Development, National Center for Rehabilitation Research (grant no. P01HD33988), and the National Institute for Disability Rehabilitation Research (grant no. H133B080024).

[a] Department of Rehabilitation Medicine, University of Washington School of Medicine, Box 356490, Seattle, WA 98195, USA
[b] 1800 Cooks Hill Road, Suite East, Centralia, WA 98531, USA
[c] Division of Neuromuscular Disorders, Department of Neurology, University of Washington School of Medicine, Box 356490, Seattle, WA 98195, USA
[d] Department of Physical Medicine and Rehabilitation, University of California at Davis, Sacramento, CA 95817, USA
[e] ALGOS, Research on pain, Rovira i Virgili University, Carretera de Valls s/n, 43007 Tarragona, Catalonia, Spain
* Corresponding author. 1800 Cooks Hill Road, Suite East, Centralia, WA 98531.
E-mail address: gtcarter@uw.edu.

general. Historically, patients with DMD and other forms of MD became orientated to expect a shortened life span. Compounding this was the stress of living every day with the anticipation that each day could be their last; this daily concern about the possibility of death could go on for as much as a decade. There is a need to reorient medical and social expectations to better serve adults with DMD and other forms of MD and an ever-growing population of geriatric patients with later-onset, slowly progressive forms of MD.

The purpose of this review article is to provide an overview of the pathophysiology of dystrophic myofiber in the context of aging and a discussion of clinical care needs of aging MD patients, with an emphasis on management strategies for the neuromuscular medicine specialist.

ADAPTATIONS OF SKELETAL MUSCLE TO DISEASE AND AGE

Skeletal muscle is a dynamic tissue with a remarkable ability to continuously respond to environmental stimuli. Among its adaptive responses is the widely investigated ability of skeletal muscle to regenerate after loading, injury, or both. Although significant research efforts have been dedicated to better understanding the underlying mechanisms controlling skeletal muscle regeneration, there has yet to be a significant impact of knowledge from this research on the clinical approaches used to treat aging dystrophic skeletal muscle.

The stem cell of skeletal muscle (also known as satellite cell) allows for muscle fiber growth in response to injury, including exercise-induced injury. This enables fiber hypertrophy and is responsible for the efficient repair of muscle fibers. This normally efficient process is greatly disrupted in patients with any form of MD, in whom this otherwise powerful repair capacity is challenged by the fragility of dystrophic skeletal muscle fibers. Even passive stretching of dystrophic muscle may cause diffuse microdamage.[1,2] In dystrophic muscle, this microdamage causes Ca^{2+}-induced injury, which ultimately produces a cascade of events in the myofiber, including degeneration, inflammation, attempted repair, and ultimately replacement with scar tissue and formation of fibrosis.[2–4] Recently it has been shown that dystrophic muscles not only are more susceptible to mechanical stress and influx of extracelluar Ca^2 but also develop contracture-induced myoplasmic separations and hypercontraction clots associated with increased intracellular Ca^{2+} at rest and subsequent damage to the dystrophin-deficient fibers, whereas control fibers do not.[5] Although these disruptions lead to irreversible damage in dystrophic muscles, the damage is not as severe, or the repair process of normal tissue is vital enough to overcome this damage and generate new healthy muscle tissue.[5–7]

The disruption of the plasma membrane and basal lamina is a critical component to stimulating repair. Within the first day of muscle injury, the tissue is invaded by inflammatory cells, including mononuclear cells and macrophages. The subsequent secretion of growth factors and cytokines further promotes increased blood flow to the area and enhances the inflammatory response.[5] Muscle regeneration begins once the phagocytic inflammatory cells have cleared away necrotic tissue. This step must occur before muscle regeneration can occur, given the fact that inflammatory cells impair muscle regeneration. In normal muscle, active muscle regeneration typically occurs within 7 to 10 days from the time of injury, peaks at 2 weeks, and gradually declines until 3 to 4 weeks.[8] In dystrophic muscle, however, the healing/regeneration process may never occur completely. In otherwise healthy individuals who are older, the muscle healing and regeneration process is delayed.[9] It is reasonable to hypothesize that this process is markedly delayed in aging dystrophic muscle.[8,9] It is not known whether or not this response is due to increased fragility of the membrane, greater susceptibility to extracellular calcium, or reduction in the repair and regeneration process.[10]

Significant efforts have focused on the development of pharmaceutical or molecular genetic therapies that could help dystrophic muscle maximize regeneration and minimize muscle scar-tissue formation, with the goal of improving enhanced regeneration. Although little is known about aging dystrophic skeletal muscle in humans, in all cases of muscle growth and repair, the proliferation of muscle stem cells is critical to the process. In tissue culture, human stem cells proliferate more and more slowly over time, until they stop dividing completely. It has been assumed that a similar event occurs, on a grander scale, during the process of aging. Supporting this hypothesis, recent studies where human muscle stem cells, obtained from biopsy, were grown in vitro and in vivo (by implanting them into skeletal muscles of immunoincompetent mice), have shown that growth correlates negatively with age of the donor. In addition, data from Pietrangelo and colleagues[11] suggest that aging human muscle (1) exhibits increased oxidative damage accumulation in molecular substrates that is probably due to impaired antioxidant activity and insufficient repair capability; (2) has myoblasts with limited ability to execute a complete differentiation program; (3) has restricted fusion, possibly due to altered cytoskeleton turnover and extracellular matrix degradation; and (4) shows evidence of increased activation of atrophic mechanisms through a specific FOXO-dependent program.[12] Between ages 2 and approximately 70 years, an average of two divisions are performed by each satellite cell in human vastus lateralis and biceps brachii muscle every 10 years.[12] For humans, by age 75, there are probably only a dozen divisions remaining in muscle stem cells before the process is completely exhausted, although this remains the subject of debate in the scientific community.

In diseases, such as DMD, the muscle fibers lack a structural protein, dystrophin, that creates enhanced vulnerability to mechanical stress. In many of the MDs, including most forms of limb-girdle MD, there are also structural proteins missing. Myotonic MD (MMD) is different, however, in that it is associated with aberrant splicing of RNA in muscle-specific chloride channel (ClC-1), producing reduced conductance of chloride ions in the sarcolemma.[13] Thus, satellite cells in children with MD may have the remaining growth capacity as low as might be found in those in their eighth decade of life. The implantation of genetically intact myoblasts obtained from healthy relatives had been proposed as a treatment of DMD. Given what is known about muscle regenerative capacity, however, it is reasonable to expect that local implantation of a fixed numbers of cells is not likely to rescue the complete musculature or even the muscles of breathing, which are perhaps the most vital in terms of survival.

The absence of dystrophin and the dystrophin-glycoprotein complex from the sarcolemma is the ultimate cause of muscle deterioration, ultimately leading to respiratory or cardiac failure. Until this problem can be definitively treated, DMD will continue to be a severe, and ultimately fatal, disease. Chamberlain and colleagues[14-16] have shown that increase expression of utrophin, a dystrophin paralog, holds significant promise as a treatment for DMD. Using an adeno-associated viral (AAV) vector, these investigators were able to show that intravenous administration of recombinant AAV (rAAV2/6) harboring a murine codon optimized microutrophin (DeltaR4-R21/DeltaCT) transgene to adult mice with complete absence of dystrophin.[14] Five-month-old mice demonstrated localization of microutrophin to the sarcolemma in all the muscles tested. These muscles displayed restoration of the dystrophin-glycoprotein complex, increased myofiber size, and a considerable improvement in physiologic performance when compared with untreated mice.[15]

Overall, microutrophin delivery alleviated most of the pathophysiologic abnormalities associated with the dystrophy in the treated mice. This approach may hold promise as a treatment option for DMD because it avoids the potential immune responses associated with the delivery of exogenous dystrophin. It also shows promise for significant prolongation of life expectancy if these results can be duplicated in humans with DMD. Restoring dystrophin expression in the muscles of patients with DMD may, therefore, halt or reverse the degenerative wasting and weakness that causes premature death.

The therapeutic efficacy of an intervention, however, may be limited by the extent of disease progression before treatment. Investigators have considered the potential for ameliorating the pathology in a mouse model of advanced-stage MD by systemic administration of rAAV6 vectors encoding a microdystrophin expression construct.[15,16] The treatment of 20-month-old mdx mice restored body-wide expression of a dystrophin-based protein in striated musculature. In aged mice that received treatment, the resultant dystrophin expression was associated with improved hindlimb and respiratory muscle morphology and function, concomitant with reduced muscle fiber degeneration. The findings demonstrate that an established dystrophic state remains amenable to improvement with appropriate intervention and, by some measures, may achieve benefits similar to those observed with intervention early in disease progression. The capacity to ameliorate the pathology in an animal model of advanced-stage MD suggests that interventions that ultimately proved to exert a therapeutic effect in young patients may offer benefits to older patients or those with advanced conditions of progressive MD.

Exercise is another intervention proposed to forestall the effects of aging in normal muscle. Although the effects of exercise on humans aging with MD is not well understood, the effects of long-term voluntary exercise on mdx mice and sedentary aging mice have been studied. Although the mdx mouse is the genetic homolog for DMD, it does not demonstrate the same progression in limb muscle dysfunction as boys with DMD do as they age.[8] Many investigators have postulated that the sedentary lifestyle of this animal plays an important role in its minimal phenotypic expression. To examine the effect of exercise, eight C57BL/10 (C57) and eight mdx mice were allowed to run ad libitum for 1 year. Forty sedentary mdx mice and 40 sedentary C57 mice from 1 month to 18 months of age were used as controls.[9] Contractile characteristics of the extensor digitorum longus and soleus muscles and morphometric characteristics of the mice were examined. The mdx mice ran approximately 45% fewer kilometers per day than the C57 mice. Long-term voluntary running had beneficial training effects on the old mdx mice and their C57 controls. The exercise ameliorated the age-associated loss in tension production that was observed in the soleus of sedentary mdx and sedentary C57 mice. There was a 9% reduction in the fatigability of the extensor digitorum longus muscle of the old mdx mice after the exercise. Despite these improvements, the old mdx mice exhibited significant functional deficits compared with their C57 controls. Thus, the hypothesis that long-term voluntary exercise would have a beneficial training effect on control mice and a deleterious effect on mdx mice as they aged was not supported by this study. Rather, this study showed that dystrophin-less muscles from sedentary mice display significant signs of muscle damage, yet can still benefit from low-level voluntary running in a manner similar to that of the C57 controls.

Part of the pathogenesis of MD shows some overlap with current theories of aging. The disruption of the muscle membrane down-regulates neuronal nitric oxide synthase (nNOS), which disrupts the exercise-induced cell signaling pathway that regulates blood flow to the muscle and results in functional muscle ischemia.[17] More recent studies have shown that when nNOS is not present at its normal location on the muscle membrane, the blood vessels that supply active muscles do not relax normally and show signs of fatigue.[18] The nNOS species has also been implicated in the normal aging of skeletal muscle.[10] Thus, much like in aging, the pathophysiology of the dystrophy may significantly affect its response to exercise. Exercise, especially exercise that places a large amount of stress on the muscle fibers, such as high-resistive and eccentric exercise, damages skeletal muscle in the dystrophies. Even mild exercise has been implicated in causing functional muscle ischemia and fatigue in MD patients due to disruptions in nNOS signaling.[17,18]

Human Studies of Aging in Individuals with Muscular Dystrophy

Parker and colleagues[19] reviewed the management of a late adolescent and adult DMD population to identify areas in which the present service provisions may be inadequate to the needs of this patient population. In 25 patients with DMD, reviewed over a 7-year period, they reported nine patient deaths. There was no significant correlation between age of wheelchair confinement and age of death. Sixteen patients received noninvasive positive pressure support. Twelve attended mainstream schools and 12 attended residential special schools. All of the patients lived at home for some or all of the time, when their main caregivers were one or both of the parents. The most striking difficulties were with the provision of practical aids, including appropriate hoists and belts, feeding and toileting aids, and the conversion of accommodation. Patients rarely wished to discuss the later stages of their disease, and death was often more precipitated than expected. Death usually occurred outside hospital and the final cause was often difficult to establish. In this study, the investigators reported that the adult patients with DMD frequently encountered inadequate and poorly directed social and medical support, further illustrating the need for improvements in the structure, coordination, and breadth of rehabilitation services for adults with DMD.

Wagner and colleagues[20] proposed that the needs of individuals aging with DMD is best addressed in a multidisciplinary clinic. They based this conclusion on their experience as a multidisciplinary team actively caring for 23 men aged 19 to 38 years of age. In their study, approximately one-fourth of the participants remained on moderate-dose corticosteroids. They recommended daily stretching exercises, particularly of the distal upper extremities.

Health-Related Quality of Life: A Target for Treating Aging Individuals with Muscular Dystrophy

There is incredible diversity in individuals who have MD, and this diversity likely increases as these patients age. Few quality-of-life (QOL) studies have been performed to help understand the effects of having a MD on QOL, and there are no specific studies examining the effect of age on QOL. Two common criticisms of the few QOL studies that have been performed are (1) they frequently lump individuals with different MDs together in a single poorly defined study group and (2) the studies predominately used generic instruments to define QOL.[21,22] Thus, the available research rarely includes measures of highly clinically relevant domains, such as physical and emotional functioning, and instead tend to focus on the extreme manifestations of dysfunction, such as severe pain and morbidity.[23]

Recently, several disease-specific QOL assessment tools have been developed for use in MD populations.[24] These disease-specific measures are especially useful in differentiating QOL and psychosocial functioning of patients as their MD progresses. The results of studies using such measures suggests that the pain of persons with

MD is undertreated.[24–30] This finding may be even more significant in individuals who are aging with MD, as pain is also undertreated in aged adults.[31]

CLINICAL PARADIGMS FOR AGING PATIENTS WITH MUSCULAR DYSTROPHY
Exercise Paradigms to Improve Strength

Normal human aging is associated with skeletal muscle atrophy and functional impairment (sarcopenia). Multiple lines of evidence suggest that mitochondrial dysfunction is a major contributor to sarcopenia.[10] Aging is associated with a transcriptional profile reflecting mitochondrial impairment. Studies show, however, that resistance exercise may reverse this signature, allowing the muscle in an older individual to approximate that in someone who is younger. Thus, healthy older adults with evidence of mitochondrial impairment and muscle weakness can partially reverse this at the phenotypic level and at the transcriptome level after longer-term resistance exercise.[32–36] Aging may increase risk of muscle injury, however, and studies in aged rats show impaired muscle adaptability.[36] Muscle injury (and dysfunction in subsequent repair) is also a hallmark of MD. Studies performed in normal and dystrophic animals have shown that unaccustomed eccentric exercise (lengthening of the muscle during contraction) may injure the contractile and cytoskeletal components of the muscle fibers.[37–41] Concentric exercise, which involves shortening of the muscle during contraction, does not have the deleterious effects observed in eccentric exercise.[4] During eccentric exercise, sarcomeres are stretched and the actin and myosin filaments are pulled apart, leading to disruption of the thick and thin filament array and damage to cytoskeletal proteins. Structural damage is observed by the appearance of Z-line streaming and myofibrillar disruptions.[4] Mechanical strain, the contributing factor that induces muscle injury, causes an immediate loss of force-generating capacity and initiates a cascade of processes that result in skeletal muscle damage. The inability to quickly repair a disruption of the membrane causes an elevation in intracellular calcium concentration, which triggers calcium-activated degradation pathways and further ultrastructural damage.[42–44] This damage results in fiber degeneration followed by inflammation and, eventually, fiber regeneration. Younger animals tend to benefit more from exercise studies than do older animals. High-repetitive exercise typically had no effect or it had a deleterious effect, in fast-twitch muscles that were more severely affected by disease, which makes them more vulnerable to damage by eccentric exercise.[4,43,45,46] Unfortunately, there are not enough reports examining the effect of high-resistive strength training exercises in older, dystrophic animals to allow any major conclusions to be drawn.

In humans, skeletal muscle weakness is the ultimate cause of most clinical problems in the MDs. There have been several well-controlled studies documenting the effect of exercise as a means to gain strength in MDs, although much remains to be learned in this area.[47–68] In slowly progressive MDs, a 12-week moderate resistance (30% of maximum isometric force) exercise program resulted in strength gains ranging from 4% to 20% without any notable deleterious effects.[54] In the same population, a 12-week high-resistance (training at the maximum weight a subject could lift 12 times) exercise program showed no further added beneficial effect compared with the moderate resistance program, and there was evidence of overwork weakness in some of the study participants.[52]

In one study comparing patients with MMD type 1 (DM1) to patients with Charcot-Marie-Tooth disease, only the Charcot-Marie-Tooth disease patients seemed to benefit significantly from a strengthening program.[62] Similar results were found in a second study that also included facioscapulohumeral muscular dystrophy

(FSHD).[65] These studies point out that the most effective exercise regimens for myopathies and neuropathies are most likely going to differ, although further investigation is needed to clarify which type of exercise is most beneficial for which patient population. In rapidly progressive disorders, such as DMD, there is active ongoing muscle degeneration and the risk for overwork weakness and exercise-induced muscle injury is much greater. In this population, exercise should be prescribed with caution and a common-sense approach. All of this is made more complex in aging MD patients and this is an area that needs further investigation.

Thus, it is advisable that all patients with MD, in particular aged patients, be advised not to exercise to exhaustion, due to the risk of exercised-induced muscle damage. MD patients in an exercise program should be monitored for signs of overwork weakness. Eccentric exercise should be avoided due to increased risk for muscle injury.[52] This includes excessive delayed onset muscle soreness that usually occurs 24 to 48 hours after exercise. Other warning signs include severe muscle cramping, heaviness in the extremities, and prolonged dyspnea. Despite exercise interventions, all of the major forms of MD are progressive and weakness increases over time.[63–78]

Submaximal, low-impact aerobic exercise (walking, swimming, and stationary bicycling) improve symptoms of fatigue via enhancement of cardiovascular performance and increase muscle oxygen and substrate use.[55] This is important because fatigue is a significant limiting factor in physical performance in patients with MDs.[60] Fatigue in this setting is likely multifactorial, due to deconditioning and impaired muscular activation, all made more significant by age. Improving cardiopulmonary performance through aerobic exercise improves not only physical functioning but also mood state and helps fight depression and osteoporosis, which in turn reduces fracture risk.[79] Appropriate exercise is also an effective treatment for depression. Aerobic exercise also helps achieve and maintain ideal body weight and improve pain tolerance. Non-ballistic, sustained muscle stretching is also helpful and should be routinely done after exercise.

Aging and Management of Joint Contractures

Joint contractures are a major clinical problem in MD, particularly in individuals with DMD.[71–75,80–87] Routine examination of the spine and major joints in MD patients should be performed at each clinic visit. Contractures seem to be related to prolonged static limb positioning and frequently develop shortly after patients become wheelchair dependent.[81] In ambulatory patients, upper-extremity contractures may occur and be complicated by joint subluxation, particularly in the shoulder girdle. Slings may provide support but not prevent contracture formation. Again, stretching and positional splinting may slow the progression of contractures, although the actual efficacy of this approach has not been well studied or documented in the literature. In younger patients, surgical release of contractures in the lower extremities may allow patients to be functionally braced. This may prolong ambulation although several studies have shown that weakness, not contractures, contribute most to the loss of functional ambulation.[84] As patients with MD age, contractures are best treated with gentle, static stretching and appropriated support of the joint.

Older patients with MD weakness may benefit from bracing, depending on the distribution of weakness, gait problems, and joint instability. The decision to brace should include the risk of added weight of the brace and the willingness of patients to use the brace. MD patients should be referred for a course of physical therapy after being fitted with braces to help them learn to use the devices effectively. Bracing should be done with the goal of improving function and joint stability. Otherwise, bracing may be cumbersome for many individuals aging with MD. Ankle-foot orthoses are often the most useful and are best if they are custom-made with a lightweight polymer (polypropylene or carbon fiber). They should fit intimately to avoid skin problems and provide good stability. If a pressure sore occurs, patients should be taken out of the brace until the pressure sore heals. Double metal upright ankle-foot orthoses may be built into the shoe but are often too heavy and may limit ambulation, particularly for older patients with more proximal muscle weakness.[85,87] If there is significant ankle instability noted, then the braces should be high profile (come around in front of the malleoli).

Psychosocial Issues in Aging Patients with Muscular Dystrophy

Although the literature on prevalence of depression in older adults is complicated by several health-related and demographic confounds, rates of subclinical depression seem to be between 8% and 16%, making this one of the most common mental health problems faced by older people.[88,89] Depression associated with aging has been shown to be influenced by genetic, situational, illness-related biologic, and psychosocial factors. The psychosocial model of mental health hypothesizes that late-life depression, when it occurs, arises from several significantly losses associated with aging, such as the loss of self-esteem (helplessness, powerlessness, or alienation), loss of meaningful roles (work productivity), loss of significant others, declining social contacts due to health limitations and reduced functional status, dwindling financial resources, and a decreasing range of coping options. Most, if not all, of these issues are already a problem in individuals with MD.[71–75] Clinical depression may, therefore, be underdiagnosed in the MD patient population, and the effects of aging on depression become increasingly more important to investigate as this population ages. Moreover, many patients with MD already experience symptoms that could mimic a major depression, including fatigue, loss of appetite, and difficulty sleeping. Studies in patients with MD have been noted to have higher levels of depression on the Minnesota Multiphasic Personality Inventory.[71–75]

Many patients with MD also report feelings of worthlessness and self reproach, as noted in prior studies.[71–75] As discussed previously, studies on MD patients have shown elevated scores for depression on Minnesota Multiphasic Personality Inventory testing. In one investigation, depression was more closely associated with level of independent functioning than with limb strength, suggesting that good family, social, and religious support systems are critical for positive psychological functioning. Depression in other family members and caregiverrs should also not be overlooked. Individual, group, and family counseling may be beneficial.

Older patients with MD should be referred to a support group when one is available, which can be an excellent resource for psychological support and problem solving. If necessary, referral to a mental health professional should be done. Antidepressant medicine may help with mood elevation and improve appetite and sleep although the efficacy of antidepressants for the management of depression in individuals with MD has not yet been studied.

Cognitive Functioning and Aging in Patients with Muscular Dystrophy

Cognitive involvement is common in MMD and is also seen, to a lesser extent, in DMD.[71–75,90] Learning disabilities are seen in approximately one-third of boys with DMD. Beyond that, most people with MD show normal intelligence. There have been no studies to date looking at cognitive capacity or function in aging patients with MD, although studies have shown that that patients with coexisting cognitive impairment and depression required significantly more psychiatric care than patients with depression alone. Although much remains to be studied, the existing data suggest aggressively treating depression in any aging MD patient with coexisting cognitive impairment.

Modoni and colleagues[91] characterized the progression of the cognitive involvement in patients affected by DM1in a longitudinal neuropsychological follow-up study. The neuropsychological test battery included Mini-Mental State Examination, memory, linguistic, level, praxis, attentional and frontal-executive tasks. They found that, over time, the whole group of patients in their sample showed a significant deterioration in linguistic functions, together with a tendency toward decline in executive abilities, confirming a predominant involvement of cognitive functions subserved by frontotemporal areas. Moreover, they observed that their older patients obtained the lowest scores on the neuropsychological tests. A similar longitudinal study by Sansone and colleagues[92] using neuropsychological testing also demonstrated frontal lobe dysfunction, largely attentional, progressing over time in DM1 and DM2 patients. These findings support the hypothesis that cognitive damage, when it occurs, tends to be confined to frontotemporal functions in adult DM1 patients, and that frontotemporal functions tend to decline with aging. Further studies are needed to determine best treatment approaches to help reduce morbidity and improve care for patients with coexisting depression and cognitive impairment, such as might be found in aging DM1 patients.

Vocational Issues in Aging Patients with Muscular Dystrophy

Employment rates for people with MDs are significantly less than for the able-bodied population, although in the MD population, higher levels of education correlate more closely with employment rate than does functional level or physical performance.[93] Level of self-esteem noted on personality testing has also been shown associated positively with education and employment.[93] These findings suggest that altered personality profiles in MD patients may be a factor in the ability to integrate into mainstream society and hold steady employment. In this regard, education seems as important as physical abilities with respect to employability and self-esteem in people with MDs. This may become more pertinent as boys with DMD grow old enough to consider employment. This is yet another area that is in need of further investigation.

Restrictive Lung Disease

Despite the frequent reference of having restrictive lung disease, the lung in MD is often normal. The problem is with a "weak bellows" (ie, weakened diaphragm, chest wall, and abdominal muscles) and is well described in the literature.[94–101] This causes patients with MD to have problems getting air into and out of the lungs, including coughing. The most severe respiratory complications are usually seen in DMD and DM1.[71–75,94–96,98] Although respiratory failure in FSHD is unusual, a recent study identified 10 FSHD patients on nocturnal ventilatory support at home, representing approximately 1% of the Dutch FSHD population.[96] Severe muscle disease, wheelchair dependency, and kyphoscoliosis seemed to be risk factors for respiratory failure in FSHD.[96] Given the risk factors for lung disease, periodic assessment of respiratory function is indicated in all patients with MD; this is likely to be even more important as patients with MD age. This has been shown in longitudinal studies of pulmonary function in large MD populations.[71–75]

If better airway access becomes absolutely necessary, informed MD patients may choose to have a tracheotomy.[97] This does not eliminate the possibility of aspiration and does require deep suctioning and judicious care of the tracheostomy tube. Although preserving the ability to phonate, a tracheostomy can actually increase aspiration risk, along with other complications, including bleeding.[98] It is critical that MD patients understand that tracheostomy, while making it easier to use mechanical ventilation, may not necessarily improve their overall QOL. Fortunately, with the advancements in noninvasive ventilation, these options are used only infrequently.[94] As this patient population ages, this will likely become a bigger issue. Simple interventions, including pursed lip breathing and attention to pulmonary toilet, have proved effective at decreasing morbidity in patients with MD.[99,100]

Cardiac Complications

Cardiac involvement may occur in many of the hereditary muscular dystrophies, including DMD, Becker MD (BMD), MMD, and some cases of limb-girdle MD.[102] A high (60%–80%) occurrence of cardiac involvement is present in DMD and BMD subjects of all ages.[71–75,102,103] Dystrophin has been localized to the membrane surface of cardiac Purkinje fibers, perhaps contributing to the high incidence of electrocardiogram (ECG) and echocardiographic abnormalities in DMD and BMD in the preadolescent years.[71,72] In spite of this, only approximately 30% of DMD patients have clinically significant cardiac complications. The myocardial impairment may remain clinically silent until the late stages of the disease.[71] This may be due to lack of physical activity. As patients with DMD frequently live well into the third, and sometimes fourth, decade of life, this will become an increasingly important area for research. Pulmonary hypertension also has been implicated in the cardiorespiratory insufficiency of DMD. Death has been attributed to congestive heart failure in as many as 40% of patients with DMD by some investigators.[71]

Severe cardiac involvement in BMD may occasionally precede the clinical presentation of skeletal myopathy.[72,103] Moreover, cardiac compromise can be disproportionately severe relative to respiratory compromise in some patients with BMD. Thus, ECG and echocardiography screening of all BMD patients at regular intervals is indicated. Patients with myocardial involvement need close follow-up and management by a cardiologist with expertise in this area. Successful cardiac transplantation has been reported in BMD patients with cardiac failure who remained ambulatory.[103] There is also a high incidence of ECG abnormalities in both forms of MMD. Studies have shown that approximately one-third of DM1 patients have first-degree atrioventricular block, whereas approximately one-fifth have left axis deviation.[73] Only 5% have left bundle branch block. Bundle of His conduction delays have also been rarely reported.[73] Complete heart block, requiring pacemaker placement, is rare but can occur. Patients with any form of DM should receive routine cardiac evaluations.

Pain

Pain is a significant problem for most patients with MD, although it is not typically a direct consequence of the disease.[21–26] Pain, when present, does cause significant impairment of QOL. It is most commonly caused by immobility. This may lead to adhesive capsulitis, low back pain, pressure areas on the skin, and generalized myofascial pain. There are many novel pharmaceutical agents available to treat different forms of pain associated with neuromuscular disease.[104]

Osteoporosis/Bone Density/Lean Body Mass

Patients with MD, including DMD, are living longer into adulthood.[105] Thus the risk for osteoporosis will likely increase dramatically for many reasons, including malabsorption, loss of weight bearing, and nutritional deficiencies.[106–111] This growing patient population presents new therapeutic challenges in terms of maintaining bone density. Studies suggest approximately one-quarter of adult DMD patients remain on moderate dose corticosteroids.[20,112] This increases the risk for osteoporosis even further. Prior case reports in boys with DMD and known osteoporosis have shown a favorable response to weekly alendronate and daily calcium and vitamin D.[112] Measurements of lumbar spine and proximal femur using dual-energy x-ray absorptiometry have demonstrated increases in bone mineral density, with z scores improving from baseline to 1-year follow-up. Improvements have been reported in the lumbar spine, femoral neck, and greater trochanter.[112] Although more research is indicated, there is at least anecdotal evidence that weekly oral alendronate plus daily vitamin D and calcium is effective in improving bone mineral density in patients with DMD.[112] Additionally, home-based, weight-bearing exercises may also help prevent osteoporosis and loss of lean body mass.[107–111]

Hypogonadism

Hypoganadism has been described in patients with MMD but has not been evaluated in other forms of MD. Tarnopolsky and colleagues[113] measured total and free serum testosterone levels in 59 men with MD, including MMD (N = 12), FSHD (N = 11), DMD/BMD (N = 12), metabolic myopathy (N = 7), and inclusion body myositis (N = 17), and compared these with the normal reference values. Their results showed that 32 of the 59 (54%) participants had low total testosterone, 23 (39%) had low total and free values, and 5 (8%) had low free with normal total levels. There were no significant differences in the prevalence of hypogonadism between the various forms of MD or myopathy, even after considering age as a confounder. From these data it can be presumed that hypogonadism is common in men with MD and other myopathies. This is important and will become a bigger issue in aging men with MD. The importance of testosterone in the maintenance of muscle mass is critical and if hypogonadism is present, testosterone replacement therapy should be considered.

Nutritional Management

Nutrition is a significant problem for most people with MD.[114–118] In the more severe MDs, there is a tendency toward obesity shortly after the loss of functional ambulation, even if stature is impaired. Metabolic syndrome (obesity, dyslipemia, and hypertension) will likely become increasingly prevalent in the aging MD population, due in part to immobility, impaired nutritional intake, and lack of access to appropriate medical care. Recent evidence has shown that the MD patient population is a higher risk for developing metabolic syndrome.[114] Obesity is common in MDs, in particular DMD, where a prevalence of 54% has been reported. Weight control has its primary rationale in ease of care, in particular transfers and skin care, decreasing postoperative complication risk, and decreasing risk of developing metabolic syndrome.[118]

To determine whether or not a home-based activity and dietary intervention can increase activity level, reduce caloric intake, and have a positive impact on components of metabolic syndrome in patients with MD, Kilmer and colleagues[107,110,111] did several studies examining the effects of a home-based nutritional and exercise program. After initial laboratory testing of anthropometric and metabolic variables and 3 days of home-based activity and dietary monitoring, a personally tailored activity and dietary prescription was given, based on baseline testing. Twenty adult volunteer ambulatory subjects with slowly progressive MD were given a pedometer and instructed to increase number of steps by 25% over their baseline determined from home monitoring. An individualized dietary prescription was provided focusing on problematic issues identified from the baseline dietary profile. The main outcome measures included body composition, physical activity, dietary intake, energy expenditure, gait efficiency, metabolic variables, and QOL. The results showed that, by the end of the protocol, mean step count increased approximately 27% above baseline

(P = .001), and caloric intake decreased over 300 kcal/d (P = .002). Body fat percentage significantly decreased (from 33.3% ± 1.5% to 32.6% ± 1.6%, P = .032).[111] Gait efficiency did not change, however, and metabolic variables did not show statistically significant improvement, although two of the five subjects originally meeting the criteria for metabolic syndrome at baseline no longer met the criteria at the end of the intervention period. Six months after completing the protocol, caloric intake remained significantly reduced (P = .02), but although mean step count remained elevated, it was no longer statistically significantly higher than baseline levels. The study findings indicate that using a home-based protocol, people with slowly progressive MD can increase activity and reduce caloric intake. Although this 6-month program showed positive changes, it was insufficient to affect risk factors associated with metabolic syndrome.[111] It remains to be seen if a program longer than 6 months or a more rigorous program could lead to a reduction in the risk factors associated with metabolic syndrome.

Patients with MD may be prone to nutrient deficiency due to mobility limitations or oropharyngeal weakness. Patients with DM1 may be particularly prone to nutritional deficiencies from associated dysmotility of the entire gastrointestinal tract.[106,111] Prior studies in adult patients with many forms of MD demonstrated inadequate nutrient intake of protein, energy, vitamins (water and fat soluble), and minerals (calcium and magnesium), and poor intake of antioxidant nutrients.[119–121] This is important as most MD patients have a high free-radical load (oxidative stress) due to ongoing muscle tissue breakdown.[121] Significant correlations were found between measures of strength and certain individual nutrients (eg, copper and water-soluble vitamins).[119] These data indicate that a substantial number of adults with MD do not meet current dietary intake recommendations. The potential clinical implications of this will likely increase substantially as this population ages as nutrition is also an issue for most aging, able-bodied individuals.

The advanced stages of DMD may be marked by severe malnutrition.[120] As discussed previously, if there is severe respiratory compromise, the increased work of breathing may drastically increase caloric needs. The situation is complicated by the fact that this is often a time when patients lose the ability to self-feed.[71,106] Caloric requirements should be assessed by a nutritionist and proper dietary requirements constructed for patients. This should be routinely done for all MD patients with a forced vital capacity of less than 50% predicted.[120] Placement of a percutaneous endoscopic gastrostomy tube placement may facilitate nutrition because it eases intake of large amounts of calories and fluids. Patients should be reassured that they may still eat food orally for enjoyment, provided they have intact swallowing function. Another complicating factor in DMD patients is gastroparesis, which may make feeding more difficult.[106] How gastric motility changes as patients with DMD age has not been studied.

Pharmaceuticals that May Improve Function or Prolong Life

Major pharmacologic advances have occurred over the past decade. Although a comprehensive discussion of clinical trials is beyond the scope of this article, some of the major advances that are particularly relevant with respect to aging with MD are noted. Given the severity of the disease and the rapid progression, DMD has received the most attention in terms of pharmaceuticals aimed at prolonging life. Although not Food and Drug Administration approved for this indication, prednisone (0.75 mg/kg/d), given to boys with DMD aged 4 to 8 years, has been shown to prolong the time of ambulation and at least should be considered for use in this disease.[122–127] The positive effect of glucocorticoids on muscle function in MD have been known for some time and have similar, if not more profound, effects in animal models. Major side effects of prednisone include weight gain, osteoporosis, and mood lability.[122–127] Deflazacort has similar beneficial effects and may have slightly less side effects than prednisone; however, this drug is not currently available in the United States. Recently a high-dose, weekend-only dosing regimen has shown equal efficacy with potentially less long-term side effects.[127] Patients with DMD are given 5 mg/kg body weight on Saturday and Sunday only. Whether or not continuing treatment with prednisone long term in men with DMD as they age has added benefit remains to be studied.

Oxandrolone may also have a modest beneficial effect in DMD.[128] There have also been several recent randomized, crossover, double-blind, placebo-controlled pilot studies of extended release albuterol in patients with dystrophinopathies (DMD and BMD) and FSHD.[129,130] Outcomes were isometric knee extensor and flexor strength and manual muscle testing (MMT). There was some small evidence of benefit in the dystrophinopathies but not FSHD. Larger, double-blind, randomized studies are necessary, however, to confirm these results.

There is evidence showing a modest positive benefit of the protein creatine monohydrate in DMD for transient improvement of strength.[131–135] Various neurotrophic growth factors may hold some promise, yet this remains to be studied further. Insulin-derived growth factor, commercially known as myotrophin, is the best studied of this group.[136,137]

Modafinil (Provigil) is approved by the Food and Drug Administration to treat the symptoms of fatigue and excessive daytime sleepiness in narcolepsy. Fatigue and subsequent excessive daytime sleepiness secondary to fatigue, however, are also common symptoms in many forms of MD, in particular DM1.[138] Patients with DM1 have shown efficacy with modafinil at dosing of 200 to 400 mg/d.[138] The most commonly reported side effects of modafinil include nausea, nervousness, anxiety, and insomnia.

Palliative and End-of-Life Care Issues

Although DMD is considered an ultimately fatal condition, it may take many years before patients succumb to its effects. In the other, more slowly progressive forms of MD, death is still likely to occur due to complications from the disease. In the process, the disease contributes to more and more debility for patients and leads to important ethical and humanitarian issues. Patients may have a great deal of time to think of their impending death and also the various decisions they need to make at different stages of their disease. It is imperative that a social worker be involved early after the diagnosis to aid in the various decisions facing patients. One such important choice is the decision regarding durable power of attorney. A living will may also be drafted in regards to patients' wishes for the extent of medical intervention, not only near end of life but also in the event of an unforeseen medical complication. As patients enter hospice-level care, these issues take on a greater importance.

Even though patients may have accepted the eventual death resulting from the MD, it is often difficult for them to accept hospice care, as this implies that the disease has entered its terminal stage. Therefore, it is especially important at these times to not only be sensitive to patient needs but also assist patients in making practical decisions. It is also important for patients to be referred to a support group early. The Muscular Dystrophy Association usually has local branches that can identify the most convenient support group. The importance of support groups should not be underestimated as they can provide not only psychological support but also further education and serve as a resource for problem solving and recycling of equipment, such as modified beds, lift devices, and communication equipment. Modern medicine is continually advancing and has many interventions that can prolong life. Although there are many potential medical interventions, physicians should be sensitive to the possibility that patients with an advanced MD may reject such interventions.

It is patients, and not the physicians, who determine whether or not to initiate life-sustaining therapy, artificial devices, or interventions that compensate for the failing organ or system to prevent death. Mechanical ventilation, artificial hydration, and nutritional supports are the most obvious examples. Legally and ethically, competent patients or their legal guardians have the right to refuse any prescribed intervention or treatment. The physicians' and nurses' role is to thoroughly explain the consequences of a patient's decision and to foster and respect patient autonomy.

It takes a great deal of time to explain all of the end-of-life issues, including available treatment options and choices. Without this investment of time by clinicians, patients may be unaware of the available services and choices. An appropriate level of care for end-stage MD patients may change frequently and thus necessitates a close follow-up. Even in the advanced stages of the disease, optimizing in-home care with hospice can maximize QOL for the remaining time in these patients. Effective hospice care provides an interdisciplinary team of professionals whose goal is to support patients and families through their remaining days together. It can provide invaluable psychological, emotional, and spiritual support for patients and families in a familiar and comforting setting.

Equipment

Proper equipment may significantly improve QOL for aging MD patients. Common examples include hospital beds, commode chairs, wheelchairs and wheelchair ramps, handheld showers, bathtub benches, grab bars, and raised toilet seats.[139] An occupational therapist is best qualified to determine if any of these devices are useful for MD patients. Wheelchairs are a critical component of mobility in those with severe MD. Wheelchairs need to be fitted appropriately with the right frame size, type of seat, lumbar support, and cushioning to avoid pressure ulcers.[139] Other mechanical devices, such as the Tilt-n-Space (Postural Seating Material, Lawrence, KS, USA) allow patients to independently tilt the wheelchair seat, providing improved comfort and better pressure relief for the skin. These devices can often be retrofitted on to existing chairs. Patients should be evaluated by a physical or occupational therapist to ensure proper wheelchair prescription. Simply giving patients a prescription for a wheelchair frequently results in a chair that does not fit properly or has improper components. Power wheelchairs are indicated in most MD patients who can no longer ambulate and do not have enough upper-extremity strength to independently propel a manual chair.

In patients who can ambulate, walkers or quad (4-point) canes help reduce fall risk. Pressure-relieving mattresses, with foam wedges for proper positioning, help prevent pressure skin ulcers. In some MD patients, severe weakness in neck musculature causes may produce neck pain and muscle spasms. A cervical collar, in particular the Freeman or Headmaster type, which is a wire-frame collar with padding over the pressure points, may be helpful. Stretching at home may also have pain relieving and palliative benefits.[140]

FUTURE AREAS OF RESEARCH

A comprehensive discussion of all areas of future research in the field of aging and MD is beyond the scope and intent of this article. As a whole, this field of study is under-investigated, as previously discussed. There are some areas of particular promise, however, which are highlighted here.

Although the understanding of the molecular basis of many forms of MD has greatly enhanced diagnostic accuracy, there is little known about how these genetic mutations have an impact on muscle function as MD patients go through other expected age-related changes.

As previously discussed, AAV vector systemic delivery and therapeutic benefits of the functional human minidystrophin gene hold significant promise to improve function and life span in DMD. Theoretically, this technology could be applied to other forms of MDs that are based on a gene deletion resulting in a missing protein product. The highly efficient minidystrophin gene expression seems capable of ameliorating muscle pathology, improving function, and potentially prolonging life span. A recent report suggests a possible therapeutic approach for DM.[141] Preclinical studies demonstrated reversal of myotonia in the HSALR mouse model of DM. Using an modified (morpholino) DNA antisense oligonucleotide-based binding approach, investigators were able to inhibit binding to the pathogenic mRNA carrying a CUG repeat expansion. The association of the DNA antisense oligonucleotides with the mutant mRNA caused the release of proteins normally involved in splicing of a variety of mRNAs, including CLCN1, the chloride channel mRNA. Restoration of CLCN1 mRNA splicing allows protein to be made and to function at the sarcolemma, alleviating the myotonia in the HSALR mice that is similarly caused by its absence in individuals with MMD. This study suggests that altering the pathogenic mRNA in a way that alleviates sequestration of proteins necessary for proper mRNA splicing, through displacement through morpholino binding or directed degradation of the mutant mRNA with oligonucleotides that direct its destruction or an RNA interference-targeted degradation approach, offers a potential treatment for DM, which could not only improve QOL but also lengthen life span.

Important advances in the use of reliable functional assessment tools have made it easier to judge the effectiveness of experimental interventions. The timed motor performance assessment is a good example of a simple measurement scale that can be used at routine clinic visits.[24] There are also new, better tools for assessing the impact of biochemical and biomechanical intervention, including tools that specifically measure how a novel treatment might have an impact not only on simply physical performance but also on QOL.[22]

SUMMARY

Major advances in the fields of medical science and physiology, molecular genetics, biomedical engineering, and computer science have provided individuals with MD with more functional equipment, allowing better strategies for improvement of QOL. These advances have also allowed a significant number of these patients to live much longer, thus providing new problems and challenges for clinicians. As progress continues to change management, it also changes patients' expectations. Even patients with severe childhood forms of MD are living well into adulthood, going to college, starting careers, living through childbearing years, possibly even bearing children, and expecting to enjoy a high QOL. A comprehensive medical and rehabilitative approach to management of aging MD patients can often fulfill these expectations and help them enjoy an enhanced QOL.

REFERENCES

1. Petrof BJ, Shrager JB, Stedman HH, et al. Dystrophin protects the sarcolemma from stresses developed during muscle contraction. Proc Natl Acad Sci U S A 1993;90:3710–4.

2. Abresch RT, Fowler WM, Larson DB, et al. Contractile abnormalities in dystrophin-less (mdx) mice. Med Sci Sports Exerc 1993;5:15–7.

3. Carter GT, Kikuchi N, Horasek S, et al. The use of fluorescent dextrans as a marker of sarcolemmal injury. Histol Histopathol 1994;9(3):443–7.

4. Carter GT, Kikuchi N, Abresch RT, et al. Effects of exhaustive concentric and eccentric exercise on murine skeletal muscle. Arch Phys Med Rehabil 1994; 75(5):555–9.

5. Claflin DR, Brooks SV. Direct observation of failing fibers in muscles of dystrophic mice provides mechanistic insight into muscular dystrophy. Am J Physiol, Cell Physiol 2008;294(2):C651–8.

6. Carter GT, Wineinger MA, Walsh SA, et al. Effect of voluntary wheel-running exercise on muscles of the mdx mouse. Neuromuscul Disord 1995;5(4): 323–31.

7. Carter GT, Abresch RT, Walsh SA, et al. The mdx mouse diaphragm: exercise-induced injury. Muscle Nerve 1997;20:393–4.

8. Carter GT, Abresch RT, Fowler WM. Adaptations to exercise training and contraction-induced muscle injury in animal models of neuromuscular disease. Am J Phys Med Rehabil 2002;81:151–61.

9. Wineinger MA, Abresch RT, Walsh SA, et al. Effects of aging and voluntary exercise on the function of dystrophic muscle from mdx mice. Am J Phys Med Rehabil 1998;77(1):20–7.

10. Chabi B, Ljubicic V, Menzies KJ, et al. Mitochondrial function and apoptotic susceptibility in aging skeletal muscle. Aging Cell 2008;7(1):2–12.

11. Pietrangelo T, Puglielli C, Mancinelli R, et al. Molecular basis of the myogenic profile of aged human skeletal muscle satellite cells during differentiation. Exp Gerontol 2009;44(8):523–31.

12. Beccafico S, Puglielli C, Pietrangelo T, et al. Age-dependent effects on functional aspects in human satellite cells. Ann N Y Acad Sci 2007;1100:345–52.

13. Cho DH, Tapscott SJ. Myotonic dystrophy: emerging mechanisms for DM1 and DM2. Biochim Biophys Acta 2007;1772(2):195–204.

14. Gregorevic P, Blankinship MJ, Allen JM, et al. Systemic microdystrophin gene delivery improves skeletal muscle structure and function in old dystrophic mdx mice. Mol Ther 2008;16(4):657–64.

15. Odom GL, Gregorevic P, Allen JM, et al. Microutrophin delivery through rAAV6 increases lifespan and improves muscle function in dystrophic dystrophin/utrophin-deficient mice. Mol Ther 2008;16(9):1539–45.

16. Wang B, Li J, Fu FH, et al. Systemic human minidystrophin gene transfer improves functions and life span of dystrophin and dystrophin/utrophin-deficient mice. J Orthop Res 2009;27(4):421–6.

17. Kobayashi YM, Rader EP, Crawford RW, et al. Sarcolemma-localized nNOS is required to maintain activity after mild exercise. Nature 2008;456(7221):511–5, 26.

18. Sander M, Chavoshan B, Harris S, et al. Functional muscle ischemia in neuronal nitric oxide synthase-deficient skeletal muscle of children with Duchenne muscular dystrophy. Proc Natl Acad Sci U S A 2000;97:13818–23.

19. Parker AE, Robb SA, Chambers J, et al. Analysis of an adult Duchenne MD population. QJM 2005;98(10):729–36.

20. Wagner KR, Lechtzin N, Judge DP. Current treatment of adult Duchenne MD. Biochim Biophys Acta 2007;1772(2):229–37, 40.

21. Abresch RT, Carter GT, Jensen MP, et al. Assessment of pain and health-related quality of life in slowly progressive neuromuscular disease. Am J Hosp Palliat Care 2002;19(1):39–48.

22. Carter GT, Han JJ, Abresch RT, et al. The importance of assessing quality of life in patients with neuromuscular disease. Am J Hosp Palliat Med 2007;23(6):493–7.

23. Hoffman AJ, Jensen MP, Abresch RT, et al. Chronic pain in persons with neuro-muscular disorders. Phys Med Rehabil Clin N Am 2005;16(4):1099–112.

24. Carter GT. Current trends in neuromuscular research: assessing function, enhancing performance. Phys Med Rehabil Clin N Am 2005;16(4):27–8.

25. Jensen MP, Abresch RT, Carter GT. The reliability and validity of a self-reported version of the functional independence measure in persons with neuromuscular disease and chronic pain. Arch Phys Med Rehabil 2005;86(1):116–22.

26. Jensen MP, Abresch RT, Carter GT, et al. Chronic pain in persons with neuro-muscular disorders. Arch Phys Med Rehabil 2005;86(6):1155–63.

27. Jensen MP, Hoffman AJ, Stoelb BL, et al. Chronic pain in persons with myotonic and facioscapulohumeral muscular dystrophy. Arch Phys Med Rehabil 2008; 89(2):320–8.

28. Molton I, Jensen MP, Ehde DM, et al. Coping with chronic pain among younger, middle-aged, and older adults living with neurologic injury and disease: a role for experiential wisdom. J Aging Health 2008;20:972–96.

29. Carter GT, Jensen MP, Stoelb BL, et al. Chronic pain in persons with myotonic muscular dystrophy, type 1. Arch Phys Med Rehabil 2008;89(12):2382.

30. Miro J, Raichle KA, Carter GT, et al. Impact of biopsychosocial factors on chronic pain in persons with myotonic and facioscapulohumeral muscular dystrophy. Am J Hosp Palliat Med 2009;26(4):308–19.

31. Carter GT. Pharmacologic approaches to geriatric pain management. Arch Phys Med Rehabil 2004;85(6S):50–2.

32. Henriksson J. Effects of physical training on the metabolism of skeletal muscle. Diabetes Care 1992;15(11):1701–11.

33. Favier FB, Benoit H, Freyssenet D. Cellular and molecular events controlling skeletal muscle mass in response to altered use. Pflugers Arch 2008;456: 587–600.

34. Zinna EM, Yarasheski KE. Exercise treatment to counteract protein wasting of chronic diseases. Curr Opin Clin Nutr Metab Care 2003;6:87–93.

35. Grutel M. The sarcomere and the nucleus: functional links to hypertrophy, atrophy and sarcopenia. Adv Exp Med Biol 2008;642:176–91.

36. McBride TA, Gorin FA, Carlsen RC. Prolonged recovery and reduced adaptation in aged rat muscle following eccentric exercise. Mech Ageing Dev 1995;83(3): 185–200.

37. Weiss MD, Luciano CA, Quarles RH. Nerve conduction abnormalities in aging mice deficient for myelin-associated glycoprotein. Muscle Nerve 2001;24:1380–7.

38. Wineinger MA, Carter GT, Abresch RT, et al. Effect of aging on the histological, biochemical and contractile properties of dystrophin-deficient (mdx) mice. J Cell Biochem 1994;18:525–6.

39. Johnson EW, Braddom R. Over-work weakness in facioscapulohumeral dystrophy. Arch Phys Med Rehabil 1971;52:333–62.

40. Vignos PJ Jr, Watkins MP. Effect of exercise in muscular dystrophy. JAMA 1966; 197:843–8.

41. Dubowitz V, Hyde SA, Scott OM, et al. Controlled trial of exercise in Duchenne muscular dystrophy. In: Serratrice G, editor. Neuromuscular diseases. New York: Raven Press; 1984. p. 571–5.

42. Scott OM, Hyde SA, Goddard C, et al. Effect of exercise in Duchenne muscular dystrophy: controlled six-month feasibility study of effects of two different regimes of exercises in children with Duchenne dystrophy. Physiotherapy 1981;67:174–6.

43. DeLateur BJ, Giaconi RM. Effect on maximal strength of submaximal exercise in Duchenne muscular dystrophy. Am J Phys Med 1979;58:26–36, 49.

44. Franco A Jr, Lansman JB. Calcium entry through stretch-inactivated ion channels in mdx myotubes. Nature 1990;344:670–3.

45. Turner PR, Fong PY, Denetclaw WF, et al. Increased calcium influx in dystrophic muscle. J Cell Biol 1991;115:1701–12.

46. Stedman HH, Sweeney HL, Shrager JB, et al. The mdx mouse diaphragm reproduces the degenerative changes of Duchenne muscular dystrophy. Nature 1991;352:536–9.

47. Krivickas LS, Ansved T, Suh D, et al. Contractile properties of single muscle fibers in myotonic dystrophy. Muscle Nerve 2000;23:529–37.

48. Krivickas LS, Suh D, Wilkins J, et al. Age- and gender-related differences in maximum shortening velocity of skeletal muscle fibers. Am J Phys Med Rehabil 2001;80:447–55.

49. Kilmer DD. The role of exercise in neuromuscular disease. Phys Med Rehabil Clin N Am 1998;9:115–25.

50. Kilmer DD, Aitkens S. Neuromuscular disease. In: Frontera WR, Dawson DM, Slovik DM, editors. Exercise in rehabilitation medicine. Champaign (IL): Human Kinetics; 1999. p. 253–66.

51. Kilmer DD, Aitkens SG, Wright NC, et al. Simulated work performance tasks in persons with neuropathic and myopathic weakness. Arch Phys Med Rehabil 2000;81:938–43.

52. Kilmer DD, Aitkens SG, Wright NC, et al. Response to high-intensity eccentric muscle contractions in persons with myopathic disease. Muscle Nerve 2001; 24:1181–7.

53. Kilmer DD, McCrory MA, Wright NC, et al. The effect of a high resistance exercise program in slowly progressive neuromuscular disease. Arch Phys Med Rehabil 1994;75:560–3, 37.

54. Aitkens SG, McCrory MA, Kilmer DD, et al. Moderate resistance exercise program: its effect in slowly progressive neuromuscular disease. Arch Phys Med Rehabil 1993;74:711–5.

55. Sveen ML, Jeppesen TD, Hauerslev S, et al. Endurance training improves fitness and strength in patients with Becker muscular dystrophy. Brain 2008; 131:2824–31.

56. Milner-Brown HS, Miller RG. Muscle strengthening through high-resistance weight training in patients with neuromuscular disorders. Arch Phys Med Rehabil 1988;69:14–9.

57. McCartney N, Moroz D, Garner SH, et al. The effects of strength training in patients with selected neuromuscular disorders. Med Sci Sports Exerc 1988; 20:362–8.

58. Florence JM, Hagberg JM. Effect of training on the exercise responses of neuromuscular disease patients. Med Sci Sports Exerc 1984;16:460–5.

59. Kilmer D. Response to resistive strengthening exercise training in humans with neuromuscular disease. Am J Phys Med Rehabil 2002;81:S121–6.

60. Kilmer DD. Response to aerobic exercise training in humans with neuromuscular disease. Am J Phys Med Rehabil 2002;81:S148–50.

61. Eagle M. Report on the MD campaign workshop: exercise in neuromuscular diseases Newcastle. Neuromuscul Disord 2002;2002(12):975–83.

62. Lindeman E, Leffers P, Spaans F, et al. Strength training in patients with myotonic dystrophy and hereditary motor and sensory neuropathy: a randomized clinical trial. Arch Phys Med Rehabil 1995;76:612–20.

63. Mathieu J, Boivin H, Richards CL. Quantitative motor assessment in myotonic dystrophy. Can J Neurol Sci 2003;30:129–36.

64. Aitkens S, Lord J, Bernauer E, et al. Relationship of manual muscle testing to objective strength measurements. Muscle Nerve 1989;12:173–7.

65. Kalkman JS, Zwarts MJ, Schillings ML, et al. Different types of fatigue in patients with facioscapulohumeral dystrophy, myotonic dystrophy and HMSN-I. Experienced fatigue and physiological fatigue. Neurol Sci 2008; 29(S2):S238–40.

66. Sockolov R, Irwin B, Dressendorfer RH, et al. Exercise performance in 6- to 11-year old boys with Duchenne MD. Arch Phys Med Rehabil 1977;58:195–201.

67. McDonald CM, Widman LM, Walsh DD, et al. Use of step activity monitoring for continuous physical activity assessment in boys with Duchenne MD. Arch Phys Med Rehabil 2005;86:802–8.

68. Wenneberg S, Gunnarsson LG, Ahlstrom G. Using a novel exercise programme for patients with MD. Part I: a qualitative study. Disabil Rehabil 2004;26:586–94.

69. Wenneberg S, Gunnarsson LG, Ahlstrom G. Using a novel exercise programme for patients with MD. Part II: a quantitative study. Disabil Rehabil 2004;26: 595–602.

70. Steffensen BF, Lyager S, Werge B, et al. Physical capacity in non-ambulatory people with Duchenne MD or spinal muscular atrophy: a longitudinal study. Dev Med Child Neurol 2002;44:623–32.

71. McDonald CM, Abresch RT, Carter GT, et al. Profiles of neuromuscular disease: Duchenne muscular dystrophy. Am J Phys Med Rehabil 1995;74(5):S70–92.

72. McDonald CM, Abresch RT, Carter GT, et al. Profiles of neuromuscular disease: Becker muscular dystrophy. Am J Phys Med Rehabil 1995;74(5):S93–103.

73. Johnson ER, Carter GT, Kilmer DD, et al. Profiles of neuromuscular disease: myotonic muscular dystrophy. Am J Phys Med Rehabil 1995;74(5):S104–16.

74. McDonald CM, Abresch RT, Carter GT, et al. Profiles of neuromuscular disease: limb-girdle syndromes. Am J Phys Med Rehabil 1995;74(5):S117–30.

75. Kilmer DD, Abresch RT, Aitkens SG, et al. Profiles of neuromuscular disease: facioscapulohumeral dystrophy. Am J Phys Med Rehabil 1995;74(5):S131–9.

76. Kilmer DD, Abresch RT, Fowler WM Jr. Serial manual muscle testing in Duchenne MD. Arch Phys Med Rehabil 1993;74:1168–71.

77. Brooke MH, Fenichel GM, Griggs RC, et al. Duchenne MD: patterns of clinical progression and effects of supportive therapy. Neurology 1989;39:475–81.

78. Bakker JP, De Groot IJ, Beelen A, et al. Predictive factors of cessation of ambulation in patients with Duchenne MD. Am J Phys Med Rehabil 2002;81:906–12.

79. McDonald DG, Kinali M, Gallagher AC, et al. Fracture prevalence in Duchenne MD. Dev Med Child Neurol 2002;44:695–8.

80. Johnson ER, Fowler WM Jr, Lieberman JS. Contractures in neuromuscular disease. Arch Phys Med Rehabil 1992;73:807–10.

81. Bach JR, McKeon J. Orthopedic surgery and rehabilitation for the prolongation of brace- free ambulation of patients with Duchenne MD. Am J Phys Med Rehabil 1991;70:323–31.

82. Fowler WM Jr, Carter GT, Kraft GH. Role of physiatry in the management of neuromuscular disease. Phys Med Rehabil Clin N Am 1998;9:1–8.

83. Oda T, Shimizu N, Yonenobu K, et al. Longitudinal study of spinal deformity in Duchenne MD. J Pediatr Orthop 1993;13:478–88.

84. Hart DA, McDonald CM. Spinal deformity in progressive neuromuscular disease: natural history and management. Phys Med Rehabil Clin N Am 1998; 9:213–32.

85. Heckmatt JZ, Dubowitz V, Hyde SA, et al. Prolongation of walking in Duchenne MD with lightweight orthoses: review of 57 cases. Dev Med Child Neurol 1985;27:149–57.

86. Lord J, Behrman B, Varzos N, et al. Scoliosis associated with Duchenne MD. Arch Phys Med Rehabil 1990;71:13–7.

87. McDonald CM. Limb contractures in progressive neuromuscular disease and the role of stretching, orthotics, and surgery. Phys Med Rehabil Clin N Am 1998;9:187–211.

88. Richter D, Berger K, Reker T. Are mental disorders on the increase? A systematic review. Psychiatr Prax 2008;35(7):321–30.

89. Choi NG, McDougall G. Unmet needs and depressive symptoms among low-income older adults. J Gerontol Soc Work 2009;52(6):567–83.

90. Sigford BJ, Lanham RA Jr. Cognitive, psychosocial, and educational issues in neuromuscular disease. Phys Med Rehabil Clin N Am 1998;9(1):249–70.

91. Modoni A, Silvestri G, Vita MG, et al. Cognitive impairment in myotonic dystrophy type 1 (DM1): a longitudinal follow-up study. Dep J Neurol 2008; 255(11):1737–42.

92. Sansone V, Gandossini S, Cotelli M, et al. Cognitive impairment in adult myotonic dystrophies: a longitudinal study. Neurol Sci 2007;28(1):9–15.

93. Fowler WM Jr, Abresch RT, Koch TR, et al. Employment profiles in neuromuscular diseases. Am J Phys Med Rehabil 1997;76(1):26–37.

94. Benditt JO. Management of pulmonary complications in neuromuscular disease. Phys Med Rehabil Clin N Am 1998;9:167–85.

95. Carter GT, Bird TD. Facioscapulohumeral MD presenting as respiratory failure. Neurology 2005;64:401.

96. Wohlgemuth M, van der Kooi EL, van Kesteren RG, et al. Ventilatory support in facioscapulohumeral MD. Neurology 2004;63:176–8.

97. Bach JR, Campagnolo DI, Hoeman S. Life satisfaction of individuals with Duchenne MD using long-term mechanical ventilatory support. Am J Phys Med Rehabil 1991;70:129–35.

98. Baydur A, Kanel G. Tracheobronchomalacia and tracheal hemorrhage in patients with Duchenne MD receiving long-term ventilation with uncuffed tracheostomies. Chest 2003;23:1307–11.

99. Ugalde V, Breslin EH, Walsh SA, et al. Pursed lip breathing improves ventilation in myotonic MD. Arch Phys Med Rehabil 2000;81:472–8.

100. Hahn A, Bach JR, Delaubier A, et al. Clinical implications of maximal respiratory pressure determinations for individuals with Duchenne MD. Arch Phys Med Rehabil 1997;78:1–12.

101. Topin N, Matecki S, Le Bris S, et al. Dose-dependent effect of individualized respiratory muscle training in children with Duchenne MD. Neuromuscul Disord 2002;12:576–83.

102. Lewis W, Yadlapalli S. Management of cardiac complications in neuromuscular disease. Phys Med Rehabil Clin N Am 1998;9:145–66.

103. Sakata C, Sunohara N, Nonaka I, et al. A case of Becker MD presenting with cardiac failure as an initial symptom. Rinsho Shinkeigaku 1990;30:210–3.

104. Carter GT, Galer BS. Advances in the management of neuropathic pain. Phys Med Rehabil Clin N Am 2001;12:447–59.

105. Eagle M, Baudouin SV, Chandler C, et al. Survival in Duchenne MD: improvement in life expectancy since 1967 and the impact of home nocturnal ventilation. Neuromuscul Disord 2002;12:926–9.

106. Jaffe KM, McDonald CM, Ingman E, et al. Symptoms of upper gastrointestinal dysfunction: case-control study. Arch Phys Med Rehabil 1990;71:742–4.

107. McCrory MA, Kim HR, Wright NC, et al. Energy expenditure, physical activity, and body composition of ambulatory adults with hereditary neuromuscular disease. Am J Clin Nutr 1998;67:1162–9.

108. McDonald CM, Carter GT, Abresch RT, et al. Body composition and water compartment measurements in boys with Duchenne MD. Am J Phys Med Rehabil 2005;84:483–91.

109. Uchikawa K, Liu M, Hanayama K, et al. Functional status and muscle strength in people with Duchenne MD living in the community. J Rehabil Med 2004;36:124–9.

110. Kilmer DD, Zhao HH. Obesity, physical activity, and the metabolic syndrome in adult neuromuscular disease. Phys Med Rehabil Clin N Am 2005;16(4):1053–62.

111. Kilmer DD, Wright NC, Aitkens S. Impact of a home-based activity and dietary intervention in people with slowly progressive neuromuscular diseases. Arch Phys Med Rehabil 2005;86(11):2150–6.

112. Apkon S, Coll J. Use of weekly alendronate to treat osteoporosis in boys with muscular dystrophy. Am J Phys Med Rehabil 2008;87(2):139–43.

113. Al-Harbi TM, Bainbridge LJ, McQueen MJ, et al. Hypogonadism is common in men with myopathies. J Clin Neuromuscul Dis 2008;9(4):397–401.

114. Aitkens S, Kilmer DD, Wright NC, et al. Metabolic syndrome in neuromuscular disease. Arch Phys Med Rehabil 2005;86:1030–6.

115. Carter GT, Yudkowsky MP, Han JJ, et al. Topiramate for weight reduction in Duchenne MD. Muscle Nerve 2005;6:788–9.

116. Edwards RJ, Round JM, Jackson MJ, et al. Weight reduction in boys with MD. Dev Med Child Neurol 1984;26:384–90.

117. Eiholzer U, Boltshauser E, Frey D, et al. Short stature: a common feature in Duchenne MD. Eur J Pediatr 1988;147:602–5.

118. Iannaccone ST, Owens H, Scott J, et al. Postoperative malnutrition in Duchenne MD. J Child Neurol 2003;18:17–20.

119. Motlagh B, MacDonald JR, Tarnopolsky MA. Nutritional inadequacy in adults with muscular dystrophy. Muscle Nerve 2005;31(6):713–8.

120. McCrory MA, Wright NC, Kilmer DD. Nutritional aspects of neuromuscular diseases. Phys Med Rehabil Clin N Am 1998;9:127–43.

121. Rodriguez MC, Tarnopolsky MA. Patients with dystrophinopathy show evidence of increased oxidative stress. Free Radic Biol Med 2003;34:1217–20.

122. Griggs RC, Moxley RT, Mendell JR, et al. Duchenne dystrophy: randomized, controlled trial of prednisone (18 months) and azathioprine (12 months). Neurology 1993;43:520–7.

123. Carter GT, McDonald CM. Preservation of function in Duchenne dystrophy with long-term pulse prednisone therapy. Am J Phys Med Rehabil 2000;79:455–8.

124. Fenichel GM, Florence JM, Pestronk A, et al. Long-term benefit from prednisone therapy in Duchenne MD. Neurology 1991;41:1874–7.

125. Fenichel GM, Mendell JR, Moxley RT, et al. A comparison of daily and alternate-day prednisone therapy in the treatment of Duchenne MD. Arch Neurol 1991;48:575–9.

126. Alman BA, Raza SN, Biggar WD. Steroid treatment and the development of scoliosis in males with Duchenne MD. J Bone Joint Surg Am 2004;86:519–24.

127. Escolar D, McDonald CM, Korengberg A, et al. Randomized, double-blind, controlled study to compare efficacy and tolerability of standard daily prednisone regime with a novel intermittent high dose regime in ambulant boys with Duchenne muscular dystrophy. Neuromuscul Disord 2008;18(9–10):824–5.

128. Fenichel G, Pestronk A, Florence J, et al. A beneficial effect of oxandrolone in the treatment of Duchenne MD: a pilot study. Neurology 1997;48:1225–6.

129. Fowler EG, Graves MC, Wetzel GT, et al. Pilot trial of albuterol in Duchenne and Becker MD. Neurology 2004;62(6):1006–8.

130. Rose MR, Tawil R. Drug treatment for facioscapulohumeral MD. Cochrane Database Syst Rev 2004:CD002276.

131. Tarnopolsky MA, Bourgeois JM, Snow R, et al. Histological assessment of intermediate- and long-term creatine monohydrate supplementation in mice and rats. Am J Physiol Regul Integr Comp Physiol 2003;285:R762–S769.

132. Tarnopolsky M, Mahoney D, Thompson T, et al. Creatine monohydrate supplementation does not increase muscle strength, lean body mass, or muscle phosphocreatine in patients with myotonic dystrophy type 1. Muscle Nerve 2004;29: 51–8.

133. Tarnopolsky MA, Mahoney DJ, Vajsar J, et al. Creatine monohydrate enhances strength and body composition in Duchenne MD. Neurology 2004;62:1771–7.

134. Tarnopolsky M, Martin J. Creatine monohydrate increases strength in patients with neuromuscular disease. Neurology 1999;52:854–7.

135. Tarnopolsky MA, Roy BD, MacDonald JR. A randomized, controlled trial of creatine monohydrate in patients with mitochondrial cytopathies. Muscle Nerve 1997;20:1502–9.

136. Distad BJ, Weiss MD. Neurotrophic factors in neuromuscular disease. Phys Med Rehabil Clin N Am 2005;16(4):999–1014.

137. Weiss MD, Hammer J, Quarles RH. Oligodendrocytes in aging mice lacking myelin-associated glycoprotein are dystrophic but not apoptotic. J Neurosci Res 2000;62:772–80.

138. MacDonald JR, Hill JD, Tarnopolsky MA. Modafinil reduces excessive somnolence and enhances mood in patients with myotonic dystrophy. Neurology 2002;59:1876–80.

139. Liu M, Mineo K, Hanayama K, et al. Practical problems and management of seating through the clinical stages of Duchenne MD. Arch Phys Med Rehabil 2003;84:818–24.

140. Scott OM, Hyde SA, Goddard C, et al. Prevention of deformity in Duchenne MD. A prospective study of passive stretching and splintage. Physiotherapy 1981; 67:177–80.

141. Wheeler TM, Sobczak K, Lueck JD, et al. Reversal of RNA Dominance by displacement of protein sequestered on triplet repeat RNA. Science 2009; 325(5938):336–9.

Index

Note: Page numbers of article titles are in **boldface** type.

A

Active seating, stimulated, in pressure ulcer prevention, 349–350

Age, psychological functioning related to, in persons with disabilities, **281–297**. See also *Disability(ies), relationship of age-related factors to psychological functioning in persons with.*

Aging

  BF/PTG and, 287, 290

  cognitive effects of, **375–382**. See also *Cognition, aging effects on.*

  communication and, **309–319**. See also *Communication, aging and.*

  defined, 253

  described, 253

  falls related to, **357–373**. See also *Fall(s), by older adults.*

  functional, SCI-related, 391–393

  in general population, factors related to, 283

  in older adults, physical activity and, 300–301

  MS and, 286–289

  of brain, 376–378

  paradox of, paradox of disability and, 259–262

  psychosocial, SCI-related, 391–393

  with developmental disabilities, **419–427**. See also *Developmental disabilities, aging with.*

  with disability, **253–265**

    adjustment to, cognitive abilities central to, 379–380

    assessment of, 326–328

    biopsychosocial perspectives of, **253–265**

      described, 253–255

      life span developmental approach, 257–259

      social support network, 256–257

      socioemotional selectivity therapy, 259

      theoretical perspectives, 257–259

    described, 267–268, 321–322

    effects on health and functioning, 324–326

    falls among people with

      consequences of, 363–364

      prevalence, 358–359

      risk factors for, 360–362

    fatigue, **321–337**

    future directions in, 330

    gaps in, 330

    in workplace, **267–279**. See also *Workplace, aging with disability in.*

    maintaining functional independence, 340

Phys Med Rehabil Clin N Am 21 (2010) 451–460

doi:10.1016/S1047-9651(10)00012-4

1047-9651/10/$ – see front matter © 2010 Elsevier Inc. All rights reserved.

pmr.theclinics.com

Moving?

Make sure your subscription moves with you!

To notify us of your new address, find your **Clinics Account Number** (located on your mailing label above your name), and contact customer service at:

Email: journalscustomerservice-usa@elsevier.com

800-654-2452 (subscribers in the U.S. & Canada)
314-447-8871 (subscribers outside of the U.S. & Canada)

Fax number: 314-447-8029

Elsevier Health Sciences Division
Subscription Customer Service
3251 Riverport Lane
Maryland Heights, MO 63043

*To ensure uninterrupted delivery of your subscription, please notify us at least 4 weeks in advance of move.

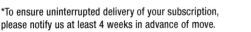

Printed and bound by CPI Group (UK) Ltd, Croydon, CR0 4YY

03/10/2024

01040452-0002